EDITORS FOR THE CHEMICAL RUBBER CO.

Editor-in-Chief

ROBERT C. WEAST, Ph.D.

Vice-President, Research, Consolidated Natural Gas Service Company, Inc.
Formerly Professor of Chemistry at Case Institute of Technology

Coordinating Editor

GEORGE L. TUVE, Sc.D.

Formerly Professor of Engineering at Case Institute of Technology

Editor-in-Chief of Mathematics

SAMUEL M. SELBY, Ph.D.

Distinguished Professor Emeritus of Mathematics
Formerly Chairman of Mathematics Department, University of Akron
Presently Chairman of Mathematics Department, Hiram College

Editor-in-Chief of Biosciences

IRVING SUNSHINE, Ph.D.

Chief Toxicologist
Cuyahoga County Coroner's Office
Cleveland, Ohio
Associate Professor of Toxicology
Case Western Reserve University

Editors

Chromatography

Gunter Zweig, Ph.D.	*Syracuse University Research Corporation*

Engineering Sciences

Ray E. Bolz, D.Eng.	*Case Western Reserve University*
Richard G. Bond, M.P.H.	*University of Minnesota*
Donald F. Gibbons, Ph.D.	*Case Western Reserve University*
W. Bruce Johnson, Ph.D.	*Case Western Reserve University*
Robert J. Pressley, Ph.D.	*RCA Laboratories*
Conrad P. Straub, Ph.D., D.Eng.	*University of Minnesota*

Laboratory Safety

Norman V. Steere	*The 3M Company*

Life Sciences

Willard R. Faulkner, Ph.D.	*Vanderbilt University Medical Center*
Thomas E. Furia	*Geigy Chemical Corporation*
John W. King, M.D., Ph.D.	*The Cleveland Clinic Foundation*
Allen I. Laskin, Ph.D.	*Esso Research and Engineering*
Aaron M. Leash, D.V.M.	*Case Western Reserve University*
Hubert A. Lechevalier, Ph.D.	*Rutgers University*
Herbert A. Sober, Ph.D.	*National Institutes of Health*

Mathematics

Brian Girling, M.Sc., F.I.M.A.	*The City University, London, England*

Nuclear Sciences

Yen Wang, M.D., D.Sc.(Med.)	*Homestead Hospital*

Organic Chemistry

Saul Patai, Ph.D.	*Hebrew University of Jerusalem*
Zvi Rappoport, Ph.D.	*Hebrew University of Jerusalem*

Statistics

William H. Beyer, Ph.D.	*University of Akron*

THE CHEMICAL RUBBER CO. HANDBOOK SERIES

Handbook of Chemistry and Physics, 50th edition
Standard Mathematical Tables, 17th edition
Handbook of Tables for Mathematics, 3rd edition
Handbook of Tables for Organic Compound Identification, 3rd edition
Handbook of Tables for Probability and Statistics, 2nd edition
Handbook of Clinical Laboratory Data, 2nd edition
Manual of Clinical Laboratory Procedures, 2nd edition
Handbook of Laboratory Safety, 1st edition
Handbook of Food Additives, 1st edition
Handbook of Biochemistry: Selected Data for Molecular Biology, 1st edition
Handbook of Radioactive Nuclides, 1st edition
Handbook of Analytical Toxicology, 1st edition
*Handbook of Tables for Applied Engineering Science, 1st edition
*Handbook of Lasers and Laser Applications, 1st edition
*Handbook of Chromatography, 1st edition
*Handbook of Properties of Engineering Materials, 1st edition
*Handbook of Environmental Polution Control, 1st edition
*CRC-Fernaroli Handbook of Flavors, 1st edition
*Handbook of Laboratory Animal Care, 1st edition
*Handbook of Microbiology, 1st edition
*Handbook of Electro-Optics, 1st edition

*Currently in preparation

Manual of Clinical Laboratory Procedures

CO-EDITORS

Willard R. Faulkner, Ph.D.
Vanderbilt University Medical Center
Nashville, Tennessee

John W. King, M.D., Ph.D.
Cleveland Clinic Foundation
Cleveland, Ohio

Published by

THE CHEMICAL RUBBER CO.

18901 Cranwood Parkway, Cleveland, Ohio 44128

Library of Congress Card No. 78–108656

Compilers

CHEMISTRY

Willard R. Faulkner, Ph.D.
Vanderbilt University Hospital
Nashville, Tennessee

John W. King, M.D., Ph.D.
Cleveland Clinic Foundation
Cleveland, Ohio

Irving Sunshine, Ph.D.
Cuyahoga County Coroner's Office
Cleveland Ohio

Robert P. Winslow, B.A.
Polyclinic Hospital
Cleveland, Ohio

ENDOCRINOLOGY

Andrew M. Michelakis, M.D., Ph.D.
Vanderbilt University School of Medicine
Nashville, Tennessee

BLOOD BANK

John W. King, M.D., Ph.D.
Cleveland Clinic Foundation
Cleveland, Ohio

HEMATOLOGY

George C. Hoffman, M.B., B.Chir., M.C.Path.
Cleveland Clinic Foundation
Cleveland, Ohio

HISTOLOGY

John W. King, M.D., Ph.D.
Cleveland Clinic Foundation
Cleveland, Ohio

BACTERIOLOGY

Thomas L. Gavan, M.D.
Cleveland Clinic Foundation
Cleveland, Ohio

SEROLOGY

Thomas L. Gavan, M.D.
Cleveland Clinic Foundation
Cleveland, Ohio

MISCELLANEOUS

John W. King, M.D., Ph.D.
Cleveland Clinic Foundation
Cleveland, Ohio

Robert P. Winslow, B.A.
Polyclinic Hospital
Cleveland, Ohio

Table of Contents

CHEMISTRY

CONTENTS

CONTENTS

CONTENTS

CONTENTS

MISCELLANEOUS

CHEMISTRY

Sectional Directory

Introduction

The purpose of this section is to provide the laboratory with a basic group of selected and proven manual procedures for carrying out many of the frequently requested analyses.

In this 2nd edition, a number of substitutions of procedures have been made with the objective of presenting those that, from the experience of the editors and authors, have certain advantages with respect to accuracy, reliability and simplicity over those of the 1st edition. Also, new procedures have been added to extend the range of analytical coverage.

It has been the intention to present each procedure in sufficient detail and completeness, so that reference to other volumes or to other section of this manual is unnecessary in carrying out any one determination.

The editors continue to welcome comments and suggestions directed toward an improvement of the procedures in the Manual.

Willard R. Faulkner, Ph.D.

Acetoacetic Acid, Urine

Gerhardt's Ferric Chloride Test

PRINCIPLE

The three acetone bodies (acetone, acetoacetic acid, and beta-hydroxybutyric acid) occur almost always together in the urine and have essentially the same significance. The usual tests are for the detection of acetone or acetoacetic acid or both; there is no satisfactory simple test for beta-hydroxybutyric acid. Of the acetone bodies, ferric chloride solution will give a positive test only with acetoacetic acid. This test is neither sensitive nor specific.

NORMAL VALUES

Acetoacetic acid is not present in normal urine.

SPECIMEN

Fresh urine.

PROCEDURE

Test

1. Pipette 5 ml of urine into a test tube.
2. Add 10% aqueous solution of ferric chloride, a few drops at a time, with agitation of test tube until the precipitate that usually forms redissolves. A deep wine-red color develops if acetoacetic acid is present. A positive reaction from the above indicates the possible presence of acetoacetic acid. Substances other than acetoacetic acid may also give a positive color (see Note 1).

Control

1. Place 5 ml of urine in a small Erlenmeyer flask and boil vigorously for 3 to 5 minutes.
2. Cool the flask and repeat the above test.
3. Compare with the test on the unboiled sample. Boiling the specimen will decompose acetoacetic acid to acetone, which does not give a positive test with ferric chloride. In the presence of acetoacetic acid only, the resulting test should be negative (or less positive than before boiling). If the test is positive, the color is due to the presence of substances other than acetoacetic acid.

NOTES

1. A similar color is produced by phenols, coal tar antipyretics, salicylates, thiocyanates, and acetophenetidine.
2. Acetoacetic acid may be extracted from urine specimens with ether, dried, dissolved in water, and tested with ferric chloride solution.

REAGENTS

1. Ferric chloride (10%).
   Dissolve 10 g of the reagent-grade salt in water and dilute to 100 ml.

REFERENCES

Free, A. H., and Free, Helen M., Nature of Nitroprusside-Reactive Material in Urine in Ketosis. Am. J. Clin. Pathol., *30*, 7, 1958.

Hawk, P. B., Oser, B. L., and Summerson, W. H., Practical Physiological Chemistry, 13th ed., p. 840. The Blakiston Co., Inc., New York, 1954.

Smith, M. J. H., Chemical Test for Ketonuria. J. Clin. Pathol., *10*, 101, 1957.

Acetoacetic Acid, Urine

Rothera's Nitroprusside Test

PRINCIPLE

The nitroprusside test is one of the most widely used tests for ketonuria. Many variations in technic have been devised. All are based on the reaction of acetone and acetoacetic acid with an alkaline solution of sodium nitroprusside to yield a violet to purple color. This reaction will detect either compound, although with quite different sensitivities. The Rothera modification of the nitroprusside test is more sensitive (five or more times) to acetoacetic acid than to acetone; hence, when applied to urine directly, the result will depend largely on the relative amounts of these two substances. A fresh urine specimen giving a positive test may on standing and after decomposition of the acetoacetic acid to acetone give a negative test.

NORMAL VALUES

No significant amount detectable.

SPECIMEN

Fresh urine.

PROCEDURE

1. Measure approximately 20 ml of urine into a test tube.
2. Add a few crystals of ammonium sulfate and shake.
3. Add 2 to 3 drops of concentrated ammonium hydroxide.
4. Add a few drops of a 5% solution of sodium nitroprusside and shake.

INTERPRETATION

1. A positive test is indicated by the development of a purple color, which gradually deepens.
2. A brown color is not a positive result.

Readings

1. A quick, strong reaction indicates about 0.25% acetoacetic acid.
2. A slow, weak reaction is given by as little as 0.0005% acetoacetic acid.

NOTES

Reagents for the nitroprusside test are available commercially.

1. "Acetone Test" powder may be obtained from the Denver Chemical Mfg. Co., Inc., New York. To use, place a few drops of urine on a small amount of the powder; a purple color indicates acetone or acetoacetic acid.
2. Acetest® Reagent Tablets may be obtained from the Ames Co., Division of Miles Laboratories, Inc., Elkhart, Indiana. To use, place 1 drop of urine on the reagent tablet; a purple color indicates acetoacetic acid and possibly acetone.

REAGENTS

1. Sodium nitroprusside (5%)
   Dissolve 5 g in 100 ml of distilled water.
2. Ammonium sulfate crystals (ACS)
3. Ammonium hydroxide (concentrated)

REFERENCE

Hawk, P. B., Oser, B. L., and Summerson, W. H., Practical Physiological Chemistry, 13th ed., p. 840. The Blakiston Co., Inc., New York, 1954.

Addis Test

PRINCIPLE

The Addis test is an attempt to estimate the number of formed elements in a urine specimen collected under standard conditions. Usually the protein content of the specimen is determined and reported along with the formed elements. The kidney has considerable functional reserve, and the constitution of the urine varies widely with conditions such as fluid intake, body temperature, exercise, and related factors. The Addis test requires the patient to be on a restricted fluid intake and, by collecting the urine at night, ensures that the patient is at minimal activity. In addition, the higher acidity of night urine ensures better preservation of the casts in the urine. The test should not be done on azotemic patients or on patients with kidney infection.

NORMAL VALUES

Casts (almost all hyaline):	0—5,000/12-hour specimen
Leukocytes and epithelial cells:	0—1,000/12-hour specimen
Erythrocytes:	0—500,000/12-hour specimen
Protein:	<100 mg/24 hours

SPECIMEN

Night urine collected over a period of 12 hours (see procedure).

PROCEDURE

Preparation of Patient

1. The patient is placed on a dry diet for 12 hours preceding the test. No fluid, frozen or fresh fruit, or vegetables are allowed. To make the diet tolerable, the patient should use no salt in his food.
2. Usually the preliminary 12-hour period is scheduled to end at 8:00 p.m., at which time the patient empties his bladder and the test proper begins.

Test Procedure

1. All urine formed between 8:00 p.m. and 8:00 a.m. is saved and pooled. The container in which the specimen is collected is kept refrigerated during the collection period. If the patient has been properly prepared, the volume of this collection should not exceed 500 ml.
2. The urine specimen is sent to the laboratory, where it is mixed by pouring from one container to another; pH, volume, and specific gravity are noted. The pH should be acid and the specific gravity above 1.022 in the properly prepared patient.
3. Pipette a 10-ml aliquot of this well-mixed urine collection into a suitable graduated centrifuge tube and centrifuge for 5 minutes at 1,800 rpm in a No. 2 International centrifuge.
4. Decant the supernatant urine, except for the final 1 ml (including the sediment). Resuspend the sediment in the residual urine. If more than 1 ml of urine is needed

to resuspend the urine, use as much as is necessary and make appropriate adjustment for the value of S in the formula.

5. Fill an ordinary hemocytometer with this material and count the number of casts in nine of the large squares on both sides of the hemocytometer. Average the two readings.
6. Calculate the number of casts by the following formula:

$$N = \frac{S}{v} \times n \times \frac{V}{10}$$

where N = casts per 12-hour specimen,
V = volume (in ml) of the 12-hour specimen,
v = volume (in ml) of the sediment suspension actually counted (0.0009 ml),
S = volume of the mixed sediment,
n = casts counted in the hemocytometer,
10 = volume (in ml) of the aliquot used.

7. The total counts for white blood cells and epithelial cells, which are usually reported together, and the count for the erythrocytes may be calculated by using the same formula.
8. The protein in the specimen is determined, using a 10-ml or 6.5-ml Addis centrifuge tube and Tsuchiya's reagent. Mix 4 ml of filtered urine and 2.5 ml of Tsuchiya's reagent in a graduated centrifuge tube. To complete mixing of urine and sediment, invert at least 3 times.
9. Allow the mixture to stand for 10 minutes.
10. Centrifuge for 15 minutes at 1,800 rpm, then read the volume of the packed precipitates.
11. Each ml of packed precipitate represents 7.2 g of protein per liter of urine. Convert this value to g/24 hours, using the following equation:

$$\text{g/liter} \times \text{total volume (in liters)} \times \frac{12}{24} = \text{total g/24 hours.}$$

12. The data for the entire test are reported as numbers of formed elements in the 12-hour specimen, as the amount of protein per liter, and as grams of protein per 24 hours. Usually volume, pH, and specific gravity of the specimen are also reported.

NOTES

1. Sometimes the clinician can gain considerable information on a quantitative study of formed elements and of protein in the urine from a patient who has not been on a fluid-restricted diet, and indeed, sometimes it is not desirable to restrict fluid to this extent in a seriously ill patient. Such "Addis" reports must be plainly marked, as the findings in such specimens may vary widely from those found in the classical test. The clinician interprets such findings according to his own experience, as differences in the state of hydration of the patient can seriously affect the values reported.
2. There are two types of Addis tubes available. One is graduated to 6.5 and 10 ml and is used for the Addis count. It may also be used for the protein determination, but the other type of tube, which is graduated only to 6.5 ml, usually has markings

in the narrow tip that are easier to read and therefore permit a more accurate estimate of the sediment to be made.

3. In children a somewhat higher limit is allowed for casts (10,000), leukocytes (2,000,000), and red blood cells (600,000).

REAGENTS

1. Tsuchiya's reagent

phosphotungstic acid, crystals	1.5 g
ethyl alcohol (95%)	93.5 ml
hydrochloric acid, concentrated	5.0 ml

Dissolve the phosphotungstic acid crystals in the alcohol, then add the acid.

Amylase, Serum and Urine

Saccharogenic Method of Henry and Chiamori, Modified by Ford and Rudolph

PRINCIPLE

The specimen is incubated with an adequately buffered starch substrate, after which the reducing substances formed from the starch are measured by a modification of the method of Folin and Wu.

NORMAL VALUES

A. Serum

Men: 38—118 units/100 ml* (95% limits)
Women: 46—141 units/100 ml (95% limits)

B. Urine

Pooled random specimens: 66—740 units/100 ml (95% limits)
6- to 24-hour samples: 43—245 units/hour

SPECIMEN

Amylase has been reported to be stable in serum and urine without preservatives for at least one week at room temperature. It may be stored for longer periods in a refrigerator.

Urine amylase, to be of the most significance, must be determined on a timed specimen of which the volume is known.

PROCEDURE

1. Place 7.0 ml of buffered starch substrate in each of two tubes, labeled "Incubated" and "Control". Place them in a water bath at 37°C.
2. After 5 minutes, add 1.0 ml of serum or 0.5 ml of urine plus 0.5 ml of 0.9% sodium chloride (NaCl) to the *incubated* tube. Mix well and note the time of specimen addition.
3. After exactly 34 minutes, remove the tubes from the bath and immediately add 1.5 ml of 2/3*N* sulfuric acid (H_2SO_4) to both tubes. Mix.
4. Add 1.0 ml of the same serum or urine-saline mixture to the *control* tube.
5. Add 0.5 ml of 10% sodium tungstate to both tubes. Mix.
6. Prepare a glucose-standard tube containing 7.0 ml of buffered starch substrate, 1.5 ml of 2/3*N* sulfuric acid, 0.5 ml of 10% sodium tungstate, and 1.0 ml of a standard containing 100 mg/100 ml of glucose. Mix.
7. Centrifuge the tubes or filter the contents through Whatman #40 filter paper. If the filtrates are not clear, filter again through the same filters.

*The unit of amylase activity is defined as the amount that will produce 0.01 mg of reducing substance, expressed as glucose, formed by 1.0 ml of specimen in the reaction.

8. Determine the amount of reducing carbohydrates in the filtrates as follows.
   (a) Place in Folin-Wu tubes the following, as indicated in the table below:

	Blank	Incubated	Control	Standard
Water (ml)	2.0	1.0	1.0	1.0
Filtrate from incubated (ml)	0	1.0	0	0
Filtrate from control (ml)	0	0	1.0	0
Filtrate from standard (ml)	0	0	0	1.0
Alkaline copper tartrate (ml)	2.0	2.0	2.0	2.0

   (b) Place all tubes in a boiling water bath and heat for exactly 15 minutes.
   (c) Immediately on taking the tubes out of the boiling water bath, add 4.0 ml of acid molybdate reagent to each.
   (d) Dilute the contents of each tube to 25 ml with water. Mix thoroughly by inverting several times.
   (e) Measure the absorbances of the contents of each tube at 540 mμ, using the blank as a reference.

CALCULATIONS

A. Serum

1. Calculate the glucose in the incubated and in the control tube as indicated below:

$$\frac{A_{\text{incubated}}}{A_{\text{standard}}} \times 100 = \text{mg glucose/100 ml unknown,}$$

$$\frac{A_{\text{control}}}{A_{\text{standard}}} \times 100 = \text{mg glucose/100 ml control,}$$

$$\text{glucose}_{\text{incubated}} - \text{glucose}_{\text{control}} = \text{amylase (Somogyi units/100 ml).}$$

2. If the amylase is above 1,500 units, repeat the test, using a 1-ml aliquot of a 1:10 serum dilution in 0.9% saline. Subtract the control from the incubated and multiply the result by 10 to obtain the units of amylase.

B. Urine

1. The calculations for urine are the same as those for serum, except that, since 0.5 ml is used instead of 1.0 ml, the difference between the control and the incubated sample is multiplied by 2 to yield units/100 ml of urine.
2. To be of any clinical significance, the urinary-amylase determination must be performed on a timed specimen of which the volume is known for that interval. To obtain the value for the interval, use the formula given below:

$$\frac{\text{volume for timed interval}}{100 \text{ ml}} \times \text{units/100 ml} = \text{amylase/timed interval.}$$

REAGENTS

1. Disodium phosphate (0.1*M*)
   Dissolve 2.68 g of disodium phosphate ($Na_2HPO_4 \cdot 7H_2O$) in water and dilute to 100 ml.
2. Potassium acid phosphate (0.1*M*)
   Dissolve 1.74 g of the anhydrous salt (KH_2PO_4) in water and dilute to 100 ml.

3. Phosphate buffer (0.1*M*, pH 7.0)
   Dissolve 4.55 g of KH_2PO_4 and 9.35 g of Na_2HPO_4 in water and make up to 1 liter. Adjust the pH to the proper value with one or the other of the above 0.1*M* phosphate solutions.
4. Starch substrate
   Place 1.5 g of soluble starch* and 100 ml of phosphate buffer in a 250-ml Erlenmeyer flask and heat at the boiling point for about 3 minutes. Cool to room temperature, transfer to a graduated cylinder, and add sufficient buffer to bring the volume to 140 ml. Store in a refrigerator.
5. Sulfuric acid (2/3*N*)
   Add slowly and with stirring 18.5 ml of concentrated sulfuric acid to approximately 500 ml water in a 1-liter volumetric flask. Cool to room temperature and dilute to 1,000 ml. Titrate with standard alkali and adjust the volume, if necessary, to obtain the correct normality.
6. Sodium tungstate (10%)
   Dissolve 10 g of sodium tungstate ($Na_2WO_4 \cdot 2H_2O$) in water and dilute to 100 ml.
7. Alkaline copper tartrate
   Dissolve the following compounds in approximately 800 ml of water and dilute to 1 liter:

sodium carbonate, anhydrous	16.0 g
sodium tartrate	12.0 g
copper sulfate, pentahydrate	5.0 g

   Mix the above solution and allow to stand in a tightly stoppered bottle for about 1 week before using. Filter, then store in a tightly stoppered bottle. If after aging and filtration any further deterioration occurs, it will be indicated by a sediment of reduced copper on the the walls of the bottle. If this is the case, filter and continue to use.
8. Acid molybdate
   Place 300 g of sodium molybdate in a 2-liter flask. Add 800 to 900 ml of water and shake until solution has taken place, except for a slight turbidity. Add with stirring 450 ml of 85% phosphoric acid. Cool in ice water and add 300 ml of a cold sulfuric acid solution (25% *V*/*V*). When cool, add 150 ml of glacial acetic acid and make up to 2000 ml in a 2-liter mixing cylinder. Store in a brown bottle.
9. Glucose stock solution (1000 mg/100 ml)
   Dissolve 1.000 g of anhydrous reagent-grade glucose in a few ml of water and dilute to 100 ml in a volumetric flask with saturated benzoic acid solution.
10. Glucose standard (100 mg/100 ml)
   Dilute 10 ml of glucose stock solution to 100 ml in a volumetric flask with saturated benzoic acid solution.

REFERENCES

Folin, O., The Determination of Sugar in Blood and Normal Urine. J. Biol. Chem., *67*, 357, 1926.

Folin, O., and Wu, H., A System of Blood Analysis. J. Biol. Chem., *38*, 81, 1919.

Ford, W. J., and Rudolph, G. G., Personal Communication.

Henry, R. J., and Chiamori, N., Study of the Saccharogenic Method for the Determination of Serum and Urine Amylase. Clin. Chem., *6*, 434, 1960.

*Argo Corn Starch, Best Foods Division, Corn Products Company, New York, New York.

Barbiturates

PRINCIPLE

Chloroform extracts of the sample are reextracted with dilute sodium hydroxide. Any barbiturate present will be found in this alkaline extract. Ultraviolet spectrophotometry is then used to determine any barbiturate present in the sodium hydroxide.

NORMAL VALUES

Barbiturates are normally never present. The concentrations found in biological samples vary with the amounts of drugs ingested. These correlations are given below as part of the test interpretation.

SPECIMEN

Unclotted blood, urine, or stomach contents.

PROCEDURE

1. Extract 3 ml of sample with 50 ml of chloroform. If urine or stomach contents are to be analyzed, adjust the pH of these samples to between 5.5 and 7.0.
2. Separate a 40-ml aliquot of the chloroform from the extracted sample.
3. Extract the clear 40-ml aliquot of chloroform with 5 ml of 0.45*N* sodium hydroxide.
4. Remove the alkaline layer and centrifuge it. The residual chloroform can be discarded, or can be reserved for a determination of any neutral drugs it may contain (e.g., meprobamate or glutethimide).
5. Transfer 3 ml of the clear alkaline solution (see step 4), whose pH is approximately 13, to a cuvette and determine its absorbance from 300 mμ to 230 mμ.
6. Adjust the pH of the solution to 10.3 $\pm$ 0.2 by adding 0.5 ml of 2.25*M* sodium dihydrogen phosphate.
7. Determine the absorbance of the solution from 300 mμ to 230 mμ.
8. Both absorbance measurements are made using a reagent blank as the reference solution. To obtain this reagent blank solution, extract 3 ml of water in the same manner as the biological sample.
9. Determine the amount of barbiturate by calculating the difference in absorbance of the two solutions at 260 mμ and comparing the difference with that obtained from a known concentration of barbiturate.

CALCULATION

1. Record the absorbance at 260 mμ of the solution whose pH is 13 (A).
2. Record 7/6* of the absorbance at 260 mμ of the solution whose pH is 10.3 (B).
3. Subtract to get the difference (C). Then,

$$\text{concentration of barbiturate} = \text{C} \times \frac{5.0}{\text{S}\dagger}$$

*The factor 7/6 is used to compensate for the addition of the 0.5 ml of buffer to the 3-ml sample.

†S is the comparable difference in absorbance that is obtained when 3 ml of a solution containing 5.0 mg of barbiturate per 100 ml is processed in a manner identical to that described above.

INTERPRETATION

The ultraviolet spectrophotometric data are easily reproducible to $\pm 5\%$ of the true value if only one barbiturate is present, and its extinction is used to calculate the concentration. If an extinction value is used that is the average extinction value for several common barbiturates, the result is $\pm 10\%$ of the true value. If more than one barbiturate is present, the total concentration is within $\pm 10\%$, but the relative concentration of each must be determined by some other technic.

Many investigators have studied the correlation between a patient's clinical condition and his blood barbiturate level. The reported data are summarized in the table below.

RELATION OF AVERAGE LEVELS* OF BARBITURATE IN THE BLOOD TO PATIENT'S CLINICAL CONDITION

Barbiturate	Clinical Stages†				
	5	4	3	2	1
Phenobarbital	—	10.0	6.5	4.4	3.5
Amobarbital	8.6	6.2	4.7	2.5	1.5
Secobarbital	—	2.5	1.5	1.0	0.8
Pentobarbital	—	3.0	2.0	1.5	—

*Milligrams of barbiturate per 100 ml of blood. Each figure represents the concentration of barbiturate at which the average nontolerant patient enters a given clinical stage. The figures are averages calculated from findings in at least four to six patients.

†The clinical conditions of the patients were grouped into five arbitrary categories, based on the following criteria.

Stage 1: awake, competent, and mildly sedated.
Stage 2: sedated, reflexes present, prefers sleep, answers questions when roused, does not cerebrate properly.
Stage 3: comatose, reflexes present.
Stage 4: comatose, areflexive.
Stage 5: comatose, circulatory and/or respiratory difficulty.

These stages do not have definitive limits, but blend into each other as the patient progresses from stage to stage. The deep tendon reflexes were used as the criteria for presence or absence of reflexes. Corneal, pupillary, and abdominal responses are subject to more variability in relation to the levels of anesthesia. Gag and cough reflexes return at approximately the same time as the deep tendon reflexes: response to pain returns at a later time. The respiratory difficulty considered in Stage 5 is that due to direct depression of the respiratory center in the medulla and should not be confused with the attendant respiratory difficulty due to pneumonia, which is always a possible complication in a heavily sedated individual.

These data indicate that spontaneous recovery from phenobarbital intoxication occurs when the blood phenobarbital level is 4.4 to 5 mg per 100 ml of blood. Stage 2, defined as the patient's ability to respond to questioning, is the criterion used for describing recovery. In amobarbital intoxication, recovery was noted in the range of 2.5 to 3.6 mg per 100 ml of blood. At blood levels of amobarbital higher than 4.4 mg, which is the recovery level for phenobarbital intoxication, patients were always severely intoxicated. The recovery levels for pentobarbital and secobarbital range from 0.5 to 1.0 mg per 100 ml of blood. Severe intoxication was noted when pentobarbital and secobarbital blood levels exceeded 1.5 mg per 100 ml. This emphasizes the need for qualitative as well as quantitative chemical analysis in all instances of barbiturate intoxication.

REAGENTS

Analytical-grade chemicals are required.

1. Sodium hydroxide (0.45*N*)

   Dissolve 18 g of reagent-grade sodium hydroxide in water and dilute to 1 liter. Store in a polyethylene bottle.

2. Sodium dihydrogen phosphate (2.25*M*)
   Dissolve 310 g of the monohydrate salt in water and dilute to 1 liter. Store in a polyethylene bottle.
3. Alkaline buffer
   Add 0.5 ml of 2.25*M* sodium dihydrogen phosphate to 3.0 ml of 0.45*N* sodium hydroxide. The pH of this buffer solution must be 10.3 $\pm$ 0.2. If it is not, suitably dilute either of the two reagents. The buffer's pH is critical within the stated limits. Once prepared, the component solutions are stable for at least 2 months if stored in polyethylene bottles.
4. Phosphate buffer (pH 7.0)
   Add 30 ml of 0.1*N* sodium hydroxide to 50 ml of 0.1*M* potassium dihydrogen phosphate and dilute to 100 ml with distilled water. Any other buffer with a pH of 7.0 will suffice.
5. Chloroform
   All chloroform should be obtained in glass containers. An aliquot of each new lot should be extracted with 0.45*N* sodium hydroxide. The absorbance of this alkaline solution should be compared with 0.45*N* sodium hydroxide. There should be no significant absorption between 240 μ and 300 μ. If there is, the chloroform must be washed with dilute alkali, dilute acid, and water.
6. Barbiturate solutions of known concentrations
   Dissolve and dilute 50.0 mg of a given barbiturate to 100 ml in a 100-ml volumetric flask. If the free acid is used, add a trace of alkali to help dissolve the solid, add 50 ml of water, then acidify the solution. A 1:10 dilution of the 50-mg % solution, 5.0 mg %, is used as a working reference solution. The solutions of known concentrations should be stored in glass-stoppered bottles in a refrigerator. If just enough acid is added to bring the pH to 4 or lower, these solutions are stable for at least 5 months. If improperly stored in alkaline solutions, the short-acting barbiturates are the first to deteriorate. A solution of sodium secobarbital deteriorates measurably after 4 days at room temperature.

REFERENCES

Broughton, P. M. G., A Rapid Ultraviolet Spectrophotometric Method for the Determination and Identification of Barbiturates in Biological Material. Biochem. J., *63*, 207, 1956.

Goldbaum, L. R., Analytical Determination of Barbiturates with Differentiation of Several Barbiturates. Anal. Chem., *24*, 1604, 1952.

Sunshine, I., Maes, R., and Finkle, B., An Evaluation of Methods for the Determination of Barbiturates in Biological Materials. Clin. Toxicol., *1*, 281, 1968.

Bilirubin, Blood, Conjugated and Total

Method of Malloy and Evelyn

PRINCIPLE

Serum is treated with diazotized sulfanilic acid in a hydrochloric acid solution. In this medium, bilirubin is released from its binding with albumin and is split into two 2-pyrrole moieties, each of which subsequently couples with the diazotized sulfanilic acid to form the pigment azobilirubin. The color produced after reaction for 1 minute in an aqueous solution represents the conjugated (direct-reacting) bilirubin. When methanol is substituted for water and the reaction is allowed to proceed for 30 minutes, the color developed provides a measure of the total bilirubin present.

NORMAL VALUES

Adults:

conjugated (direct)	0.05—0.25 mg/100 ml
total	0.20—1.50 mg/100 ml

SPECIMEN

Either plasma or serum may be used. Hemolysis is to be avoided, as it gives rise to falsely low values.

PROCEDURE

1. Make a 1:20 dilution of the specimen by adding 0.5 ml to 9.5 ml of water.
2. Pipette the reagents into cuvettes in the order given below:

	Conjugated Bilirubin		Total Bilirubin	
	Blank	Unknown	Blank	Unknown
Water (ml)	2.5	2.5	0	0
Methanol (ml)	0	0	2.5	2.5
Blank reagent (ml)	0.5	0	0.5	0
Diazo reagent (ml)	0	0.5	0	0.5

3. Add 2.0 ml of the diluted serum to each of the two tubes in the Total Bilirubin column. Mix and allow to stand for 30 minutes.
4. During the 30-minute wait for the total bilirubin, determine the conjugated bilirubin as follows:
   (a) place the tubes near a spectrophotometer; add 2.0 ml of the diluted serum to the *blank tube* and mix; set the spectrophotometer to 100 percent transmittance with this tube at a wavelength of 540 mμ;
   (b) add 2.0 ml of the diluted serum to the *unknown tube* and mix; read the percent transmittance at *exactly 1 minute after adding the serum.*
5. Read the percent transmittance of the total bilirubin after the 30-minute reaction period.
6. Determine the concentration of the unknown from a previously constructed standard curve.

Standardization

1. Preparation of stock bilirubin standard:
   (a) weigh 3.0 mg of an "acceptable bilirubin" on a watch glass;
   (b) add 2.0 ml of 1*M* sodium carbonate directly to the watch glass; agitate until solution is complete;
   (c) transfer to a volumetric flask, rinsing the watch glass with an "acceptable serum diluent" until all the bilirubin has been transferred; dilute with the serum diluent to 100 ml.
2. Preparation of working standards from the stock solution: make up the working standards as given below, using the same serum diluent that was used to make the stock solution.

Stock Bilirubin Solution	Dilute (with "acceptable serum diluent") to	Equivalent to (mg bilirubin per 100 ml serum)
1.0 ml	20.0 ml	3.0
3.0	24.0	7.5
5.0	20.0	15.0
7.0	21.0	21.0
10.0	20.0	30.0
14.0	21.0	42.0

3. Diazotization of standards:
   (a) place a set of suitable Coleman cuvettes in a rack as shown below, label them, and pipette into them the reagent as indicated;

	Blank	Standard
Methanol (ml)	2.5	2.5
Blank reagent (ml)	0.5	0
Diazo reagent (ml)	0	0.5

   (b) add 2.0 ml of the working standard solution to both the blank and the standard for each of the concentrations prepared above; mix thoroughly after the addition of the standard solutions; allow the tubes to stand for 30 minutes;
   (d) read the percent transmittance for each concentration at 540 mμ, with the corresponding blank set at 100 percent transmittance;
   (e) plot a transmittance–concentration curve on semi-log paper, with the transmittance on the log scale.

NOTES

1. An "acceptable bilirubin" has a 1-cm molar absorptivity of 60,000 $\pm$ 800 (mean $\pm$ S.D.) at 453 mμ in chloroform at 25°C.
2. An "acceptable serum diluent" is a pooled serum having an absorbance of less than 0.100 at 414 mμ and less than 0.040 at a dilution of 1:25 in 0.85% sodium chloride.
3. The acceptability of the bilirubin and serum diluent has been tentatively defined by a committee composed of representatives from the American Academy of Pediatrics, the College of American Pathologists, the American Association of Clinical Chemists, and the National Institutes of Health (see Standard Methods of Clinical Chemistry, *5*, 75, S. Meites, ed., Academic Press, New York, 1965).

4. The free bilirubin (indirect) can be found by subtracting the conjugated bilirubin from the total.

REAGENTS

1. Sodium nitrite stock solution (10%)
   Dissolve 10 g of sodium nitrite in water and dilute to 100 ml. Store in a refrigerator.
2. Sodium nitrite working solution (0.5%)
   Dilute 0.5 ml of the stock solution with water to 10 ml.
3. Sulfanilic acid solution
   To 1.0 g of sulfanilic acid add 15 ml of concentrated hydrochloric acid and about 300 ml of water. When the sulfanilic acid has dissolved, dilute with water to 1 liter.
4. Diazo reagent
   To 5.0 ml of sulfanilic acid solution add 0.15 ml of sodium nitrite working solution. Mix. *Make up just before use.*
5. Blank reagent
   Dilute 15 ml of concentrated hydrochloric acid with water to 1 liter.
6. Bilirubin control serum
   Establish the total bilirubin concentration of a pooled serum sample by repeated analyses, or obtain a reliable commercial serum control such as Versatol Pediatric.*

REFERENCES

Ducci, H., and Watson, C. J., The Quantitative Determination of the Serum Bilirubin with Special Reference to the Prompt-Reacting and the Chloroform-Soluble Types. J. Lab. Clin. Med., *30*, 293, 1945.

Malloy, H. T., and Evelyn, K. A., The Determination of Bilirubin with a Photoelectric Colorimeter. J. Biol. Chem., *119*, 481, 1937.

Recommendation on a Uniform Bilirubin Standard. Standard Methods of Clinical Chemistry, *5*, 75, Meites, S., ed. Academic Press, New York, 1965.

White, F. D., and Duncan, D., Photometric Studies on the Diazo Reaction for Serum Bilirubin, Can. J. Med. Sci., *30*, 552, 1952.

*Warner-Chilcott Laboratories, Morris Plains, New Jersey 07950.

Bilirubin, Urine

Gmelin's Test

PRINCIPLE

Bilirubin in urine is oxidized with concentrated or fuming nitric acid to a number of colored derivatives, e.g., mesobilirubin (yellow), mesobiliverdin (green to blue), and mesobilicyanin (blue to violet).

NORMAL VALUES

Bilirubin is normally not present.

SPECIMEN

Random urine.

PROCEDURE

1. Pipette about 5 ml of nitric acid into a test tube.
2. Carefully add an equal volume of urine so that the two fluids do not mix.
3. Note the various colored rings at the point of contact (green, blue, violet, red, and reddish yellow) if bilirubin is present.

REAGENTS

1. Nitric acid (concentrated, or preferably fuming nitric acid)

REFERENCE

Foord, A. G., and Baisinger, C. F., Comparison of Tests for Bilirubin in Urine. Am. J. Clin. Pathol., *10*, 238, 1940.

Bilirubin, Urine

Ictotest®*

PRINCIPLE

This test is semiquantitative for bilirubin in urine. The Ictotest® tablets contain *p*-nitrobenzenediazonium, *p*-toluenesulfonate, sodium bicarbonate, sulfosalicylic acid, and boric acid. They react with bilirubin in a highly specific manner, producing the violet azobilirubin, the intensity of which is compared with a color chart to provide a semiquantitative measure of the amount present.

NORMAL VALUES

Bilirubin is normally not present.

SPECIMEN

Random urine.

PROCEDURE

1. Place 5 drops of urine on one square of special test mat.
2. Place an Ictotest® reagent tablet in the center of the moistened area.
3. Flow 2 drops of water onto the tablet.
4. If the mat around the tablet turns blue or purple within 30 seconds, the test is positive. Ignore any color produced after 30 seconds. The amount of bilirubin is proportional to the speed and intensity of the color reaction.

REAGENTS

1. Ictotest® reagent tablets and test mats
   Available from the Ames Company, Division of Miles Laboratories, Inc., Elkhart, Indiana.

REFERENCE

Free, A. H., and Free, Helen M., A Simple Test for Urine Bilirubin. Gastroenterology, *24*, 414, 1953.

*Ames Company, Division of Miles Laboratories, Elkhart, Indiana.

Blood, Occult, Urine

Benzidine Reaction

PRINCIPLE

This test depends on the action of hemoglobin, which catalytically decomposes hydrogen peroxide, thereby liberating oxygen, which oxidizes benzidine to a blue or green derivative.

NORMAL VALUES

Negative.

SPECIMEN

Random urine.

PROCEDURE

1. Pipette 2 ml of urine into a test tube.
2. Set up a positive control consisting of 2 ml of water with an extremely small amount of blood (0.01 ml).
3. Add 3 ml of a saturated solution of benzidine in glacial acetic acid to the test specimen and to the control.
4. Pipette 1 ml of 3% hydrogen peroxide into each tube and mix.
5. A blue or green color indicates a positive test.

Confirmatory Test

1. Add 1 or 2 drops of glacial acetic acid to 10 ml of urine.
2. Extract by shaking with 5 ml of ether.
3. Pour ether extract into a small evaporating dish.
4. Place the dish on a hot water bath (with flame turned out) and evaporate to dryness.
5. To the residue add a few drops of water, a drop of benzidine solution, and a drop of hydrogen peroxide.
6. A blue or green color indicates blood.

NOTES

1. Benzidine solution changes readily upon contact with light; it must, therefore, be kept in the dark.
2. An excess of hydrogen peroxide may interfere with the reaction; it is, therefore, essential that the details of the procedure be followed closely. Since benzidine has been implicated as possibly carcinogenic for humans, it should be handled carefully, to avoid any contact with the skin.

REAGENTS

1. Benzidine-saturated solution in glacial acetic acid

   Place a small amount of benzidine in a test tube. Add 3 ml of glacial acetic acid and shake until the acetic acid is saturated. If necessary, add more benzidine. Prepare fresh daily.

2. Hydrogen peroxide (3%)

   Dilute 1 volume of 30% hydrogen peroxide with 9 volumes of distilled water. Commercial 3% hydrogen peroxide is also acceptable, if fresh. Hydrogen peroxide should be kept stoppered and in the dark, to avoid loss of potency.

REFERENCES

Hawk, P. B., Oser, B. L., and Summerson, W. H., Practical Physiological Chemistry, 13th ed., p. 835. The Blakiston Co., Inc., New York, 1954.

Ingham, J., An Improved and Simplified Benzidine Test for Blood in Urine and Other Clinical Materials. Biochem. J., *26*, 1124, 1932.

Bromide

PRINCIPLE

Blood proteins are precipitated with trichloroacetic acid and removed, leaving the bromide in the filtrate. The clear filtrate is then assayed for its bromide content. If bromides are present, a typical orange-brown color forms when gold chloride is added to an aliquot of the protein-free filtrate.

SPECIMEN

Clear serum free of red cells.

PROCEDURE

1. Place 2.0 ml of serum in a test tube and slowly add 8.0 ml of 10% trichloroacetic acid. Mix well and shake the contents vigorously.
2. Centrifuge the tube and contents.
3. Place 4.0 ml of the supernatant into a cuvette and add 1.0 ml of 0.5% gold chloride solution.
4. Compare the resulting color with that of the standard bromide solutions treated in an identical fashion, or determine the absorbance of the sample at 440 mμ, using a suitable photoelectric photometer, and compare this absorbance with that obtained by processing the bromide standards in a similar manner.

INTERPRETATION

Serum bromide concentrations greater than 50 mg of bromide per 100 ml are compatible with incipient toxicity, and many patients with this concentration appear confused. With concentrations between 150 and 250 mg of bromide per 100 ml, incoordination and emotional outbursts may be seen; about 300 mg of bromide per 100 ml may be fatal. Subsequent to discontinuance of bromide therapy, bromides are excreted slowly over a long period. Serum bromide concentrations drop slowly and have a half-life of about 30 days unless efforts are made to increase the bromide excretion rate.

REAGENTS

All reagents should be ACS analytical grade.

1. Gold chloride (0.5% *W/V*)
   Dissolve 0.5 g of gold chloride in water and dilute to 100 ml.
2. Trichloroacetic acid (10% *W/V*)
   Dissolve 10 g of trichloroacetic acid in water and dilute to 100 ml.
3. Reference bromide solutions
   Dissolve 0.386 g of potassium bromide in water and dilute to 100 ml. This 300 mg/100 solution should be diluted to 90 and 150 mg per 100 ml by diluting 15 ml and 25 ml of the concentrated standard respectively to 50 ml with distilled water.

Calcium, Serum

Method of Bachra, Dauer and Sobel

PRINCIPLE

The total calcium in serum is titrated in an alkaline medium with a standard EDTA reagent, using Cal-Red* as the indicator. EDTA chelates the calcium, and as the end point is approached, the color changes from violet-red to blue, indicating the complete complexing of the calcium by EDTA. The amount of calcium in the unknown serum is calculated from the volume of EDTA reagent required in comparison to that required by a standard serum of known calcium content.

NORMAL VALUES

9.0—11.0 mg/100 ml.

PROCEDURE

1. With a 1-ml pipette measure 0.5 ml of potassium hydroxide solution into each of four 10 × 35 mm vials.
2. Add 0.1 ml of standard serum with a micropipette and 1 drop of Cal-Red indicator from a dropping bottle to two of the four vials.
3. Using a microburette (the Syringe Microburet† or the Gilmont Ultramicroburet‡ are satisfactory), titrate one of the vials with EDTA until no further color change is detectable (blue). Add 10 lambdas excess. Titrate the second vial just to the color of the first and record this value.
4. Add 0.1 ml of unknown serum and 1 drop of indicator to each of the other two vials.
5. Titrate one unknown vial to the color of the standard, or as near to it as possible. Add 10 lambdas excess. Titrate the second unknown vial just to the color of the first and record this value.

CALCULATION

$$\frac{\text{vol EDTA}_{\text{unknown}}}{\text{vol EDTA}_{\text{standard}}} \times \text{conc. of Ca in standard (mg)} = \text{mg Ca/100 ml unknown.}$$

NOTES

1. The purpose of the duplicate titration is twofold. It ensures reaching the true end point, and it also allows a valid comparison of color when the serum is icteric or hemolyzed.

REAGENTS

1. Potassium hydroxide solution (1.25*N*)

   Dissolve 7.0 g of reagent-grade potassium hydroxide in water and dilute to 100 ml. Titrate with standard acid and adjust to 1.25*N*. Store in a polyethylene bottle.

*Obtainable from Instru-Chem, 204 Haskell, Dallas, Texas.
†Micro-Metric Instrument Co., Cleveland, Ohio.
‡The Emil Greiner Co., New York, New York.

2. Disodium ethylenediaminetetraacetate (EDTA), dihydrate (0.005*M*)
   Dissolve exactly 1.861 g of the salt in 100 ml of water by warming while stirring. Dilute to 1 liter and mix. Store in a polyethylene bottle.
3. Cal-Red indicator
   Dissolve 100 mg of the powder in 100 ml of water. Store in a refrigerator. Make up every 3 weeks.
4. Standard serum
   Establish the calcium content of a pooled serum specimen by the Clark-Collip Method, or use a commercial lyophilized serum control for which the calcium content is known.

REFERENCE

Bachra, B. N., Dauer, A., and Sobel, A. E., The Complexometric Titration of Micro and Ultramicro Quantities of Calcium in Blood, Serum, Urine and Inorganic Salt Solutions. Clin. Chem., *4*, 107, 1958.

Calcium, Urine

Sulkowitch Test

PRINCIPLE

The turbidity produced when a buffered oxalate solution is added to a urine specimen allows a semiquantitative estimate of the calcium present. This, in turn, presumably allows an inference to be made regarding the serum calcium level.

Since the daily urinary output of calcium depends partly upon the diet, this source of possible variation should be stabilized, supplying the patient with enough for his nutritional requirements.

This test should be replaced whenever possible by a quantitative assay of urine and/or serum calcium.

SPECIMEN

24-hour urine.

PROCEDURE

1. Pipette 5 ml of the mixed urine into a test tube.
2. Add 2 ml of Sulkowitch reagent drop by drop. If a precipitate does not form immediately, mix the contents of the tube thoroughly, allow to stand, and observe.
3. In routine examinations, the precipitates may be graded 1, 2, 3, or 4.

INTERPRETATION

1. No precipitate: the serum probably contains not more than 5 to 7.5 mg of calcium per 100 ml.
2. Fine white cloud: serum calcium content is within the normal range of 9 to 11 mg per 100 ml.
3. Heavy milk-like precipitate: serum concentration is probably above 12.5 mg per 100 ml.

REAGENTS

1. Sulkowitch's reagent

oxalic acid	2.5 g
ammonium oxalate	2.5 g
glacial acetic acid	5.0 ml

Dissolve in approximately 100 ml water, then dilute to 150 ml.

REFERENCE

Ritter, S., Spencer, H., Samachson, J., The Sulkowitch Test and Quantitative Urinary Calcium Excretion. J. Lab. Clin. Med. *56*, 314, 1960.

Carbon Dioxide Content

Natelson's Microgasometric Method

PRINCIPLE

Blood is collected and maintained without exposure to the atmosphere. Plasma or serum is obtained by centrifugation of the specimen with a minimum of agitation and then introduced into the pipette of the microgasometer (see illustration).

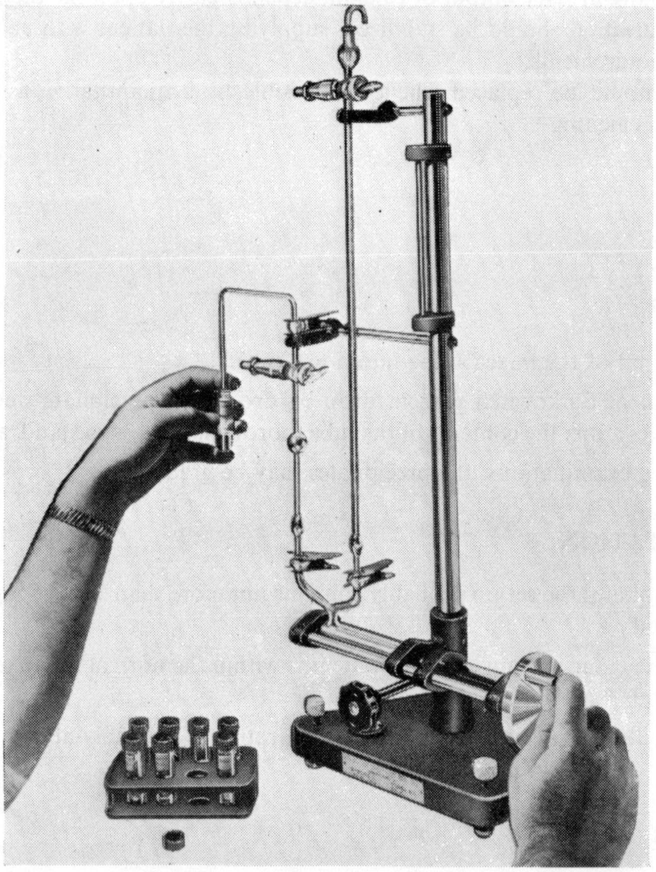

Carbon dioxide and other blood gases are released by the combined action of acidification, agitation, and the establishment of a partial vacuum over the sample. The pressure produced is then measured. The carbon dioxide is absorbed with alkali, and a second pressure reading is taken. The difference of the two pressure readings represents the carbon dioxide, which is reduced to standard conditions of pressure and temperature by the use of appropriate factors.

NORMAL VALUES

22—32 m*M*/liter.

SPECIMEN

Blood should be collected with minimal exposure to air and maintained in this condition until analyzed. Serum is suitable, as is plasma in which any of the common anticoagulants have been used.

PROCEDURE

1. Advance the drive of the microgasometer until a small bead of mercury forms on the pipette tip.
2. Draw in carefully and successively the following to the indicated marks on the tip:

   0.03 ml of sample (wipe tip)
   0.01 ml of mercury
   0.03 ml of lactic acid
   0.01 ml of mercury
   0.01 ml of caprylic or other antifoam reagent
   0.01 ml of mercury
   0.10 ml of water
   0.12 ml of mercury

3. Close the reaction chamber stopcock and retract the drive until the aqueous liquid level is at the bottom of the reaction chamber.
4. Shake the reaction mixture for about 1 minute.
5. Advance the drive until the aqueous meniscus is at the 0.12-ml mark.
6. Record the pressure (P_1) and the temperature.
7. Advance the drive until the mercury is at the top of the manometer column.
8. Immerse the pipette tip in the sodium hydroxide contained in the vial, then open the stopcock. Advance the drive to expel air from the tip and draw in sodium hydroxide to the 0.10-ml mark. Lower the tip into the mercury and draw in to the 0.12-ml mark.
9. Close the reaction chamber stopcock and retract the drive until the aqueous liquid level is at the bottom of the chamber. Shaking is not required.
10. Advance the drive to bring the aqueous meniscus to the 0.12-ml mark. Read the pressure (P_2).
11. Advance the drive until the mercury is at the top of the manometer column.
12. Open the stopcock and advance the drive to eject all aqueous liquid from the tip.
13. Wash the reaction chamber successively with lactic acid rinse solution and with water. Expel the water wash. Fill again with water and allow this to remain in the instrument while it is not in use.
14. Make sure that the reagents are prepared properly and that the instrument is operating satisfactorily by making a determination on the standard.

CALCULATION

Carbon dioxide content = $(P_1 - P_2)f$

FACTORS FOR ESTIMATION OF CARBON DIOXIDE CONTENT

Temperature (°C)	f (mEq/l)	Temperature (°C)	f (mEq/l)
17	0.242	25	0.232
18	0.240	26	0.231
19	0.238	27	0.230
20	0.237	28	0.229
21	0.236	29	0.228
22	0.235	30	0.227
23	0.234	31	0.225
24	0.233	32	0.224

REAGENTS

1. Lactic acid (approximately 8%)
   Dilute 9 ml of 85% lactic acid with water to 100 ml. Place clean mercury in a 5-ml screw-capped vial to a depth of about 5 mm. Add about 4 ml of the lactic acid.
2. Sodium hydroxide (approximately 3*N*)
   Dissolve 12 g of reagent-grade sodium hydroxide in water and dilute to 100 ml. Place clean mercury to a depth of about 15 mm in a 5-ml screw-capped vial, then add about 4 ml of the reagent. Keep mercury to a depth of at least 10 mm in the vial.
3. Distilled water
   Place clean mercury to a depth of about 15 mm in a 5-ml screw-capped vial. Add about 4 ml of distilled water that has been deaerated by vacuum or by boiling. Add mercury as needed to maintain the depth at about 10 mm.
4. Carbon dioxide standard (22.5 m*M*/liter)
   Dry reagent-grade sodium carbonate at 100°C for 2 hours, then cool. Dissolve 0.2382 g of the salt in deaerated water and dilute to 100 ml in a volumetric flask. This standard must be kept in an airtight container.
5. Lactic acid rinse
   Fill a 25-ml Erlenmeyer flask with lactic acid (approximately 1*N*) and add a few drops of 1% alcoholic bromphenol blue indicator.
6. Rinse water
   Fill a 25-ml Erlenmeyer flask with distilled water.

REFERENCES

Instruction Booklet No. 5, Natelson Microgasometer Models 600 and 650. Scientific Industries, Inc., 220–05 97th Avenue, Queens Village, New York 11429.

Natelson, S., Routine Use of Ultramicro Methods in the Clinical Laboratory. Am. J. Clin. Pathol., *21*, 1153, 1951.

Van Slyke, D. D., and Neill, J. M., The Determination of Gases in Blood and Other Solutions by Vacuum Extraction and Manometric Measurement. J. Biol. Chem., *61*, 523, 1924.

Van Slyke, D. D., and Sendroy, J., Carbon Dioxide Factors for the Manometric Blood Gas Apparatus. J. Biol. Chem., *73*, 127, 1927.

Cephalin Cholesterol Flocculation Test

Method of Hanger

PRINCIPLE

Flocculation in a cephalin-cholesterol emulsion is brought about by serum in which there are alterations from normal in the quantities of albumin and globulin and in their ratio.

NORMAL VALUES

Up to 1+ in 48 hours.

SPECIMEN

Fresh serum from a patient in a fasting state is used. The serum must not be exposed to direct sunlight.

PROCEDURE

Run the test in duplicate.

1. Pipette 0.2 ml of the unknown serum into each of two tubes.
2. Add 4.0 ml of 0.85% saline to each tube. Mix well by tapping. Do not invert. Set up a control tube and pipette 4.0 ml of 0.85% saline into it.
3. Add 1.0 ml of the cephalin-cholesterol antigen to each tube. Mix again by tapping.
4. Stopper the tubes with clean corks and place them in a dark place at room temperature.
5. Observe the degree of flocculation in each tube at 24 and 48 hours.

INTERPRETATION

1. There should be no flocculation or settling out of the emulsion in the control tube. If the control does exhibit flocculation, it is probable that all tests in this run will include some positive errors; under these circumstances the test must be repeated with a freshly prepared emulsion.
2. Report results as 0, ±, 1+, 2+, 3+, or 4+. Report both the 24- and 48-hour readings.
3. Flocculation is graded according to the description below:
   - 0 = no change in the appearance of the emulsion, same as control tube;
   - ± = a doubtful result, exhibiting a slight amount of precipitate, but little difference from the control;
   - 1+ = a small amount of precipitate, but not much change in the emulsion;
   - 2+ = a definite precipitate and a turbid emulsion;
   - 3+ = a larger amount of precipitate, with definite flocculation in the emulsion;
   - 4+ = complete precipitation of emulsified material, leaving the supernatant clear.

   If there is a difference between duplicate tubes, report the least positive result.

REAGENTS

1. Saline (0.85%)
   Dissolve 8.5 g of reagent-grade sodium chloride and 20 ml of Merthiolate®* (1 mg/ml) solution in water and dilute to 1 liter.
2. Ethyl ether (anaesthetic)
3. Cephalin-cholesterol antigen stock solution
   Add 5.0 ml of ether to a vial of the dried antigen,† cap the vial, and swirl to effect solution. If turbidity persists, add a drop of water, which should clarify the solution. Stopper tightly to prevent evaporation.
4. Emulsion
   Warm 35 ml of water to 65—70°C and add 1.0 ml of the antigen stock solution slowly and with stirring. Heat the emulsion until it simmers gently. Maintain this temperature until the volume has decreased to 30 ml. Cool to room temperature and store in a refrigerator. Discard after 1 month.

REFERENCES

Hanger, F. M., The Flocculation of Cephalin-Cholesterol Emulsion by Pathological Sera. Trans. Assoc. Am. Physicians, *53*, 148, 1938.

Knowlton, M., Cephalin-Cholesterol Flocculation Test. Standard Methods of Clinical Chemistry, *2*, 12, Seligson, D., ed. Academic Press, New York, 1958.

*A brand of sodium ethylmercurithiosalicylate. Eli Lilly and Company, Indianapolis, Indiana.
†Cephalin-Cholesterol Antigen, Difco Laboratories, Detroit, Michigan.

Chloride

Method of Schales and Schales

PRINCIPLE

The chloride of a biological specimen is titrated in an acid medium with standard mercuric nitrate, using *s*-diphenylcarbazone* as an indicator. Chloride ion reacts with mercuric ion to form the soluble but non-dissociated mercuric chloride. At the end point, when a slight excess of mercuric ion is present, a stable violet-blue complex is formed with the indicator.

NORMAL VALUES

Serum:	97—107 mEq/liter
Urine:	83—375 mEq/24 hrs
Cerebrospinal fluid:	122—129 mEq/liter

SPECIMEN

Chloride can be measured directly in plasma, serum, cerebrospinal fluid, or urine. If whole blood is used, it must first be deproteinized, in which case a Folin-Wu tungstic acid filtrate is suitable. Whole-blood chloride concentration, however, is not generally as clinically meaningful as that of plasma or serum because of the cell volume factors not usually known.

PROCEDURE

1. Place in 13 × 45 mm shell vials the following:

	Micro Modification		Macro Modification	
	Specimen	Standard	Specimen	Standard
Water	1.0 ml	1.0 ml	5.0	5.0 ml
Standard	0	0.1 ml	0	0.5 ml
Specimen	0.1 ml	0	0.5 ml	0
Indicator	2 drops	2 drops	4 drops	4 drops

2. Titrate the contents of each vial with standard mercuric nitrate solution to the first faint trace of violet-blue color.

CALCULATION

$$\frac{\text{ml for unknown}}{\text{ml for standard}} \times 100 = \text{mEq/liter of chloride}$$

REAGENTS

1. Chloride standard (100 mEq/liter)
   Dry reagent-grade sodium chloride by heating at 110—120°C for several hours. Cool in a desiccator, then dissolve 0.5845 g in water. Transfer quantitatively to a 100-ml volumetric flask and dilute to the mark. Mix.

*Distillation Products Industries, Eastman Organic Chemicals Department, Rochester, New York 14603 (Cat. No. 4459).

2. Mercuric nitrate standard (10 mEq/liter)
   Dissolve 0.81 g of anhydrous mercuric nitrate ($Hg(NO_3)_2$) in about 200 ml of water in a 500-ml volumetric flask. Add 10 ml of 2*N* nitric acid and dilute to the mark with water. Mix. Place 1.0 ml of chloride standard in a 13 × 45 mm shell vial. Add 2 drops of indicator and titrate with the mercuric nitrate solution to the first trace of a violet-blue color (10.0 ml should be required). Adjust the concentration of the mercuric nitrate solution by adding water so that 10.0 ml is exactly equivalent to 1.0 ml of chloride standard.
3. Indicator
   Dissolve 100 mg of *s*-diphenylcarbazone in 100 ml of 95% ethanol. Place in an amber dropping bottle and store in a refrigerator to delay deterioration. Discard after 1 month.

REFERENCES

Caraway, W. T., and Fanger, H., Ultramicro Procedure in Clinical Chemistry. Am. J. Clin. Pathol., *25*, 317, 1955.

Schales, O., and Schales, S. S., A Simple and Accurate Method for the Determination of Chloride in Biological Fluid. J. Biol. Chem., *140*, 879, 1941.

Cholesterol

Method of Zak,
Modified by Bauman and Wolf

PRINCIPLE

The proteins of serum are precipitated, and the cholesterol is extracted with ethanol. An aliquot of the extract is then subjected to a modified Zak reaction in which ethanol replaces glacial acetic acid. This modification eliminates the necessity of drying the extract and redissolving the residue. After color development, the absorbance is measured at 550 mμ.

NORMAL VALUES*

Age (years)	Cholesterol, Mean			
	Male (mg/100 ml)	(S.E.)	Female (mg/100 ml)	(S.E.)
16—20	199.2	3.6	199.2	2.1
21—25	225.3	7.1	219.1	4.2
26—30	230.6	5.2	216.9	5.9
31—35	238.4	4.9	222.0	5.5
36—40	244.7	4.3	235.8	4.4
41—45	250.5	5.2	236.7	4.4
46—50	250.3	5.7	258.6	4.3
51—55	257.6	4.5	278.2	4.4
56—60	262.1	4.1	276.4	4.3
61—65	252.2	5.6	283.5	5.7

SPECIMEN

Serum is the most commonly used specimen. Plasma may be used when heparin is the anticoagulant, as it does not cause shifts of water between cells and plasma. Other anticoagulants, such as the oxalates, can cause large errors.

No preservatives are ordinarily needed. Cholesterol has been reported to be stable up to 5 days at room temperature, for considerably longer periods if refrigerated, and up to 5 years if maintained at $-20°C$.

PROCEDURE

1. Place 0.10 ml of serum in a clean 15-ml screw-cap test tube. With constant shaking, rapidly add exactly 10.0 ml of ethanol. Mix immediately. A finely divided protein precipitate should be obtained, which is conducive to good accuracy and precision of results. Cap the tube and shake it vigorously for 10 seconds.
2. Centrifuge the tube for 5 minutes to remove the precipitate, then measure 2.0 ml of the ethanolic supernatant extract into a 50-ml Erlenmeyer flask.
3. Carefully add 2.0 ml of the color reagent down the side of the flask, held at an angle, so that a layer is formed under the ethanol. When this addition is complete, which should take 40 seconds, rapidly mix the contents of the flask by swirling it for 10 seconds.
4. Stopper the flask and allow it to stand for 30 minutes.

*See References: Schilling et al.

5. Prepare a standard by substituting 2.0 ml of the 200 mg/100 ml working standard for the ethanolic serum extract. Treat with color reagent in the same manner as described for serum.
6. Prepare a blank by substituting 2.0 ml of ethanol for the extract. Treat in the same manner as the serum or standard.
7. Measure the absorbance of the unknown and of the standard at 550 mμ, using the blank as a reference. The unknown and the standard should be read within 30 and 60 minutes of adding the color reagent.

CALCULATION

$$\frac{A_{unknown}}{A_{standard}} \times 200 = \text{mg cholesterol/100 ml serum}$$

Standard Curve

Alternatively, serum concentration of cholesterol may be read from a standard curve prepared by treating 2.0 ml of each of the working standards as an ethanolic extract. Plot absorbances against concentration on ordinary graph paper.

REAGENTS

1. Iron stock reagent
   Dissolve 2.5 g of ferric chloride ($FeCl_3 \cdot 6H_2O$*) in 100 ml of 87% phosphoric acid (H_3PO_4*). This reagent is stable indefinitely.
2. Color reagent
   Dilute 8 ml of the iron stock reagent to 100 ml with concentrated sulfuric acid. This reagent may be used until a precipitate forms (usually 6 to 8 weeks).
3. Cholesterol stock standard
   Dissolve 100 mg of dry certified cholesterol in 100 ml of absolute ethanol.
4. Cholesterol working standards
   Prepare working standards by diluting the stock as indicated below:

Cholesterol Stock (ml)	Absolute Ethanol (ml)	Water (ml)	Equivalent to Serum Concentration of (mg/100 ml)
1.0	99.0	1.0	100
2.0	98.0	1.0	200
3.0	97.0	1.0	300
4.0	96.0	1.0	400
5.0	95.0	1.0	500
6.0	94.0	1.0	600

5. Absolute ethanol
   Test the ethanol for the presence of reacting aldehyde by subjecting 0.10 ml of a saturated aqueous solution to the Zak color reaction as described above. Absence of an absorption peak indicates a satisfactory grade of alcohol. If the test is positive for aldehyde, redistill it and test again.

REFERENCES

Anderson, J. T., and Keys, A., Cholesterol in Serum and Lipoprotein Fractions; Its Measurement and Stability. Clin. Chem., *2*, 145, 1956.

*Fisher Scientific Company.

Bowman, R. E., and Wolf, R. C., A Rapid and Specific Ultramicro Method for Total Serum Cholesterol. Clin. Chem., *8*, 302, 1962.

De Traverse, P. M., Lavergne, G. H., and Depraitere, R., Les Incertitudes de la Mesure du Cholesterôl Total du Serum; Choix d'une Technique Fidèle. Ann. Biol. Clin., *14*, 236, 1956.

Keys, A., Mickelsen, O., Miller, E. v. O., Hayes, E. R., and Todd, R. L., The Concentration of Cholesterol in the Blood Serum of Normal Man, and Its Relation to Age. J. Clin. Invest., *29*, 1347, 1950.

Rice, E. W., Standard Methods of Clinical Chemistry, *3*, 39, Seligson, D., ed. Academic Press, New York, 1961.

Schilling, F. J., Christakis, G., Orbach, A., and Becker, W. H., Serum Cholesterol and Triglyceride: An Epidemiological and Pathogenic Interpretation. Am. J. Clin. Nutr., *22*, 133, 1969.

Creatinine, Serum and Urine

PRINCIPLE

Creatinine reacts with sodium picrate in an alkaline solution to form a red complex. The reaction is not completely specific for creatinine, but because most of the non-creatinine chromogenic substances occur in the erythrocytes, much of their interference can be avoided by performing the determination on plasma or serum rather than on whole blood. Urine contains very little non-creatinine chromogenic material.

NORMAL VALUES

Serum: 0.8—1.5 mg/100 ml
Urine: 1.0—2.0 g/24 hours

SPECIMEN

Plasma, serum, and urine are the usual specimens upon which the creatinine content has been found clinically most useful. Whole blood is seldom used because of the interference mentioned above. Because of a slow equilibrium reaction between creatinine and creatine, it is advisable to make analyses on fresh specimens. When this is not possible, adjustment of the pH to 7.0 and refrigeration may delay the change.

PROCEDURE

1. Place 1.0 ml of plasma or serum into a test tube.
2. Add 8.0 ml of *N*/12 sulfuric acid and 1.0 ml of 10% sodium tungstate.
3. Mix well, then centrifuge at moderate speed for 5 to 10 minutes.
4. Place the following in cuvettes:

	Blank	Standard	Unknown
Water (ml)	5.0	4.0	0
Creatinine working solution (ml)	0	1.0	0
Supernatant fluid from step 3, or 1:20 dilution of urine (ml)	0	0	5.0
Alkaline picrate solution (ml)	2.5	2.5	2.5

5. Mix the contents of each cuvette by inversion and allow to stand for 10 minutes.
6. At a wavelength in the region of 490 mμ, measure the percent transmittances of the standard and the unknown against the blank.
7. Find the concentration of the unknown by reference to a previously prepared calibration chart. A single standard (equivalent to 2 mg per 100 ml serum) is made up and carried through the procedure with each run to verify the fact that the reagents and photometer have not undergone change since the time the calibration curve was prepared.

Standardization

1. Place creatinine working standards in cuvettes as indicated in the table:

Tube	Creatinine Working Standard (ml)	Water (ml)	Equivalent to (mg creatinine per 100 ml serum)
1	02.5	4.75	1
2	0.50	4.50	2
3	1.00	4.00	4
4	2.00	3.00	8
5	3.00	2.00	12
6	4.00	1.00	16
7	5.00	0	20
Blank	0	5.00	0

2. Add 2.5 ml of alkaline picrate solution to each tube and proceed as directed in step 6 of the test procedure.
3. Plot %T reading on the log scale against mg/100 ml on semi-log paper.
4. Draw a smooth curve through the points. The curve will not be a straight line, as the reaction does not follow Beer's law.
5. Prepare a chart relating the creatinine concentrations to the percent transmittance readings.
6. For plasma or serum, read values directly from chart; for urine, multiply chart readings by 2.

REAGENTS

1. Picric acid solution (1.17% *W/V*)
2. Alkaline picrate solution

   Mix 1 volume of 10% sodium hydroxide and 5 volumes of picric acid solution. Prepare this reagent just before use.
3. Creatinine stock standard (100 mg/100 ml)

   Dissolve 100 mg of reagent-grade creatinine in 100 ml of 0.1*N* hydrochloric acid. Store in a refrigerator.
4. Creatinine working standard (2 mg/100 ml)

   Dilute 1.0 ml of the stock standard to 50 ml with water in a volumetric flask. Add a few drops of chloroform as a preservative.
5. Sulfuric acid (*N*/12)

   Dilute 2.32 ml of concentrated sulfuric acid with water to 1 liter.
6. Sodium tungstate (10%)

   Dissolve 100 g of the reagent-grade salt in water and make up to 1 liter.

REFERENCES

Clark, L. C., and Thompson, H. L., Determination of Creatine and Creatinine in Urine. Anal. Chem., *21*, 1218, 1949.

Peters, J. H., The Determination of Creatinine and Creatine in Blood and Urine with the Photoelectric Colorimeter. J. Biol. Chem., *146*, 176, 1942.

Ethyl Alcohol

PRINCIPLE

Ethanol is volatile at room temperature and is a reducing agent. Both of these properties are used in the microdiffusion screening test. The rugged, inexpensive porcelain Conway cell* is preferred to many other similar units designed to accomplish the same purpose. The sample is placed in one of the two concentric compartments of the cell. Potassium dichromate is put in the other compartment, and the unit is sealed by placing a lubricated ground-glass cover over the cell's lip. In the cell any ethanol present diffuses from the sample and reacts with the potassium dichromate. The reduction of the dichromate produces a color change from orange to green to blue. This color change is a function of the ethanol present and can be used to estimate the approximate ethanol concentration.

SPECIMEN

1 ml of unclotted blood or urine.

PROCEDURE

1. Spread a thin layer of Ucon®† in a 2½-inch circle on the ground-glass surface of the Conway dish's lid. Spread a 1-inch circle in the center of the same lid.
2. Place the lubricated lid against the lip of its Conway dish.
3. Add 2 ml of 20% sodium carbonate to the outer well of each Conway dish.
4. Place 3 ml of potassium dichromate solution in the center well.
5. Add 1 ml of the sample blood, urine, or standard ethanol solution to the outer well.
6. Place the lid over the lip of the cell and slide it around to ensure that both the lip and the lid are lubricated with the Ucon® sealant.
7. Carefully tilt the dish back and forth twice through a 15° angle to the dish top, thus mixing the contents of the outer well.
8. Observe the color of the center well 10 minutes after the analysis was started. If no green color is apparent, continue this check for another 10 minutes.
9. The time when the appearance of a green color in the center well in the unknown is compared with that of the reference ethanol solutions and gives a semiquantitative result.

NOTES

1. Each sample requires its own Conway dish. The solution containing 0.08 g of ethanol per 100 ml should be included in each series of samples that are analyzed.
2. If more precise information is desired, it is possible, but not desirable, to make this procedure quantitative by careful control of all steps. All volumes must be measured with suitable pipettes. After diffusion is complete (3 hours), transfer the contents of the center well to a 5-ml volumetric flask. The center well should be rinsed at least twice with small volumes of 50% (V/V) sulfuric acid. The rinsings are added to the flask, and then sufficient 50% sulfuric acid is added to adjust the volume to 5.0 ml. Determine the absorbance of this solution at 600 mμ.

*Available from Arthur H. Thomas Co., P.O. Box 779, Philadelphia, Pennsylvania 19105.
†Trademark of Union Carbide Corporation.

Compare these results with those obtained by processing the reference solutions in a similar manner at the same time. Data obtained from the reference solutions yield a linear relationship between concentration and absorbance.

INTERPRETATION

This test is nonspecific and will detect any volatile reducing substance that may be present in the sample. Ethanol is the most common of these substances, and seldom are others involved. Of all the reducing substances other than ethanol, methanol is the one most likely to be implicated. On the infrequent occasions when this is so, a specific test for methanol can be performed. If present, its dichromate reduction equivalent can be calculated and this value subtracted from the result of the dichromate test; the difference would probably be due to ethanol. If, when the test is performed on a sample of blood, a green color begins to appear in 20 minutes or less, the patient from whom the sample was taken can probably be presumed to be under the influence of ethanol. If the patient has symptoms usually associated with ethanol intoxication and the green color does not begin to appear in the center well in 25 to 30 minutes, the probability is that the symptoms are not due to ethanol.

REAGENTS

1. Potassium dichromate reagent
   Dissolve 1.667 g of reagent-grade potassium dichromate ($K_2Cr_2O_7$) in 500 ml of water in a 1-liter volumetric flask. Slowly add in small increments, allowing the mixture to cool before adding additional amounts, a total of 520 ml of reagent-grade concentrated sulfuric acid (H_2SO_4). Dilute this mixture with water to 1 liter, cool the mixture to room temperature, then add water to dilute the mixture to exactly 1 liter. A dark glass-stoppered bottle should be used. This solution is stable for 6 months if stored in a refrigerator. Before use, allow the solution to come to room temperature. Polyethylene bottles are undesirable, because they cause a reduction of the dichromate solution.
2. Sodium carbonate solution (20%)
   Dissolve 20 g of sodium carbonate in water and dilute to 100 ml.
3. Sealant
   Ucon® 75H-90,000, available from Union Carbide Corporation, 270 Park Avenue, New York, New York 10017.
4. Reference ethanol solutions
   Add absolute alcohol in quantities of 0.5 ml, 1.00 ml, and 2.00 ml respectively to each of three 1-liter volumetric flasks containing 500 ml of water and dilute to volume with water. At 20°C the concentrations of the reference solutions as prepared are 0.04, 0.08, and 0.16 g ethanol/100 ml solution (*W/V*) respectively. Preparation of the reference solutions at room temperatures between 17° and 30°C will produce solutions of slightly different ethanol concentrations, but these variations are so slight that they may be disregarded, since this test is only semiquantitative. The reference solutions, if stored in glass-stoppered bottles, are stable for 3 months.

Glucose

Glucose Oxidase (FermcoTEST*) Method

PRINCIPLE

Glucose in serum, plasma, cerebrospinal fluid, or in an aqueous standard is oxidized to gluconic acid and hydrogen peroxide by molecular oxygen. Glucose oxidase catalyzes this reaction. The hydrogen peroxide yielded in stoichiometric quantities oxidizes a chromogen to an amber-colored compound under the catalytic influence of peroxidase. This colored compound is converted by sulfuric acid to a stable red pigment that is proportional in intensity to the glucose initially present. The final measurement is made colorimetrically.

1. $\text{Glucose} + O_2 + H_2O \xrightarrow[\text{oxidase}]{\text{glucose}} \text{gluconic acid} + H_2O_2$
2. $H_2O_2 + \text{chromogen} \xrightarrow{\text{peroxidase}} \text{amber compound}$
3. $\text{Amber compound} + H_2SO_4 \longrightarrow \text{stable red pigment}$

NORMAL VALUES

Serum or plasma (fasting):	70—110 mg/100 ml
Cerebrospinal fluid (fasting):	45—80 mg/100 ml

SPECIMEN

Hemolysis should be avoided, as glycolytic enzymes in the erythrocytes decrease the glucose content. Heparinized or fluoridated plasma may be used. However, fluoride is not recommended, as it may cause some hemolysis and also depress the enzymatic reactions of the analytic procedure. For best results, serum or plasma is separated from the cells within a few minutes of collection. In this state the glucose is stable for several days at room temperature.

Cerebrospinal fluid should be free of erythrocytes. The same general conditions for preservation of serum or plasma apply to cerebrospinal fluid.

PROCEDURE

1. With a 1.0-ml volumetric pipette measure 1.0-ml portions of the mixed enzyme reagent into 13 × 120 mm tubes. Warm to 37°C in a water bath.
2. At zero time, quickly pipette 20 μl of the unknown serum into a correspondingly labeled tube and mix. Allowing sufficient time (30 seconds) for this pipetting step, continue for other specimens and for the glucose standards. Prepare a blank containing only the mixed reagent.
3. Stop the reaction after exactly 10 minutes for each tube in the series by quickly adding and mixing 4.0 ml of 7.2*N* sulfuric acid.
4. Measure the absorbance of the unknowns and of the standards at 540 mμ, using the blank as a reference.

CALCULATION

Calculate the glucose in the unknown specimens by the formula below, using a standard that is in the same region of glucose concentration as the unknown.

$$\frac{A_{\text{unknown}}}{A_{\text{standard}}} \times \text{conc. of standard} = \text{glucose (mg/100 ml)}$$

*Fermco Laboratories, Inc., P.O. Box 5110, Chicago, Illinois 60680.

Standard Curve

Alternatively, the concentration may be read from a standard calibration curve prepared by plotting absorbance against concentration on rectangular coordinate paper.

NOTES

1. The final color is formed immediately after adding sulfuric acid and is stable for several hours.
2. If the color is sufficiently intense to indicate a concentration of over 300 mg/100 ml, dilute the specimen with 1 volume of saline and repeat the determination. Multiply the results by 2.

REAGENTS

1. Mixed enzyme-chromogen-buffer reagent*

   Reconstitute the reagent by adding deionized water in a volume appropriate for the bottle size (30 ml for the 30-test size, etc.). Cap the bottle tightly and mix. Store the unused portion in a refrigerator. Do not freeze.
2. Sulfuric acid (7.2*N*)

   With stirring and cooling, add 250 ml of concentrated reagent-grade sulfuric acid slowly to 1000 ml of deionized water.
3. Glucose standards

   Prepare a 300 mg/100 ml standard by dissolving 300 mg of anhydrous reagent-grade glucose (dextrose) in about 80 ml of deionized water in a 100-ml volumetric flask. Add about 0.25 g of benzoic acid (not sodium benzoate). Mix to insure complete solution of the glucose and benzoic acid. Add water to the mark and mix again. Make working standards containing 60, 120, and 240 mg/100 ml by diluting 20, 40, and 80 ml of stock standard respectively to 100 ml with saturated benzoic acid solution.

REFERENCES

Kingsley, G. R., and Getchell, G., Direct Ultramicro Glucose Oxidase Method for Determination of Glucose in Biologic Fluids. Clin. Chem., *6*, 466, 1960.

Martinek, R. G., Preliminary Report on the Evaluation of a Stable Glucose Oxidase-Peroxidase-Chromogen Testing System for Glucose. Clin. Chem., *12*, 541, 1966.

Technical Bulletin No. 10. Fermco Laboratories, Inc., P.O. Box 5110, Chicago, Illinois 60680, 1967.

*Available as FermcoTEST in 30-, 60-, and 125-test size from Fermco Laboratories, Inc., P.O. Box 5110, Chicago, Illinois 60680.

Glucose, Blood

Somogyi-Nelson Method, Modified

PRINCIPLE

Whole blood, plasma, or serum is deproteinized with zinc hydroxide (mixture of sodium hydroxide and zinc sulfate), which yields a filtrate or centrifugate low in reducing substances other than glucose. The protein-free fluid is heated with an alkaline copper solution. Cupric ion oxidizes the glucose and in the process is converted to cuprous ion. The cuprous ion thus formed reduces an equivalent quantity of arsenomolybdate. The intensity of color of this solution is measured colorimetrically, which allows a quantitation of the glucose initially present in the specimen.

NORMAL VALUES

Whole blood (fasting): 65—110 mg/100 ml

SPECIMEN

The assay method may be applied to whole blood, plasma, serum, or cerebrospinal fluid. Any anticoagulant may be used. If the determination is to be performed on whole-blood specimens, either sodium fluoride should be added to inhibit glycolysis or the specimens should be refrigerated until they can be analyzed.

PROCEDURE

Standard Calibration Curve

1. Dilute 0.5, 1.0, 2.0, 3.0, and 4.0 ml of the stock standard to 10 ml in volumetric flasks. These working standards are equivalent to 50, 100, 200, 300, and 400 mg glucose/100 ml of solution respectively. Treat 1.0 ml of each standard in the same manner as blood, beginning at step 1 in the test procedure.
2. Measure the absorbance of each solution at 530 mμ, using the blank for a reference.
3. Prepare a standard curve by plotting absorbance against corresponding concentrations on rectangular coordinate paper.

Test Procedure

1. Place the volumes indicated below in 15 × 125 mm tubes in the order given. Mix thoroughly after each addition. Allow the tubes to stand for 5 minutes after adding and mixing the sodium hydroxide.

	Blank	Unknown	Standard
Water (ml)	1.0	0	0
Standard (ml)	0	0	1.0
Blood, plasma, serum, or CSF (ml)	0	1.0	0
Sodium hydroxide, 0.08*N* (ml)	7.0	7.0	7.0
Zinc sulfate (ml)	2.0	2.0	2.0

2. Centrifuge all tubes for 5 minutes.
3. Transfer 1.0 ml of supernatant fluid into correspondingly labeled sugar tubes marked at 12.5 ml and at 25.0 ml (Folin-Wu tubes may be used).
4. Add 2.0 ml of alkaline copper solution to each tube and mix.

5. Heat the tubes in a boiling water bath for 15 minutes. Remove the tubes and cool in several changes of cold tap water.
6. Add 1.0 ml of arsenomolybdate reagent to each tube and mix. Dilute to the 25-m mark with distilled water. Mix by inversion.
7. Measure the absorbance at 530 mμ.
8. Determine the glucose concentration by reference to the standard curve.
9. Run the 100 mg/100 ml glucose standard as a check on the procedure. Treat it exactly as the specimen.

REAGENTS

1. Sodium hydroxide (1*N*)

   Dissolve 8 g of reagent-grade sodium hydroxide in about 100 ml of water. When cool, dilute to 200 ml and mix.
2. Zinc sulfate (5% *W*/*V*)

   Dissolve 50.0 g of anhydrous zinc sulfate ($ZnSO_4$) in water. Dilute to 1 liter and mix.
3. Phenolphthalein (1% *W*/*V* in 95% ethanol)
4. Sodium hydroxide (0.08*N*)

   Dissolve 3.15 g of reagent-grade sodium hydroxide pellets in 1 liter of water. Adjust the strength so that 7 ml of this solution are required to produce a permanent pink color when titrated against 2 ml of the 5% zinc sulfate solution, using phenolphthalein as the indicator.
5. Copper sulfate (10% *W*/*V*)

   Dissolve 10 g of pulverized copper sulfate ($CuSO_4 \cdot 5H_2O$) in water and dilute to 100 ml.
6. Alkaline copper reagent

   Dissolve 28 g of anhydrous disodium phosphate and 40 g of Rochelle salt ($KNaC_4H_4O_6 \cdot 4H_2O$) in about 700 ml of water. While stirring, slowly add 100 ml of the 1*N* sodium hydroxide and 80 ml of the 10% copper sulfate solution. To this solution add 180 g of anhydrous sodium sulfate. When dissolved, dilute the solution to 1 liter. If a precipitate is observed after a few days, decant the clear top portion and filter the remainder through a coarse filter paper. Combine and mix the supernatant fluid and the filtrate. The solution is stable indefinitely.
7. Arsenomolybdate reagent

   Dissolve 25 g of ammonium molybdate in 450 ml of water. Add 21 ml of concentrated sulfuric acid and 25 ml of a solution containing 3.0 g of sodium arsenate, dibasic ($Na_2HAsO_4 \cdot 7H_2O$). Incubate this solution at 37°C for 48 hours. Store in a brown glass-stoppered bottle; discard if a green or blue color develops.
8. Benzoic acid (sat. aq.)

   Dissolve 2.0 g of benzoic acid in 500 ml of water. Apply heat and occasional stirring to effect solution. A small amount of the acid may precipitate from solution, indicating a saturated solution.
9. Glucose stock standard (1000 mg/100 ml)

   Dissolve 1.0 g of anhydrous reagent-grade glucose (dextrose) in a few ml of water. Quantitatively transfer the solution to a 100-ml volumetric flask, dilute to the mark with the saturated benzoic acid, and mix thoroughly.

REFERENCES

Nelson, N., A Photometric Adaptation of the Somogyi Method for the Determination of Glucose. J. Biol. Chem., *153*, 375, 1944.

Somogyi, M., A New Reagent for the Determination of Sugars. J. Biol. Chem., *160*, 61, 1945.

Somogyi, M., Determination of Blood Sugar. J. Biol. Chem., *160*, 69, 1945.

Glucose, Cerebrospinal Fluid

Rapid Screening Method

PRINCIPLE

This semiquantitative estimation is accomplished by the use of a Clinitest® tablet,* designed primarily for reducing substances in the urine. Tablets consisting of copper sulfate, sodium carbonate, sodium hydroxide and citric acid are placed in test tubes containing either cerebrospinal fluid or glucose standards. The action of citrate on sodium carbonate causes an effervescence that facilitates rapid solution of the tablet. Sodium hydroxide provides an alkaline medium and heat necessary for the oxidizing action of copper sulfate to take place. Reducing substances in cerebrospinal fluid (chiefly glucose) or in the standards react with the copper sulfate to yield cuprous oxide, which in the test ranges in color from green to orange. If none is present, the solution remains blue. Semiquantitative estimations are made by comparing the color, after reaction, with six color blocks on a chart enclosed with the bottle of Clinitest® tablets.

NORMAL VALUES

50—70 mg/100 ml (postabsorptively).

SPECIMEN

Because of the utilization of glucose by bacteria that may be present in the fluid, the test should be carried out as soon as possible after collection. A crystal of thymol in the fluid will inhibit bacterial action.

PROCEDURE

1. Pipette 0.5 ml of cerebrospinal fluid into a test tube.
2. Pipette 0.5 ml of glucose standards, 25, 50, 75, and 100 mg/100 ml, into similar tubes.
3. To each tube add 2 drops of caprylic alcohol and 1 Clinitest® tablet.
4. Permit the reaction to proceed until bubbling ceases.
5. Shake the tubes gently, add 1 ml of water to each, and shake again.
6. Compare the color in the cerebrospinal-fluid tube with that of the standards.
7. Report the fluid glucose concentration as a range between the two nearest standards; for example, 0—25 mg/100 ml.

REAGENTS

1. Clinitest® tablets
2. Glucose standards

   Dilute a 100 mg/100 ml standard (described under reagent for blood glucose) with water as shown in the table below:

Glucose Standard, 100 mg/100 ml (ml)	Water (ml)	Equivalent to (mg) glucose/100 ml
2.5	7.5	25
2.5	2.5	50
7.5	2.5	75

*Ames Company, Elkhart, Indiana.

REFERENCE

Hanock, A., and Worthy, W. L., A Rapid Screening Procedure for Sugar in Spinal Fluid. Lab. Dig., *24*, 17, 1961.

Glucose, Urine

Benedict's Qualitative Method

PRINCIPLE

Benedict's test is a nonspecific test for glucose. Cupric ion chelated by citrate is reduced to cuprous ion by glucose and other reducing compounds in urine when heated in alkaline solution. The initial blue color changes to green, to yellow, and to orange, depending upon the amount of reduction taking place.

NORMAL VALUES

Glucose is normally not detectable in urine.

SPECIMEN

Random urine.

PROCEDURE

1. Pipette 5 ml of Benedict's qualitative reagent into a test tube.
2. Add 8 drops of urine and mix well.
3. Place in a boiling water bath for 5 minutes.
4. Allow to cool at room temperature; do not hasten cooling by immersion in cold water.
5. Note the color of the final solution and of any precipitate.

INTERPRETATION

Color Reaction	Readings	Approximate Concentration (g/100 ml)
Blue	Negative	0
Green	Trace	0.25
Green with yellow precipitate	1+	0.5
Yellow to olive	2+	1.0
Brown	3+	1.5
Orange to red	4+	2.0 or more

REAGENTS

1. Benedict's qualitative sugar reagent

copper sulfate	17.3 g
sodium citrate	173.0 g
sodium carbonate	100.0 g
distilled water to make	1000.0 ml

With the aid of heat, dissolve the sodium citrate and carbonate in about 800 ml of water. Dissolve the copper sulfate in 100 ml. Add the copper sulfate solution to the carbonate-citrate solution slowly, with constant stirring. Dilute the final mixture to 1000 ml with distilled water.

REFERENCES

Hawk, P. B., Oser, B. L., and Summerson, W. H., Practical Physiological Chemistry, p. 826 and p. 1322. The Blakiston Co., Inc., New York, 1954.

Page, L. B., and Culver, P. J., A Syllabus of Laboratory Examinations in Clinical Diagnosis, p. 306. Harvard University Press, Cambridge, Massachusetts, 1962.

Glucose, Urine

Benedict's Quantitative Test

PRINCIPLE

Benedict's quantitative test for reducing substances in the urine depends upon the reduction of cupric ion to cuprous ion in an alkaline copper sulfate solution. Benedict's test is nonspecific, as it will give a positive reaction with reducing agents other than glucose. In this test, urine is titrated into the reagent. The end point is indicated by the loss of all blue color and the formation of a white precipitate, showing that all copper has been reduced.

This method is simple and reliable, and the reagent has the advantage of being stable for an indefinite length of time.

NORMAL VALUES

No measurable glucose.

SPECIMEN

Urine. To be meaningful, the specimen must be collected over a timed period. The urine should be refrigerated during the collection period.

PROCEDURE

1. Prepare a 1:10 dilution of urine with distilled water.
2. Fill a 50-ml burette with the diluted urine.
3. Pipette exactly 25 ml of Benedict's reagent into a porcelain evaporating dish. Add 20 g of crystalline sodium carbonate (or one half the weight of anhydrous salt) and a small quantity of talc. Heat the mixture to dissolve the sodium carbonate; continue to heat at the boiling point throughout the titration.
4. While stirring, add the urine from the burette rapidly at the beginning until a chalk-white precipitation forms and the blue color of the mixture begins to fade; then run in a few drops at a time until the last trace of blue color disappears. This marks the end point. If the mixture becomes too concentrated during the process, water may be added from time to time to replace the volume lost by evaporation.

CALCULATION

The 25 ml of Benedict's solution is reduced by exactly 50 mg of glucose. The formula for calculating the percentage of glucose is the following:

$$\%\ \text{glucose in original sample} = \frac{0.05}{X} \times D \times 100,$$

where X = ml of urine required to reduce 25 ml of copper solution,
D = dilution factor: 1 equals undiluted urine, and 10 equals 1:10 dilution of urine.

REAGENTS

1. Benedict's quantitative reagent

copper sulfate ($CuSO_4 \cdot 7H_2O$)	18 g

sodium carbonate (anhydrous)	100 g
sodium or potassium citrate	200 g
potassium thiocynate	125 g
potassium ferrocyanide (5% aqueous)	5 ml

With the aid of heat, dissolve the carbonate, citrate and thiocyanate in approximately 800 ml of distilled water; filter, if necessary. Dissolve the copper sulfate separately in about 100 ml of water. Pour this solution into the first with constant stirring. Add the ferrocyanide solution, cool, and dilute to exactly 1000 ml. The weight of the copper sulfate must be exact.

REFERENCES

Hawk, P. B., Oser, B. L., and Summerson, W. H., Practical Physiological Chemistry, 13th ed., p. 918. The Blakiston Co., Inc., New York, 1954.

Henry, R. J., Clinical Chemistry: Principles and Technics, p. 653. Hoeber Medical Division, Harper and Row, New York, 1967.

Glucose, Urine

Clinistix® *Reagent Strips

PRINCIPLE

Glucose oxidase promotes the oxidation of glucose to gluconic acid and hydrogen peroxide in the first of two reactions. In the second step, hydrogen peroxide in the presence of peroxidase oxidizes *o*-tolidine to a colored compound. The reagents are buffered, and impregnated into absorbent paper.

This test is sensitive and quite specific for glucose. However, it is subject to false positive reactions by such substances as hydrogen peroxide and hypochlorite. Ascorbic acid will cause false negative results.

NORMAL VALUES

No significant amount detectable.

SPECIMEN

Freshly voided random urine.

PROCEDURE

1. Dip test area of the strip into fresh urine, or pass it briefly through urine stream. Remove immediately.
2. Shake off excess urine.
3. Ten seconds after wetting, compare color of test area with color chart (see Notes).

NOTES

1. The sensitivity and speed of the reaction are affected by urine pH, temperature, concentrations of inhibitors present, and the concentration of ascorbic acid. For this reason, the test is read as either positive or negative, without attempt to estimate the amount of glucose present.

REAGENTS

1. Clinistix® reagent strips
   Available from the Ames Company, Division of Miles Laboratories, Inc., Elkhart, Indiana.

*Trademark of Ames Company, Division of Miles Laboratories, Inc., Elkhart, Indiana.

Glucose, Urine

Clinitest® *Reagent Tablets

PRINCIPLE

Clinitest® tablets contain anhydrous copper sulfate, anhydrous sodium hydroxide, citric acid, and sodium bicarbonate, and constitute a nonspecific test for reducing substances, having reactions similar to those described for Benedict's qualitative test.

NORMAL VALUES

No significant amounts detectable.

SPECIMEN

Random urine.

PROCEDURE

1. With a dropper in an upright position, place 5 drops of urine in a test tube.
2. Add 10 drops of water.
3. Drop 1 Clinitest® tablet into the tube.
4. Do not shake the tube during the reaction. 15 seconds after boiling has stopped, shake the tube gently, then compare with color chart. Chart colors are given corresponding to approximately 0, 0.25, 0.5, 0.75, 1, and 2 g/100 ml.

NOTES

1. Clinitest® tablets are hygroscopic and must be kept in a tightly closed bottle. If they absorb moisture, they may react less vigorously and give false negative reactions.

REAGENTS

1. Clinitest® reagent tablets
   Available from the Ames Company, Division of Miles Laboratories, Inc., Elkhart, Indiana.

REFERENCE

Kasper, J. A., and Jeffrey, Isabelle, A., A Simplified Benedict Test for Glycosuria. Am. J. Clin. Pathol., Tech. Sec., *14*, 117, 1944.

*Trademark of Ames Company, Division of Miles Laboratories, Inc., Elkhart, Indiana.

Hemoglobin, Plasma

Method of Crosby and Furth, Modified

PRINCIPLE

Benzidine in an acid solution and hydrogen peroxide in the presence of heme pigments combine to give a green color that changes to blue and finally to a reddish violet. The intensity of the color may be compared photoelectrically with that produced by a solution of known hemoglobin content. The test is an important measure of hemolysis, as free hemoglobin appears in the plasma only when the rate of hemolysis is relatively rapid.

NORMAL VALUES

Normally the plasma contains 1 to 4 mg of hemoglobin per 100 ml.

SPECIMEN

Plasma from heparinized or versenated blood.

PROCEDURE

1. Using a cuvette with a capacity of at least 30 ml, set up the unknown tube as follows:

plasma	0.1 ml
benzidine reagent	2.0 ml
hydrogen peroxide	1.0 ml

   Also prepare a blank tube, substituting 0.1 ml of water for the plasma.
2. Allow both mixtures to stand at room temperature for 1 hour.
3. Add 20.0 ml of 20% (*V*/*V*) aqueous solution of glacial acetic acid to each tube and shake gently to mix.
4. As soon as the colors are developed, compare the unknown against the blank by means of a photoelectric colorimeter. A blue-green filter is suitable (500 mμ).
5. Determine the results, using the standard curve prepared according to the directions given below.

Standard Curve

1. In four flasks place the following:

Flask No.	Stock Solution (ml)	Distilled Water (ml)	Concentration (mg/100 ml)
1	1	99	1.5
2	3	97	4.5
3	5	95	7.5

2. Prepare a chart on ordinary graph paper, using the three points determined by flasks 1, 2, and 3.

NOTES

1. Plasma having levels above 5 mg is usually colored enough to be noticeable.

REAGENTS

1. Benzidine solution

   Dissolve 0.50 mg of pure benzidine dihydrochloride (Merck) in 15 ml of hot (not boiling) distilled water. Add 25 ml of 95% ethanol and 10 ml of glacial acetic acid. This solution will keep several weeks if stored in a glass bottle under refrigeration.

2. Hydrogen peroxide (0.6% *V*/*V*)

   Dilute 1 volume of 30% hydrogen peroxide with 50 volumes of distilled water. This solution must be prepared fresh each time it is used.

3. Aqueous solution of glacial acetic acid (20% *V*/*V*)

4. Hemoglobin stock solution

   Add 1 ml of blood with a known hemoglobin concentration of 15 g/100 ml to 100 ml of distilled water to give a hemoglobin concentration of 150 mg/100 ml.

REFERENCE

Crosby, W. H., and Furth, F. W., A Modification of the Benzidine Method for Measurement of Hemoglobin in Plasma and Urine. Blood, *11*, 380, 1956.

Lactic Dehydrogenase

PRINCIPLE

Lactic dehydrogenase is an enzyme that catalyzes the following reaction:

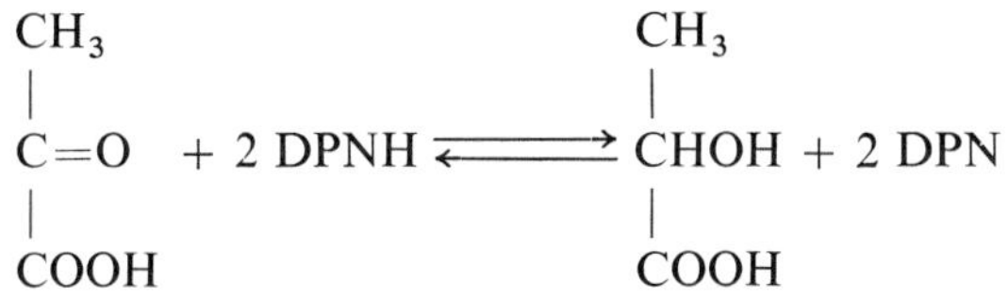

pyruvic acid — lactic acid

This reaction is reversible, and the rate in either direction can be used to assay the concentration of lactic dehydrogenase (LDH).

This procedure measures the amount of pyruvate remaining after incubation, which is inversely proportional to the amount of lactic dehydrogenase enzyme present in the reaction.

NORMAL VALUES

200—500 units.

SPECIMEN

Serum.

PROCEDURE

1. Prepare a 1:6 dilution of serum with water (1 volume of serum plus 5 volumes of water).
2. Pipette 0.1 ml of reduced beta-diphosphopyridine nucleotide (DPNH)* solution into a 13 × 150 mm test tube.
3. Add 1 ml of pyruvate acid-buffered substrate.
4. Place the tube in a 30°C constant water bath for 10 minutes.
5. Leaving the tube in the water bath, add 0.1 ml of diluted serum and start an interval timer.
6. After exactly 30 minutes, add 1 ml of dinitrophenylhydrazine solution, mix by swirling, and let stand for 20 minutes.
7. Add 10 ml of 0.4*N* sodium hydroxide and mix by inversion. Allow to stand for 5 to 10 minutes, then read the absorbance, using water as a blank at the same wavelength used for preparation of the calibration curve.
8. If the reading shows a value greater than 2,000 units, dilute the diluted serum with volumes of water (1:5) and repeat the test. Multiply the result by 5 to determine the enzyme concentration.

Calibration Curve

1. Prepare six test tubes as follows:

*Stock No. 500L-1, available from Sigma Chemical Company, 3500 De Kalb Street, St. Louis, Missouri 63118.

Tube No.	Pyruvate Substrate (ml)	Water (ml)	Units/ml
1	1.0	0.1	0
2	0.8	0.3	280
3	0.6	0.5	640
4	0.4	0.7	1,040
5	0.2	0.9	1,530
6	0.1	1.0	2,000

2. Add 1 ml of dinitrophenylhydrazine, mix gently, and allow to stand for 20 minutes.
3. Add 10 ml of 0.4*N* sodium hydroxide and mix gently.
4. Wait at least 5 minutes, then read the absorbances at 400—500 mμ against a water blank.
5. Plot the reading against the corresponding values of lactic dehydrogenase. Be sure to plot the highest optical density (OD) obtained (tube 1) against zero units of lactic dehydrogenase; similarly, the lowest OD reading is plotted against 2,000 units of lactic dehydrogenase.

NOTES

1. Hemolysis must be avoided. A trace in the serum specimen may give falsely elevated values.

REAGENTS

1. Pyruvic acid-buffered substrate (pH 7.8—8.0)

   Weigh 0.2 g of pyruvic acid and dilute with water to 1 liter. Add 10 g of potassium phosphate dibasic ($K_2HPO_4 \cdot 3H_2O$). This reagent is stable for at least 2 weeks, if stored under refrigeration.

2. Reduced beta-diphosphopyridine nucleotide (DPNH) solution

   Prepare a solution of 10 mg DPNH per 1 ml of distilled water. 0.1 ml of this solution is needed for each determination. This solution is unstable and must be prepared fresh before each determination.

3. Dinitrophenylhydrazine solution

   Dissolve 200 mg of 2-4-dinitrophenylhydrazine with 85 ml of concentrated hydrochloric acid in a 1000-ml volumetric flask. Dilute with distilled water to 1000 ml. This solution is stable for several weeks, if kept under refrigeration.

4. Sodium hydroxide (0.4*N*)

   In a 1000-ml volumetric flask dissolve 16 g of sodium hydroxide with enough distilled water to make 1000 ml. Filter, if necessary, to remove any trace of turbidity.

REFERENCES

Sigma Technical Bulletin No. 500 (published 1957, revised April 1964, reissued June 1965). Sigma Chemical Company, 3500 De Kalb Street, St. Louis, Missouri 63118.

Cabaud, P. G., and Wroblewski, F., Colorimetric Measurement of Lactic Dehydrogenase Activity of Body Fluids. Am. J. Clin. Pathol., *30*, 234, 1958.

Magnesium

Method of Orange and Rhein

PRINCIPLE

Titan yellow dye (Clayton yellow) complexes with the magnesium of a protein-free filtrate of plasma or serum in an alkaline medium to form an orange-pink magnesium-hydroxide-titan yellow lake, which is stabilized with polyvinyl alcohol. The intensity of color of the lake, which is measured colorimetrically, is proportional to the magnesium concentration.

NORMAL VALUES

Plasma or Serum	
Mean	**Range**
2.0 mg/100 ml 1.7 mEq/liter	1.7—2.3 mg/100 ml 1.4—1.9 mEq/liter

SPECIMEN

Plasma or serum are the specimens most commonly assayed. Whole blood is also suitable, but the values will be higher, as magnesium concentration is greater in erythrocytes than in plasma. Plasma or serum should be separated from the cells as soon as possible to avoid errors due to passage of magnesium out of the cells. This procedure is not applicable to urine.

PROCEDURE

1. Pipette the following into 13 × 100 mm tubes:

	Blank	Standard	Unknown
Trichloroacetic acid (ml)	5.0	5.0	5.0
Magnesium working standard (ml)	0	1.0	0
Unknown serum (ml)	0	0	1.0
Water (ml)	1.0	0	0

2. Mix the contents of the tubes by tapping. Centrifuge the unknown.
3. Measure the following into a suitable cuvette:

	Blank	Standard	Unknown
Supernatant from serum (ml)	0	0	2.0
Standard from step 2 (ml)	0	2.0	0
Blank from step 2 (ml)	2.0	0	0
Polyvinyl alcohol, 0.2% (ml)	1.0	1.0	1.0
Titan yellow solution (ml)	2.0	2.0	2.0
Sodium hydroxide, 15% (ml)	1.0	1.0	1.0

4. After addition of the sodium hydroxide, mix each tube by inverting several times. Color development is immediate and is stable for several hours.
5. Measure the absorbances of the standard and the unknown at 535 mμ, using the blank as a reference.

CALCULATION

$$\frac{A_{unknown}}{A_{standard}} \times 2 = \text{mg of magnesium/100 ml serum}$$

Standard Curve

Alternatively, the magnesium concentration may be determined by reference to a standard calibration curve prepared as outlined below:

1. Prepare the following standards from the magnesium stock solution:

Magnesium Stock (ml)	Diluted to (ml)	Magnesium Concentration (mg/100 ml)
1.0	100	1
2.0	100	2
3.0	100	3
4.0	100	4
5.0	100	5

2. Treat each standard as outlined in steps 1 through 5 of the test procedure.
3. Plot magnesium concentrations against absorbances on rectangular coordinate paper.

NOTES

1. When suitable instruments become available, atomic absorption spectrophotometry may come to be considered the method of choice for the measurement of magnesium in biological fluids and tissues.

REAGENTS

1. Trichloroacetic acid (TCA, 10% *W/V*)
2. Polyvinyl alcohol* (PVA, 0.2% *W/V*)

   Place 0.2 g of polyvinyl alcohol in a beaker and dissolve in 5 ml of water with the aid of heat and stirring. Make up to 100 ml and add a few drops of chloroform.
3. Titan yellow (Clayton yellow) solution (7.5 mg/100 ml *W/V*)

   Place 7.5 mg of the dye† in a beaker and dissolve in a few ml of water. Transfer quantitatively to a 100-ml volumetric flask; dilute to the mark and mix. Store in a refrigerator. Discard after about 3 months.
4. Sodium hydroxide (15% *W/V*)

   Place 15 g of reagent-grade sodium hydroxide in a beaker. Dissolve in a few ml of water. When cool, dilute to 100 ml.
5. Magnesium stock standard (1 mg/ml)

   Place exactly 100 mg of reagent-grade magnesium ribbon in a beaker and

*Dupanol, E. I. du Pont de Nemours & Co., Wilmington, Delaware 19898.
†Distillation Products Industries, Eastman Kodak, Co., Rochester, NY 14603.

add a mixture consisting of 2.5 ml of concentrated hydrochloric acid and 5.0 ml of water. Cover the beaker with a watch glass. When the reaction is complete, wash off the bottom of the glass with a stream of water from a wash bottle, adding the washings to the beaker. Transfer the contents of the beaker to a 100-ml volumetric flask and dilute to the mark with water. Mix thoroughly. Add 2.0 ml of chloroform and store in a refrigerator.

6. Magnesium working standard (2 mg/100 ml)
   Dilute 2.0 ml of the stock standard to 100 ml with water in a volumetric flask. Store in a refrigerator. Discard after a few weeks.

REFERENCE

Orange, M., and Rhein, H. C., Microestimation of Magnesium in Body Fluids. J. Biol. Chem., *189*, 379, 1951.

Phenothiazines

PRINCIPLE

The phenothiazines are easily oxidized. Their oxidation products are usually colored. A relatively sensitive test for the presumptive presence of phenothiazines was developed by Forest and Forest, and it has been used extensively. This test permits the detection of therapeutic amounts of phenothiazines in urine, but not in blood.

NORMAL VALUES

See interpretation.

SPECIMEN

1 ml of urine or stomach contents.

PROCEDURE

1. Add 2.0 ml of FPN reagent (see below) to the 1-ml sample.
2. Observe the intensity and color produced in 10 seconds. Disregard any change that takes longer than 10 seconds.

INTERPRETATION

The intensity of the blue, purple, or red color that forms within 10 seconds may be an indication that phenothiazines are present. The limits of detection are such that the test is not useful on blood samples. The color and intensity vary with the particular phenothiazine involved. After use of therapeutic amounts of the more potent phenothiazines or fluorinated derivatives, false negatives may occur. Thus the test may not be optimal as an indication of whether or not a patient is taking a prescribed phenothiazine. However, it is a good indication of gross overdosage and seldom yields false negatives following the ingestion of relatively large amounts of the drug. The limited value of this test must be recognized.

REAGENTS

1. FPN reagent

   Prepare the following solutions as indicated below, then mix, using the amount specified for each ingredient:

ferric chloride (5%)	5 ml
perchloric acid (20% *V*/*V*)	45 ml
nitric acid (50% *V*/*V*)	50 ml

   Dissolve 5 g of ferric chloride in 100 ml of water. Dilute 20 ml of 70% perchloric acid to 100 ml with water. Dilute 50 ml of concentrated nitric acid to 100 ml with water.

Phenylalanine

PRINCIPLE

A protein-free supernatant fluid of plasma or serum is treated with ninhydrin to produce a fluorescent reaction product with phenylalanine, the intensity of which is enhanced in the presence of the peptide L-leucyl-L-alanine. This reaction is made highly specific for phenylalanine, even when other amino acids are present, by maintaining the pH at 5.8.

NORMAL VALUES

Newborn: mean ± S.D. = 1.51 mg/100 ml ± 0.82
8 months to 13 years: mean ± S.D. = 1.83 mg/100 ml ± 0.94

SPECIMEN

Serum is most often used for this determination, but plasma may also be suitable. Phenylalanine is stable for several months in serum specimens stored in a refrigerator at 5—10°C.

PROCEDURE

1. Deproteinize plasma or serum by adding 0.1 ml of 0.6*N* trichloroacetic acid to 0.1 ml of specimen. Mix well and centrifuge.
2. To 10 × 100 mm tubes add the following:

	Blank	Standard	Unknown
Succinate buffer (ml)	0.5	0.5	0.5
Ninhydrin solution (ml)	0.2	0.2	0.2
Peptide solution (ml)	0.1	0.1	0.1
Working standards, each of the 6 concentrations (ml)	0	0.05	0
Supernatant fluid from specimen (ml)	0	0	0.05
Trichloroacetic acid, 0.3*N* (ml)	0.05	0	0

3. Cover the tubes with parafilm and mix by inversion.
4. Incubate the tubes for 2 hours in a water bath at 60°C.
5. Cool the tubes in an ice bath. Add 5.0 ml of the copper reagent to each. Mix thoroughly.
6. Measure the fluorescence of the standards and the unknown sample, setting the blank at zero fluorescence. Use filters approximating the optimum wavelengths (primary 390 mμ, secondary 485 mμ).
7. Plot the fluorescence values of the standards against their corresponding concentration on rectangular coordinate paper and draw a curve of "best fit" through the points.
8. Read the values of the unknowns from the calibration curve.

REAGENTS

1. Succinate buffer (0.3*M*, pH 5.8)

   Dissolve 4.94 g of disodium succinate ($NaOCOCH_2CH_2$–$COONa \cdot 2H_2O$) in water, add 4.0 ml of 1*N* HCl, and dilute to 100 ml. Adjust pH to 5.8 with either HCl or NaOH, using a pH meter. Store in a refrigerator.

2. Ninhydrin solution (30 m*M*)
   Dissolve 0.534 g in water and dilute to 100 ml. Store in a brown bottle at room temperature.
3. Peptide solution (L-leucyl-L-alanine, 5 m*M*)
   Dissolve 0.1011 g of the peptide in water and dilute to 100 ml. Dispense in small tubes in volumes of approximately 1 ml and store in a freezer. Discard any remaining thawed reagent.
4. Copper reagent
   Dissolve each compound separately in about 100 ml of water. Add the solutions in the order listed, mixing after each addition. Dilute with water to 1 liter.

sodium carbonate, anhydrous	1.6 g
potassium sodium tartrate	0.1 g
copper sulfate, heptahydrate	0.06 g

   Store at room temperature. The reagent is stable for several weeks.
5. Trichloroacetic acid (0.6*N*)
   Dissolve 98.0 g of trichloroacetic acid in water and dilute to 1 liter.
6. Trichloroacetic acid (0.3*N*)
   Dilute 1 volume of the 0.6*N* acid with 1 volume of water.
7. Phenylalanine stock standard (100 mg/100 ml)
   Dissolve 100 mg of L-phenylalanine in 0.3*N* trichloroacetic acid and dilute to 100 ml with the acid. Store in a refrigerator.
8. Phenylalanine working standards
   Dilute the stock standard with 0.3*N* trichloroacetic acid according to the table below:

Stock (ml)	Dilute to (ml)	Phenylalanine (ml)	Equivalent to (mg phenylalanine per 100 ml serum)
5.0	50	10	20
3.0	50	8	16
2.0	50	4	8
1.0	50	2	4
1.0	100	1	2
0.5	100	0.5	1

REFERENCES

Faulkner, W. R., Phenylalanine. Standard Methods of Clinical Chemistry, *5*, 199, Meites, S., ed. Academic Press, New York, 1965.

McCaman, M. W., and Robins, E., Fluorimetric Method for the Determination of Phenylalanine in Serum. J. Lab. Clin. Med., *59*, 885, 1962.

Phenylpyruvic Acid, Urine

Method of Meulemans
(Qualitative Test)

PRINCIPLE

Phenylpyruvic acid is detected in the urine by first acidifying with hydrochloric acid and then adding ferric chloride. There are a number of other substances found in the urine that may react with ferric chloride, but this does not limit the usefulness of the test as a screening procedure. Phenylpyruvic acid reacts with Fe^{+++} to form a green or blue-green color. Phosphate ions, which could cause false negative results if present, are removed by precipitation as $MgNH_4PO_4$.

NORMAL VALUES

Not normally detectable in urine.

PROCEDURE

1. Add 1 ml of magnesium reagent to 4 ml of urine.
2. Mix, let stand for 5 minutes, then filter.
3. Acidify the filtrate with 2 drops of 10% hydrochloric acid and add 2 drops of 10% ferric chloride.
4. A positive reaction yields a green or blue-green color that eventually fades to yellow.

NOTES

1. Phenylpyruvic acid decomposes rapidly in urine at room temperature.
2. Urine can be preserved for several days by adding thymol or 1 ml of 5% sulfuric acid and refrigerating the specimen.

REAGENTS

1. Magnesium reagent

magnesium chloride	11 g
ammonium chloride	14 g
ammonium hydroxide (concentrated)	20 ml

Dissolve the above ingredients and dilute with distilled water to 1 liter.

REFERENCES

Henry, R. J., Clinical Chemistry: Principles and Technics. Hoeber Medical Division, Harper and Row, New York, 1967.

Meulemans, O., Phenylpyruvic Acid in Urine. Clin. Chim. Acta, *5*, 48, 1960.

Phosphatase, Acid

Method of Bodansky, Modified

PRINCIPLE

Serum is incubated with a sodium beta-glycerophosphate substrate buffered at pH 5.0. The inorganic phosphate liberated is measured and is expressed in Bodansky units, which are defined as the number of mg of phosphorus liberated by 100 ml of serum incubated for 1 hour at 37°C.

NORMAL VALUES

0.5—2.0 Bodansky units.

SPECIMEN

Acid phosphatase is unstable, being readily inactivated at room temperature. If the assay cannot be made soon after collection, the sample can be preserved for up to 2 hours in an ice bath. Hemolyzed samples are unsuitable for analysis because of the large positive errors that will occur.

PROCEDURE

1. Pipette 5.0 ml of beta-glycerophosphate buffer into each of three tubes, labeled "Blank", "Incubated", and "Control" respectively.
2. Place the tubes in a 37°C water bath for a few minutes.
3. Pipette 0.5 ml of water into the blank, and 0.5 ml of serum into the incubated tube. Do not add anything to the control tube at this time. Mix well and begin timing.
4. Remove all three tubes after exactly 1 hour and pipette 0.5 ml of 60% trichloroacetic acid solution into each of them.
5. Pipette 0.5 ml of serum into the control tube.
6. Cover the tubes with parafilm and mix well by inversion. Centrifuge the serum mixture, then filter the supernatant fluid through Whatman #42 filter paper.
7. Transfer 3.0 ml of the filtrates to three correspondingly labeled tubes.
8. Add 2.0 ml of acid molybdate and 1.0 ml of Elon®* (methylaminophenol sulfate) to each tube. Mix thoroughly and allow to stand for 15 minutes at room temperature.
9. Measure the absorbance of the incubated and control reaction mixtures at 660 mμ, using the blank as a reference.
10. Obtain the inorganic phosphorus concentration by reference to a previously constructed calibration curve. If the phosphorus in the incubated tube exceeds 10 mg/100 ml, repeat the assay, using 1.0 ml of the filtrate and diluting it with 2.0 ml of the blank filtrate. Proceed from step 8 and multiply the results by 3.

*Eastman Kodak Co., 343 State Street, Rochester, New York, 14650.

Calibration

1. Prepare a series of standards as shown in the table below:

Phosphorus (ml)	Water (ml)	60% Trichloro-acetic Acid (ml)	Phosphorus Contained (mg)	Equivalent to (mg inorganic phosphorus per 100 ml serum)
0.05	5.45	0.5	0.010	2.0
0.10	5.40	0.5	0.020	4.0
0.15	5.35	0.5	0.030	6.0
0.20	5.30	0.5	0.040	8.0
0.25	5.25	0.5	0.050	10.0
0.30	5.20	0.5	0.060	12.0
0	5.50	0.5	0	0 (blank)

2. Treat each standard according to the test procedure as outlined in steps 3 through 9.
3. Plot absorbances against concentration on rectangular coordinate paper, using the blank as reference.

CALCULATION

Subtract the control value from the incubated value and report the difference as Bodansky units of acid phosphatase. If the number of units is greater than 25, repeat the procedure, using 0.1 ml of serum and 0.4 ml of saline for the incubated tube, multiplying the result by 5. Subtract the control value from that of the incubated and report the difference as Bodansky units.

REAGENTS

1. Beta-glycerophosphate buffer (pH 5.0 ± 0.05)
   Dissolve 2.500 g of reagent-grade sodium beta-glycerophosphate and 2.120 g of sodium diethyl barbiturate in water. Add 25.0 ml of 1*N* acetic acid and dilute with water to 500 ml. Adjust the pH, if necessary, with either 0.1*N* sodium hydroxide or hydrochloric acid to obtain the correct value. Add a few ml of chloroform and mix. Store in a glass-stoppered bottle in a refrigerator. Discard after 1 month.
2. Trichloroacetic acid (60%)
   Dissolve 60 g of trichloroacetic acid in water and dilute to 100 ml.
3. Elon® (*p*-methyl-aminophenol sulfate)
   Dissolve 1.0 g of Elon® and 3.0 g of sodium bisulfite in 100 ml of distilled water. Store in a brown bottle in a refrigerator. Discard after 2 months.
4. Acid molybdate
   Dissolve 7.5 g of ammonium molybdate in approximately 800 ml of distilled water. Add slowly and with stirring 53 ml of concentrated sulfuric acid. Dilute with water to 1 liter.
5. Phosphorus standard (0.2 mg/ml)
   Dissolve 0.4394 g of potassium dihydrogen phosphate (KH_2PO_4) in water and dilute to the mark in a 500-ml volumetric flask.

REFERENCES

Bodansky, A., Phosphatase Studies. II. Determination of Serum Phosphatase. Factors Influencing the Accuracy of the Determination. J. Biol. Chem., *101*, 93, 1933.

Gomori, G., A Modification of the Colorimetric Phosphorus Determination for Use with the Photoelectric Colorimeter. J. Lab. Clin. Med., *27*, 955, 1941—1942.

Kaser, M. M., and Baker, J., Alkaline and Acid Phosphatases. Standard Methods of Clinical Chemistry, *2*, Seligson, D., ed. Academic Press, New York, 1958.

Phosphatase, Alkaline

Method of Bodansky
Modified by Kaplan and del Carmen

PRINCIPLE

Inorganic phosphate is liberated from a phosphate substrate by the action of serum phosphatase at an alkaline pH. The inorganic phosphate is measured before and after incubation. The difference is reported in Bodansky units, which are defined as the amount of activity that will liberate 1 mg of inorganic phosphate substrate at pH 8.6 during the first hour of incubation at 37°C.

NORMAL VALUES

Adults: 1.5—4.0 units/100 ml
Children: 5.0—12.0 units/100 ml

SPECIMEN

Serum is the most commonly used specimen. Plasma is, however, just as satisfactory, if heparin is used. Fluoride and oxalate inhibit alkaline phosphatase activity. Other anticoagulants may affect the activity also.

Activity has been reported to increase up to 30% in serum kept at room temperature or in a refrigerator for 24 hours. Because of this, it is best to assay the specimen within a few hours after collection.

PROCEDURE

Incubated Sample

1. Place 9.0 ml of substrate in a 13 × 100 mm test tube and equilibrate to 37°C.
2. Add 1.0 ml serum, mix, and incubate at 37°C for exactly 1 hour.
3. Quickly add 2.0 ml of 30% trichloroacetic acid and mix, then allow to stand for a few minutes. Centrifuge for 10 minutes at moderate speed.

Control Sample

1. Near the end of the incubation period, measure 9.0 ml of substrate into another tube and add 2.0 ml of 30% trichloroacetic acid.
2. With mixing, add 1.0 ml of serum. Allow to stand for a few minutes, then centrifuge as for the incubated sample.

Incubated and Control Sample

1. Place in 10 × 75 mm cuvettes the following, mixing after each addition.

	Blank	Standard	Incubated Sample	Control Sample
Trichloroacetic acid, 5% (ml)	8.0	0	0	0
Working standard (ml)	0	8.0	0	0
Incubated supernatant (ml)	0	0	8.0	0
Control supernatant (ml)	0	0	0	8.0
Molybdate reagent (ml)	1.0	1.0	1.0	1.0
Aminonaphtholsulfonic acid (ml)	0.5	0.5	0.5	0.5

2. Allow the tubes to stand 10 minutes for color development.
3. Measure the absorbance of the standard, incubated, and control samples at 660 mμ, using the blank as a reference. The color is stable for at least 1 hour.

CALCULATION

$$\frac{A_{incubated} - A_{control}}{A_{standard}} \times 6 = \text{Bodansky units/100 ml serum}$$

REAGENTS

1. Trichloroacetic acid (30% *W/V*)
   Dissolve 30 g of reagent-grade trichloroacetic acid in water and dilute to 100 ml. This solution is stable indefinitely.
2. Trichloroacetic acid (5%)
   Dilute 10 ml of the 30% solution with water to 60 ml.
3. Sulfuric acid (10*N*)
   Carefully add 55.5 ml of concentrated reagent-grade sulfuric acid to about 100 ml of water. Mix, allow to cool, then dilute with water to 200 ml. Check the normality by titration against standard sodium hydroxide. Adjust the solution, if necessary, to make it exactly 10*N*.
4. Molybdate reagent
   Dissolve 12.5 g of reagent-grade ammonium molybdate in about 100 ml of water. Place 150 ml of the 10*N* sulfuric acid in a 500-ml volumetric flask. Add the molybdate solution and dilute to the mark with water. This solution is stable indefinitely.
5. Aminonaphtholsulfonic acid reagent
   Place the following reagents in a mortar, grind to a powder, and mix thoroughly:

sodium bisulfite	142.5 g
sodium sulfite	10.0 g
1, 2, 4-aminonaphtholsulfonic acid	2.5 g

   Dispense the powder in 1.5-g quantities into 10 × 75 mm test tubes and stopper tightly. Make up the working solution by dissolving the contents of a tube in 10 ml of water. Store in a refrigerator. Prepare fresh about every 2 weeks.
6. Phosphate stock standard (0.4 mg phosphorus/5 ml)
   Dissolve 0.351 g of dry reagent-grade monopotassium phosphate in water and transfer quantitatively to a 1-liter volumetric flask. Add 10 ml of 10*N* sulfuric acid, then dilute to the mark and mix thoroughly. This standard is stable indefinitely at room temperature.
7. Phosphate working standard (0.04 mg phosphorus/8 ml)
   Place 6.25 ml of the stock standard in a 100-ml volumetric flask. Add 16.7 ml of 30% trichloroacetic acid solution, then dilute to the mark and mix. This standard is stable indefinitely in a refrigerator.
8. Alkaline phosphatase substrate
   Place in a 100-ml volumetric flask the following:

sodium ß-glycerophosphate	0.5 g
sodium diethylbarbiturate	0.424 g

Add water and dissolve these two compounds. Dilute to the mark with water, mix, then add about 3 ml of petroleum ether (B.P. 20—40°C). Store in a glass-stoppered bottle containing a 1-inch layer of petroleum ether and refrigerate.

REFERENCES

Bodansky, A., Phosphatase Studies. II. Determination of Serum Phosphatase. Factors Influencing the Accuracy of the Determination. J. Biol. Chem., *101*, 93, 1933.

Fiske, C. H., and Subbarow, Y., The Colorimetric Determination of Phosphorus. J. Biol. Chem., *66*, 375, 1925.

Kaplan, S. A., and del Carmen, F. T., Quantitative Ultramicroanalysis for the Clinical Laboratory. Pediatrics, *17*, 857, 1956.

Phosphorus, Inorganic

Method of Fiske and Subbarow, Modified by Kaplan and del Carmen

PRINCIPLE

The inorganic phosphate of a trichloroacetic acid filtrate of serum is reacted with an acid molybdate solution to form phosphomolybdic acid. The phosphomolybdic acid is then reduced by 1, 2, 4-aminonaphtholsulfonic acid to produce a blue color proportional in intensity to the phosphate present. The final measurement is made colorimetrically, and the results reported as inorganic phosphorus.

NORMAL VALUES

Adults: 3.0—4.5 mg/100 ml
Children: 4.5—6.5 mg/100 ml

SPECIMEN

Serum is preferred to whole blood because of the susceptibility to hydrolysis of organic phosphate present in the erythrocytes, followed by diffusion into the serum. This source of error can be large, if blood is allowed to stand for several hours. Since very little inorganic phosphate resides in erythrocytes, the hematocrit will affect the whole-blood concentration. If plasma rather than serum is used, oxalates should be avoided, as they may interfere with color development. The inorganic-phosphate concentration is quite stable in plasma or serum, remaining unchanged after several hours at room temperature and for at least 1 week in a refrigerator.

PROCEDURE

1. Place 4.5 ml of water in a test tube.
2. Add 0.5 ml of serum and mix.
3. Add 1.0 ml of 30% trichloroacetic acid. Mix by vigorous shaking, allow to stand for a few minutes, then centrifuge for 10 minutes at moderate speed.
4. Place in suitable cuvettes the following, mixing after each addition:

	Blank	Standard	Unknown
Trichloroacetic acid, 5% (ml)	4.0	0	0
Working standard (ml)	0	4.0	0
Supernatant from step 3 (ml)	0	0	4.0
Molybdate reagent (ml)	0.5	0.5	0.5
Aminonaphtholsulfonic acid (ml)	0.25	0.25	0.25

5. Allow the tubes to stand for 10 minutes. The color is stable for at least 1 hour.
6. Measure the absorbances at 660 mμ, using the blank as reference.

CALCULATION

$$\frac{A_{unknown}}{A_{standard}} \times 6.0 = \text{mg inorganic phosphorus/100 ml serum}$$

REAGENTS

1. Trichloroacetic acid (30% *W/V*)
   Dissolve 30 g of reagent-grade trichloroacetic acid in water and dilute to 100 ml.
2. Trichloroacetic acid (5% *W/V*)
   Dilute 10 ml of the 30% solution with water to 60 ml.
3. Sulfuric acid (10*N*)
   Carefully add 55.5 ml of concentrated reagent-grade sulfuric acid to about 100 ml of water. Mix, allow to cool, then dilute with water to 200 ml. Check the normality by titration with standard sodium hydroxide. Adjust the solution, if necessary, to make it exactly 10*N*.
4. Molybdate reagent
   Dissolve 2.5 g of reagent-grade ammonium molybdate in about 20 ml of water. Place 30 ml of the 10*N* sulfuric acid in a 100-ml volumetric flask. Add the molybdate solution and dilute to the mark with water. This reagent is stable indefinitely.
5. Aminonaphtholsulfonic acid reagent
   Place the following reagents in a mortar, grind to a powder, and mix thoroughly:

sodium bisulfite	142.5 g
sodium sulfite, anhydrous	10.0 g
1,2,4-aminonapththolsulfonic acid	2.5 g

   Dispense in quantities of 1.5 g into 10 × 75 mm test tubes and stopper tightly. Make up the working reagent by dissolving the contents of a tube in 10 ml of water. Store in a refrigerator. Prepare fresh about every 2 weeks.
6. Phosphate stock standard (0.4 mg phosphorus/5 ml)
   Dissolve 0.351 g of dry reagent-grade anhydrous monopotassium phosphate (KH_2PO_4) crystals in water and transfer quantitatively to a 1-liter volumetric flask. Add 10 ml of 10*N* sulfuric acid, dilute to the mark with water, and mix thoroughly. This standard is stable indefinitely.
7. Phosphate working standard (0.04 mg phosphorus/8 ml)
   Place 6.25 ml of the stock standard in a 100-ml volumetric flask. Add 16.7 ml of 30% trichloroacetic acid solution, dilute to the mark with water, and mix. This standard is stable indefinitely in a refrigerator.

REFERENCES

Fiske, C. H., and Subbarow, Y., The Colorimetric Determination of Phosphorus. J. Biol. Chem., *66*, 375, 1925.

Kaplan, S. A., and del Carman, F. T., Quantitative Ultramicroanalysis for the Clinical Laboratory. Pediatrics, *17*, 857, 1956.

Porphyrins

Method of Schlenker and Kitchell

PRINCIPLE

The porphyrins are a group of cyclic compounds composed of four pyrrole units united to form a ring structure. This ring is modified by the addition of many different types of linkages and side chains, so that a host of such compounds is possible. One of the most important of these compounds is porphyrin, which is able to form complexes with iron to form heme and, subsequently, a whole family of compounds involved in the oxidation-reduction reactions so essential to cellular life. Among these compounds are hemoglobin, myoglobin, cytochrome, and the peroxidase enzymes.

When red cells are destroyed, the hemoglobin released is broken down by the body. The iron and certain other parts of the molecule are conserved, but the protoporphyrins are not utilized by the body; they are eventually broken down further and excreted in the urine and feces. Abnormal increases in any of the porphyrins may result in detectable amounts being excreted in the urine. Such conditions are known collectively as porphyriurias. Increases in urinary porphyrin may occur in congenital disorders, in lead poisoning, liver diseases, and blood dyscrasias of many kinds.

NORMAL VALUES

Uroporphyrins:	20 μg/24 hours
Coproporphyrins:	95 μg/24 hours
Protoporphyrins:	15 μg/24 hours

SPECIMEN

Urine, 24-hour collection preserved by refrigeration.

PROCEDURE

1. Prepare the urine specimen by filtering through filter paper.
2. To a separatory funnel add 15 ml of urine, 1 ml of glacial acetic acid, and 30 ml of ethyl ether.
3. Extract the coproporphyrins and protoporphyrins by shaking the above mixture for 3 minutes. Separate the aqueous portion containing the uroporphyrins.
4. Rewash the aqueous portion with 5 ml of ether and check the wash for fluorescence; if positive, wash again. Combine the ether fractions.
5. Wash the ether fraction with 2-ml portions of distilled water until the water extracts are free of fluorescence. This usually takes at least 2 washes. Combine the aqueous portions with the aqueous portion from step 3.
6. Extract coproporphyrins from the ether fractions by washing with successive 1-ml portions of 0.1*N* hydrochloric acid until the extract is free of fluorescence. This usually takes 5 extractions or more. Combine the acid extracts and make to a definite volume (V_1) with 0.1*N* hydrochloric acid.
7. Extract the protoporphyrins in the same manner, using 2.8*N* hydrochloric acid. This is volume V_2.

8. To the aqueous uroporphyrins add 1.4 ml of concentrated hydrochloric acid and dilute to 30 ml. This gives an acid concentration of about 0.5*N*. 2 ml of this solution are equivalent to 1 ml of original urine.
9. Read the absorbances (A) in a spectrophotometer, using a blank of 0.5*N* hydrochloric acid. Apply the readings to the following formulas.
   (a) Coproporphyrins
   The Soret maximum is 401 mμ; however, readings should be taken at 399, 401, 402, and 403 mμ, and the maximum absorbance used.

$$\mu g/ml = \frac{2 \times A_{max} - (A_{430} + A_{380})}{0.667 \times 1.835} \times \frac{V_1}{V_{urine}}$$

   (b) Protoporphyrins
   The Soret maximum is 406 mμ; however, readings should be taken at 405, 406, 407, and 408 mμ, and the maximum absorbance used.

$$\mu g/ml = \frac{2 \times A_{max} - (A_{430} + A_{380})}{0.489 \times 1.668} \times \frac{V_2}{V_{urine}}$$

   (c) Uroporphyrins
   The Soret maximum is 405 mμ; however, readings should be taken at 404, 405, 406, and 407 mμ, and the maximum absorbance used.

$$\mu g/ml = \frac{2 \times A_{max} - (A_{430} + A_{380})}{0.653 \times 1.844} \times \frac{30}{V_{urine}}$$

REAGENTS

1. Hydrochloric acid (0.1*N*, 2.8*N*, 0.5*N*, concentrated)
2. Ethyl ether
3. Glacial acetic acid

REFERENCE

Schlenker, F. S., and Kitchell, Cynthia L., Analysis of Porphyrins in the Clinical Laboratory. Am. J. Clin. Pathol., *29*, 593, 1958.

Proteins, Total, Cerebrospinal Fluid

Folin-Ciocalteau Colorimetric Method

PRINCIPLE

Cerebrospinal fluid is treated with an alkaline copper tartrate solution, which forms cupric complexes with amino acid residues of the protein. Folin-Ciocalteau phenol reagent (phosphotungstomolybdic acid) is added, which is reduced by both tyrosine and cupric amino acid complexes of the protein. The intensity of color is proportional to the protein concentration of the specimen and is measured colorimetrically.

NORMAL VALUES

Adults:	15—50 mg/100 ml
Newborn infants:	60—90 mg/100 ml

SPECIMEN

The fluid should be centrifuged to eliminate cells and other particulate matter. Bloody specimens are not suitable for protein estimation.

PROCEDURE

1. Place in 25-ml Erlenmeyer flasks the following:

	Blank	Standard	Unknown
Alkaline copper reagent (ml)	10.0	10.0	10.0
Standard serum, about 50 mg per 100 ml (ml)	0	0.1	0
Unknown specimen (ml)	0	0	0.1
Water (ml)	0.1	0	0

2. Mix and allow to stand at room temperature for 15 minutes.
3. Using a different 1-ml serological pipette for each flask, add rapidly and with stirring 1 ml of Folin-Ciocalteau reagent. (Blow air into the mixture to assure rapid and complete mixing.)
4. Allow the flasks to stand at room temperature for 30 minutes. (The color is stable for about 15 minutes after development and then slowly increases.)
5. Measure the absorbance of each mixture at 700 mμ, using the blank as a reference.

CALCULATION

1. $$\left(\frac{A_{\text{unknown}}}{A_{\text{standard}}} \times \text{concentration of standard}\right) - 6 = \text{mg protein/100 ml.}$$

2. Alternatively, the concentration may be read from a calibration graph prepared according to the instructions below:
   (a) carry each of the protein working standards through the procedure; include a blank;
   (b) plot absorbance against concentration on rectangular coordinate paper;

(c) subtract 6 mg from the graph reading for an unknown (to compensate for nonprotein color-producing material) to obtain CSF protein concentration.

NOTES

1. Wavelengths between 600 and 700 mμ may be used, provided that the calibration chart is prepared at the same wavelength. Greater sensitivity is obtained at higher wavelengths.
2. An average value of 6 mg is used to correct for the nonprotein color-producing material.

REAGENTS

1. Alkaline carbonate solution

   Dissolve the following in 1 liter of 0.1*N* sodium hydroxide:

sodium carbonate, anhydrous	20.0 g
potassium sodium tartrate (Rochelle salt)	0.5 g

   Store at room temperature in a polyethylene bottle. Discard after 6 months, or sooner if turbidity develops.
2. Copper sulfate solution (0.1% *W*/*V*)

   Dissolve 1.0 g of cupric sulfate pentahydrate in 1 liter of water. Store at room temperature in a polyethylene bottle. Discard after 3 months.
3. Alkaline copper reagent

   Mix 9 volumes of the alkaline carbonate solution and 1 volume of copper sulfate solution. Prepare on day of use.
4. Folin-Ciocalteau phenol reagent

   This reagent is available commercially.* The product listed in the footnote has been found satisfactory after adjustment of the acidity, which should be $0.9 \pm 0.1N$. To check the acidity, titrate 1.0 ml (diluted with 10 ml water) with standard alkali to pH 8.5, using a pH meter. Phenolphthalein gives a very poor end point. If the normality is too high to bring it to proper volume, dilute the reagent with water, using the following formula:

   $$\text{water to add to 100 ml of phenol reagent} = \left[\frac{N_{\text{phenol regent}} \times 100}{0.9}\right] - 100.$$

   Alternatively, this reagent may be prepared as indicated below.

   (a) Reflux the following materials gently for 10 hours in an all-glass apparatus:

sodium tungstate, dihydrate	100.0 g
sodium molybdate, dihydrate	25.0 g
phosphoric acid (85%)	50.0 ml
hydrochloric acid, concentrated	100.0 ml
water	700.0 ml

   (b) Add 150 g of lithium sulfate, 50 ml of water, and a few drops of bromine (or 50 ml of bromine water). Boil the solution without a condenser for 15 minutes or until it becomes yellow. If a green tint remains, add another drop of bromine (or 10 ml of bromine water) and boil for another 15 minutes. When cool, dilute to 1 liter with water.

*Phenol reagent (Folin & Ciocalteau), Item No. 2690, Hartmann-Leddon Company, Inc., Philadelphia, Pennsylvania.

(c) Check the titratable acidity, which should be $0.9 \pm 0.1N$, as for the commercial product.

5. Protein stock standard

Purchase a serum standard of known protein concentration, or establish the value on a serum pool by Kjeldahl analysis. The product listed in the footnote has been found to be satisfactory.*

6. Protein working standards

Dilute the protein stock standard with 0.25% benzoic acid solution as indicated below:

Tube No.	Contents	Benzoic Acid, 0.25% (ml)	Equivalent to Protein in Stock Concentration (mg/100 ml)
1	0.5 ml stock	4.5	0.1
2	2.5 ml of tube 1	2.5	0.05
3	2.5 ml of tube 2	2.5	0.025
4	2.5 ml of tube 3	2.5	0.0125
5	2.5 ml of tube 4	2.5	0.00625

REFERENCES

Daughaday, W. H., Lowry, O. H., Rosebrough, N. J., and Fields, W. S., Determination of Cerebrospinal Fluid Protein with Folin Phenol Reagent. J. Lab. Clin. Med., *39*, 663, 1952.

Lowry, O. H., Rosebrough, N. J., Farr, A. L., and Randall, Rose J., Protein Measurement with Folin Phenol Reagent. J. Biol. Chem., *193*, 265, 1951.

Rice, E. W., Total Proteins in Cerebrospinal Fluid (Colorimetric). Standard Methods of Clinical Chemistry, *5*, 223, Meites, S., ed. Academic Press, New York, 1965.

*Normal clinical-chemical control serum, dried, Hyland Division of Travenol Laboratories, Inc., P.O. Box 2214, Costa Mesa, California 92926.

Proteins, Total, Plasma or Serum

Method of Gornall, Bardawill and David

PRINCIPLE

The proteins of plasma or serum are reacted with cupric ion in an alkaline medium to produce a violet complex. The intensity of the color, which is proportional to the protein concentration, is measured colorimetrically.

NORMAL VALUES

6.4—8.0 g/100 ml.

SPECIMEN

Serum may be used, or plasma in which any of the common anticoagulants have been employed. Bilirubin does not interfere, but marked hemolysis causes a large positive error.

PROCEDURE

1. Measure 0.1 ml of serum protein and of standard into 15 × 125 mm tubes and add 10 ml of the biuret reagent to each. Mix thoroughly and allow to stand for 30 minutes.
2. Set a colorimeter to zero absorbance at 540 mμ, using biuret reagent as a reference.
3. Read the absorbances of the unknowns and the standard.

CALCULATION

$$\frac{A_{\text{unknown}}}{A_{\text{standard}}} \times \text{g protein in standard} = \text{g protein/100 ml in unknown}$$

NOTES

1. If turbidity is present after color development has taken place (30 minutes), clarify the sample according to the instructions below.
   (a) Pour the sample into a glass-stoppered centrifuge tube and add 3 ml of ether. Stopper, shake for a few seconds, then centrifuge the aspirate and discard the ether layer. Read the absorbance of the aqueous layer.
   (b) If turbidity persists, repeat the ether extraction.
   (c) Extraction with ether results in about 3% increase in volume and a corresponding decrease in the absorbance.

REAGENTS

1. Sodium chloride (0.9%)
   Dissolve 9.0 g of reagent-grade sodium chloride in distilled water and dilute to 1000 ml.
2. Sodium hydroxide (2.5*N*)
   Dissolve 30 g of reagent-grade pellets in water and dilute to 300 ml.

3. Biuret reagent

Place 1.5 g of copper sulfate ($CuSO_4 \cdot 5H_2O$) and 6 g of sodium potassium tartrate ($NaKC_4H_4O_6 \cdot 4H_2O$) in a 1-liter volumetric flask. Add about 500 ml of water and shake until dissolved. Add slowly, with constant swirling, 300 ml of 2.5*N* sodium hydroxide. Add 1 g of potassium iodide, shake until dissolved, then dilute to volume with water. Store in a polyethylene bottle. This reagent is stable indefinitely.

4. Protein standard

Versatol, Hyland Laboratories serum, and Dade normal protein standard have been found to be satisfactory. If a pooled serum is used, establish the protein content by comparison with one of the known concentrations or by Kjeldahl analysis.

REFERENCES

Gornall, A. G., Bardawill, C. J., and David, M. M., Determination of Serum Proteins by Means of the Biuret Reaction. J. Biol. Chem., *177*, 751, 1949.

Henry, R. J., Sobel, C., and Berkman, S., Interferences with the Biuret Methods for Serum Proteins; Use of Benedict's Qualitation Glucose Reagent as a Biuret Reagent. Anal. Chem., *29*, 1491, 1957.

Robinson, H. W., and Hogden, G. C., The Biuret Reaction in the Determination of Serum Proteins. J. Biol. Chem., *135*, 707, 1940.

Salicylate, Serum or Urine

Method of Trinder, Modified by MacDonald

PRINCIPLE

Proteins are precipitated from the specimen with mercuric chloride and hydrochloric acid. A purple complex is formed by reaction of ferric ions with salicylate in the protein-free fluid. Interferences of oxalate and phosphates are eliminated by the high concentration of ferric nitrate.

NORMAL VALUES

Normally there is no salicylate in the body fluids. After medication with aspirin or other salicylates, the salicylate ion will be present in serum and urine. Toxic effects may be observed when the level attains 50 mg/100 ml serum.

SPECIMEN

Serum, plasma, or urine may be used. No special precautions need to be taken with the specimens.

PROCEDURE

A. Serum

1. To 15-ml centrifuge tubes make the additions indicated below:

	Blank	Standard	Unknown
Water (ml)	5.0	5.0	5.0
Serum (ml)	0	0	0.5
Working standard (ml)	0	0.5	0
Trinder's reagent (ml)	5.0	5.0	5.0

2. Mix well and allow to stand for 5 minutes.
3. Centrifuge the unknown for 10 minutes, then decant the supernatant fluid into a cuvette.
4. Measure the absorbances of the standard and the unknown at 540 mμ, using the blank as a reference.

B. Urine

1. Perform the analysis in the same manner as for serum, except include a urine blank. If the salicylate concentration exceeds 40 mg/100 ml, dilute the specimen appropriately and repeat the procedure.
2. To 15-ml centrifuge tubes make the additions indicated below:

	Blank	Urine Blank	Standard	Unknown
Water (ml	5.0	4.5	5.0	5.0
Urine (ml)	0	0.5	0	0.5
Working standard (ml)	0	0	0.5	0
Trinder's reagent (ml)	5.0	5.0	5.0	5.0
Phosphoric acid (ml)	0	0.5	0	0

3. Centrifuge the urine blank and the unknown tube. Transfer the supernatant fluids to correspondingly labeled cuvettes.
4. Measure the absorbances at 540 mμ, using the blank as a reference.

CALCULATION

A. Serum

$$\frac{A_{unknown}}{A_{standard}} \times 20 = \text{mg salicylate/100 ml serum}$$

B. Urine

$$\frac{A_{urine} - A_{urine\ blank}}{A_{standard}} \times 20 = \text{mg salicylate/100 ml urine}$$

NOTES

1. The color produced is stable for at least 1 hour.
2. If a dilution was made in the urine assay, apply an appropriate correction factor in the calculation.

REAGENTS

1. Trinder's reagent
   Transfer 4.0 g of ferric nitrate ($Fe(NO_3)_3 \cdot 9H_2O$) and 4.0 g of mercuric chloride into a 100-ml volumetric flask. Add 12.0 ml of 1*N* hydrochloric acid, dissolve the salts, dilute to the mark with water, then filter. Store at room temperature.
2. Salicylic acid stock standard (200 mg/100 ml)
   Transfer 232.0 mg of sodium salicylate into a 100-ml volumetric flask. Dissolve, then dilute to the mark with water. Add a few drops of chloroform as a preservative and store in a refrigerator. Discard after 6 months.
3. Salicylic acid working standard (20 mg/100 ml)
   Dilute 10 ml of the stock solution with water to 100 ml. Add a few drops of chloroform and store in a refrigerator. Discard after 6 months.
4. Phosphoric acid (reagent grade H_3PO_4, 85%)

REFERENCES

MacDonald, R. P., Salicylate. Standard Methods of Clinical Chemistry, *5*, Meites, S., ed Academic Press, New York, 1965.

Trinder, P., Rapid Determination of Salicylate in Biological Materials. Biochem. J., *57*, 301, 1954.

Thymol Turbidity

PRINCIPLE

The turbidity resulting from the addition of a buffered thymol reagent to serum is not completely understood, but appears to arise through alterations from normal in the concentration of albumin and globulin and in their ratio. The test, although empiric, has proven its worth as a laboratory aid in the diagnosis of liver disease involving the parenchyma.

NORMAL VALUES

0—6 Shank-Hoagland units.

SPECIMEN

Serum rather than plasma should be used. Lipemia has been reported to cause false reactions. Specimens appear to be stable for several days if stored in a refrigerator.

PROCEDURE

1. Measure 6.0 ml of the buffered thymol reagent into a cuvette and add 0.1 ml of serum. Mix gently. Allow to stand at room temperature.
2. After 20 minutes, but less than 30 minutes, measure the percent transmittance of the mixture at 650 mμ, using water as a reference.
3. Read the units from a previously prepared standard.

Standardization

1. Cool the standard and six cuvettes to 10°C.
2. Place 0, 2.0, 4.0, 6.0, 8.0, and 10.0 ml of the standard into the cuvettes and dilute with water to 10 ml. These will be equivalent to 0, 4.0, 8.0, 12.0, 16.0, and 20.0 units respectively.
3. Mix, then allow the tubes to stand for 30 minutes at room temperature. Shake well and measure the percent transmittance of each tube against the 0 (blank) tube at room temperature.
4. Plot percent transmittance against units on semi-log paper.

REAGENTS

1. Thymol reagent

   Dissolve 1.38 g of barbital (diethyl barbituric acid) and 1.03 g of sodium barbital (sodium diethyl barbiturate) in 500 ml of water. Add about 3 g of thymol. Heat to boiling and allow to cool overnight at room temperature. Add a few crystals of thymol. Shake well and allow to stand for a day at room temperature. Filter the solution through Whatman #1 filter paper. Adjust the pH to 7.8.
2. Barium chloride (0.0962*N*)

   Dissolve 1.173 g of barium chloride ($BaCl_2 \cdot 2H_2O$) in distilled water and dilute to 100 ml with water.

3. Sulfuric acid (0.2*N*)
   Dilute 6 ml of concentrated acid to 1 liter. Standardize with 0.1*N* sodium hydroxide and adjust to 0.2*N*.
4. Stock standard (equivalent to 20 units)
   Place 3 ml of the 0.0962*N* barium chloride standard in a 100-ml volumetric flask and dilute to within a few ml of the mark with the 0.2*N* sulfuric acid, which has been cooled to 10°C. Bring the temperature to 20°C and make the final adjustment to the mark with 0.2*N* sulfuric acid at 20°C.

REFERENCES

Maclagan, N. F., The Thymol Turbidity Test as an Indication of Liver Dysfunction. Brit. J. Exp. Pathol., *25*, 234, 1944.

Shank, R. E., and Hoagland, C. L., A Modified Method for the Quantitative Determination of the Thymol Turbidity Reaction of Serum. J. Biol. Chem., *162*, 133, 1946.

Transaminases—GOT and GPT

Method of Reitman and Frankel

PRINCIPLE

The transfer of the amino group from aspartate to alpha-ketoglutarate is catalyzed by glutamic-oxalacetic transaminase (GOT). A similar transfer of the amino group from alanine to alpha-ketoglutarate is brought about by glutamic-pyruvic transaminase (GPT).

$$\text{alpha-ketoglutarate} + \text{aspartate} \xrightleftharpoons{\text{GOT}} \text{oxalacetate} + \text{glutamate}$$
$$\text{alpha-ketoglutarate} + \text{alanine} \xrightleftharpoons{\text{GPT}} \text{pyruvate} + \text{glutamate}$$

After a suitable incubation period, 2,4-dinitrophenylhydrazine is added, which stops the reaction and forms the corresponding hydrazones of oxalacetate and pyruvate produced in the enzymatic reaction. Sodium hydroxide is subsequently added to intensify the color, which is measured colorimetrically.

NORMAL VALUES

To 30 units; borderline range 31—40 units

SPECIMEN

Serum is preferred to plasma because of the possible effect of an anticoagulant on the enzymatic activity. Serum has been reported to be stable for at least 8 hours at room temperature and for at least 1 week at 4°C. Freezing may preserve the activity for 1 month or longer.

PROCEDURE

1. Pipette exactly 1.0 ml of the desired substrate into each of two test tubes, labeled "Unknown" and "Control" respectively. (Prepare one control tube for each group of tests.)
2. Place the tubes in a constant-temperature water bath at 37°C and allow to warm for a few minutes. Add exactly 0.2 ml of serum to the *unknown* and 0.2 ml water to the *control*. (This control tube verifies the color development and should be consistent in terms of absorbance from day to day when read against water.)
3. Incubate 60 minutes for GOT and 30 minutes for GPT.
4. After the proper incubation period, remove the tubes from the water bath and immediately add exactly 1.0 ml of the 2,4-dinitrophenylhydrazine. Mix thoroughly and allow to stand at room temperature for 20 minutes.
5. Add 10.0 ml of 0.4*N* sodium hydroxide. Stopper the tube and mix the contents. Allow to stand for 5 minutes at room temperature.
6. Measure the absorbances at 505 mμ, using water as a reference.

Standard Curve

1. Pipette the following into the tubes as indicated in the following table:

Tube No.	Pyruvate Standard (ml)	GOT Substrate (ml)	Water (ml)	GOT (units per ml serum)	GPT (units per ml serum)
1	0	1.0	0.2	0	0
2	0.1	0.9	0.2	24	28
3	0.2	0.8	0.2	61	57
4	0.3	0.7	0.2	114	97
5	0.4	0.6	0.2	190	—

2. Add 1.0 ml of 2,4-dinitrophenylhydrazine to each tube and shake gently. Allow to stand at room temperature for 20 minutes.
3. Add 10.0 ml of 0.4*N* sodium hydroxide to each tube. Stopper the tubes and mix the contents. Allow to stand for 5 minutes.
4. Measure the absorbances of the standards at 505 mμ, using water as reference.
5. Plot absorbances against the corresponding units of GOT and GPT on rectangular coordinate paper.

REAGENTS

1. Phosphate buffer (0.1*M*, pH 7.4)
   Mix 420 ml of 0.1*M* disodium phosphate and 80 ml of 0.1*M* potassium dihydrogen phosphate.
2. Pyruvate standard (2m*M*)
   Dissolve 22.0 mg of sodium pyruvate in 100 ml of phosphate buffer.
3. GOT substrate (alpha-ketoglutarate 2m*M*, DL-aspartate 200m*M*)
   Place 29.2 mg of alpha-ketoglutaric acid and 2.66 g of DL-aspartic acid in a 100-ml beaker. Add sufficient 1*N* sodium hydroxide to effect solution. Adjust the pH to 7.4 with 1*N* sodium hydroxide. Transfer quantitatively to a 100-ml volumetric flask and dilute to the mark with phosphate buffer.
4. GPT substrate (alpha-ketoglutarate 2m*M*, DL-alanine 200m*M*)
   Place 29.2 mg of alpha-ketoglutaric acid and 1.78 g of DL-alanine in a 100-ml beaker. Add sufficient 1*N* sodium hydroxide to effect solution. Adjust to pH 7.4 with 1*N* sodium hydroxide. Transfer quantitatively to a 100-ml volumetric flask and dilute to the mark with phosphate buffer.
5. 2,4-dinitrophenylhydrazine (1m*M*)
   Dissolve 19.8 mg of 2,4-dinitrophenylhydrazine in 100 ml of 1*N* hydrochloric acid.
6. Sodium hydroxide (0.4*N*)

REFERENCES

Reitman, S., and Frankel, S., Colorimetric Method for the Determination of Serum Glutamic Oxalacetic and Glutamic Pyruvic Transaminases. Am. J. Clin. Pathol., *28*, 56, 1957.

Winsten, S., Collection and Preservation of Specimens, Standard Methods of Clinical Chemistry, *5*, Meites S., ed. Academic Press, New York, 1965.

Urea-Nitrogen

Alkaline-Hypochlorite Method

PRINCIPLE

Urease promotes the hydrolysis of urea to ammonium carbonate, and the ammonia, subsequently released by alkali, reacts with phenol and hypochlorite to form the blue indophenol. Sodium nitroprusside acts as a catalyst. The intensity of blue color produced is proportional to the urea present in the specimen and is measured colorimetrically.

Preformed ammonia is eliminated from urine specimens by adsorption on Permutit* (sodium aluminum silicate) before subjecting them to urease reaction.

NORMAL VALUES

A. Plasma or Serum

7—18 ml/100 ml.

B. Urine

12—20 g/24 hours.

SPECIMEN

With this method, urea-nitrogen can be determined directly on plasma, serum, and on most other biological fluids. Whole blood must be deproteinized to eliminate the hemoglobin, which would interfere in the colorimetric measurement. If plasma is the specimen, do not use an anticoagulant that contains ammonia or the ammonium ion.

Blood, plasma and serum specimens are stable for days if stored in a refrigerator. Since urine is susceptible to loss of urea through bacterial action, addition of thymol is recommended in addition to storage in a refrigerator.

PROCEDURE

1. Place about 0.5 g of Permutit in a 25-ml volumetric glass-stoppered cylinder. Wash with 2 changes of water. Decant the water and drain thoroughly.
2. Add 1 ml of urine and about 5 ml of water. Mix thoroughly by swirling for 5 minutes.
3. Add water to the mark and mix. Allow the Permutit to settle. The final urine dilution is 1:25.
4. Label 12 × 100 mm tubes and make the additions indicated below. Mix gently after each addition.

	Blank	Standard	Unknown
Urease working solution (ml)	1	1	1
Undiluted plasma or serum, or urine in 1:25 dilution (μl)	0	0	10
Water (μl)	10	0	0
Urea working standard (μl)	0	10	0

*Permutit according to Folin, 40—60 mesh, Cat. No. PX405-60, Matheson Scientific, Inc., 1735 North Ashland Avenue, Chicago, Illinois 60622.

5. Incubate all tubes for 15 minutes at 37°C.
6. Add quickly and successively, mixing after each addition, 5 ml of the phenol-nitroprusside reagent and 5 ml of the alkaline-hypochlorite reagent.
7. Incubate the tubes in a water bath at 37°C for 20 minutes.
8. Measure the absorbance of the contents of each tube at 560 mμ, using the blank as a reference solution.

CALCULATIONS

A. Plasma or Serum

$$\frac{A_{unknown}}{A_{standard}} \times 50 = \text{mg urea-nitrogen/100 ml}$$

B. Urine

1. $$\frac{A_{unknown}}{A_{standard}} \times 1250 = \text{mg urea-nitrogen/100 ml}$$

2. $$\text{urea-nitrogen/100 ml} \times \frac{\text{24-hr excretion in ml}}{100} = \text{mg urea-nitrogen/24 hrs}$$

NOTES

1. Ammonia in any of the reagents or in the room atmosphere will result in erroneously high values.

REAGENTS

1. Ammonia-free water

   Filter distilled water through a mixed-bed cation-anion exchanger and collect it in a glass-stoppered bottle. Use this water in the preparation of all reagents described below for use in the urea-nitrogen determination.

2. Phenol-nitroprusside reagent

   Dissolve 12.5 g of reagent-grade sodium nitroprusside ($Na_2Fe(CN)_5NO$) in water and dilute to 1 liter. This reagent is stable for at least 2 months in a refrigerator.

3. Alkaline-hypochlorite reagent

   Dissolve 5 g of reagent-grade sodium hydroxide and 8 ml of commercial bleach containing 5% sodium chloride (Clorox is satisfactory) in water and dilute to 1 liter. This reagent is stable for at least 2 months if stored in an amber bottle in a refrigerator.

4. Sodium ethylenediaminetetraacetate dihydrate (1.0%)

   Dissolve 5.0 g of the EDTA solution in water. Adjust the pH to 6.8 with sodium hydroxide and dilute to 500 ml.

5. Urease stock solution (approximately 40 modified Sumner units/ml)

   Dissolve 0.2 g of Type V* urease containing 3500 to 4100 units per gram in 10 ml water. Add 10 ml of glycerol and mix gently. This reagent is stable for about 4 months in a refrigerator.

*Sigma Chemical Company, 3500 DeKalb Street, St. Louis, Missouri 63118.

6. Urease working solution (approximately 0.4 units/ml)
   Dilute 1 ml of the the stock solution to 100 ml with the EDTA solution. Store in a refrigerator. Discard after 2 weeks.
7. Urea-nitrogen stock solution (5 mg/ml)
   Dissolve 1.0717 g of dry reagent-grade urea in about 50 ml of water in a 100-ml volumetric flask. Dissolve 0.1 g of sodium azide and dilute to the mark. The azide acts as a preservative and does not inhibit the action of urease. Keep this standard refrigerated. Discard within 6 months.
8. Urea-nitrogen working standard (50 mg/100 ml)
   Dilute 10.0 ml of the stock standard to about 80 ml in a 100-ml volumetric flask. Add 0.1 g of sodium azide. Dilute to the mark and mix thoroughly. Store in a refrigerator. Discard after 6 months.

REFERENCES

Annino, J. S., Clinical Chemistry: Principles and Procedures, 3rd ed. Little, Brown and Company, Boston, 1964.

Chaney, A. L., and Marbach, E. P., Modified Reagents for Determination of Urea and Ammonia. Clin. Chem., *8*, 130, 1962.

Kaplan, A., Urea Nitrogen and Urinary Ammonia. Standard Methods of Clinical Chemistry, *5*, Meites, S., ed. Academic Press, New York, 1965.

Uric Acid

PRINCIPLE

Uric acid in a protein-free filtrate reduces the hexavalent tungsten of phosphotungstic acid to a lower valence, with the formation of a blue color proportional in intensity to the concentration of uric acid. The color development belongs to a class of poorly defined oxidation-reduction reactions in which accuracy of results depends upon close adherence to empirically fixed conditions.

NORMAL VALUES

A. Plasma or Serum

	Mean	Range
Men	5.4 ± 0.82 mg/100 ml	3.8—7.1 mg/100 ml
Women	4.0 ± 0.72 mg/100 ml	2.6—5.4 mg/100 ml

B. Urine

250—750 mg/24 hours.

SPECIMEN

Uric acid in plasma, serum, or urine will remain essentially unchanged for several days at room temperature, and for longer periods in a refrigerator. A portion of the uric acid of a urine specimen may be lost as precipitated urate unless the specimen is brought to pH 7.5—8.0 and warmed to 50°C.

PROCEDURE

1. Place 1 ml plasma or serum in a 13 × 100 mm tube and add 8.0 ml of water and 0.4 ml of 0.5*N* sodium hydroxide.
2. Add 0.6 ml of phosphotungstic acid solution while shaking constantly. Allow to stand for 5 minutes.
3. Centrifuge the mixture at moderate speed, or filter it through a Whatman #42 filter paper.
4. Add the following in the order given, mixing after each addition:

	Blank	Standard	Unknown
Water (ml)	5.0	0	0
Working standard (ml)	0	5.0	0
Supernatant fluid, filtrate, or urine diluted 1:100 with water (ml)	0	0	5.0
Glycerol-silicate solution (ml)	2.5	2.5	2.5
Polyanethol sulfonate (ml)	0.5	0.5	0.5
Phosphotungstic acid (ml)	0.5	0.5	0.5

5. Mix and allow to stand for 15 minutes.
6. Measure the absorbance at 700 mμ, using the blank as a reference.

CALCULATIONS

A. Plasma or Serum

$$\frac{A_{unknown}}{A_{standard}} \times 5 = \text{mg uric acid/100 ml}$$

B. Urine

$$\frac{A_{unknown}}{A_{standard}} \times 50 = \text{mg uric acid/100 ml}$$

REAGENTS

1. Phosphotungstic acid solution
   To 100 g of reagent-grade sodium tungstate ($Na_2WO_4 \cdot 2H_2O$) add 800 ml of water and 80 ml of 85% orthophosphoric acid. Reflux gently for 2 hours. Make up to 1000 ml with water and store in a brown bottle.
2. Sodium hydroxide (0.5*N*)
   Dissolve 10.0 g of NaOH pellets in about 200 ml of water. When cool, dilute to 500 ml.
3. Glycerol-silicate solution
   Dissolve 10 g of Merck* crystalline sodium silicate, "soluble", or Fisher† sodium silicate, meta, crystal, in 100 ml of hot water. Add 20 ml of glycerol and mix. When cool, filter through Whatman #50 filter paper.
4. Polyanethol sulfonate (Liquid LaRoche‡)
   Dissolve 1 g in 50 ml of water. Store in a refrigerator.
5. Uric acid stock standard (1 mg/ml)
   Place 1.000 g of uric acid in a 250-ml Erlenmeyer flask. Dissolve 0.5 g of lithium carbonate in 150 ml of hot water. Pour this hot solution into the uric acid. Stir until all the uric acid has dissolved. When cool, transfer the solution quantitatively to a 1-liter volumetric flask. Add 25 ml of 40% formaldehyde and 3 ml of glacial acetic acid. Mix. When the evolution of carbon dioxide has ceased, bring the volume to the mark with water and store in a brown bottle in a dark place. This standard is stable up to 1 year.
6. Uric acid working standard (0.005 mg/ml)
   Dilute 0.5 ml of the stock solution to 100 ml with water in a volumetric flask. Make up this standard on the day of use.

REFERENCES

Alper, C., and Seitchik, J., Comparison of the Archibald-Kern and Stransky Colorimetric Procedure and the Praetorium Enzymatic Procedure for the Determination of Uric Acid. Clin. Chem., *3*, 95, 1957.

Archibald, R. M., Colorimetric Measurement of Uric Acid. Clin. Chem., *3*, 102, 1957.

Forsham, P. T., Thorn, G. W., Prunty, F. T. G., and Hills, A. G., Clinical Studies with Pituitary Adrenocorticotropin. J. Clin. Endocrinol., *8*, 15, 1948.

Kern, A., and Stransky, E., Beitrag zur Kolorimetrischen Bestimmung der Harnsäure. Biochem. Z., *290*, 419, 1937.

*Merck and Company, Rahway, New Jersey 07065.
†Fisher Chemical Company, 690 Miami Circle, N.E., Atlanta, Georgia 30324.
‡Hoffmann-LaRoche, Inc., Nutley, New Jersey 07110.

ENDOCRINOLOGY

Sectional Directory

Catechol Amines, Urine

PRINCIPLE

The free (nonconjugated) urinary catechol amines are isolated from urine by using aluminum oxide. Subsequently they are converted to fluorescent indole derivatives, trihydroxyindoles (THI), and measured fluorometrically as norepinephrine (NE) equivalents.

NORMAL VALUES

0—100 μg/24 hours.

SPECIMEN

Collect a 24-hour urine specimen in a glass bottle containing 15 ml of 6*N* hydrochloric acid.

PROCEDURE

1. Measure and record the volume of the 24-hour urine collection. Filter an aliquot of urine equivalent to 10% of the total 24-hour collection through a double layer of Whatman #1 filter paper and record the exact volume used. Transfer the filtrate to a 500-ml beaker. If the volume of the filtrate is less than 200 ml, dilute with deionized water to 200 ml. Add 3 g of alumina and 5 ml of 0.2*M* EDTA.
2. Place the beaker on a magnetic stirrer and stir just fast enough to keep the alumina suspended. Using a pH meter, adjust the pH of the mixture to 7—7.5 by dropwise addition of 5*N* sodium hydroxide. By further dropwise addition of 5*N* sodium hydroxide, bring the pH to 8.4 and maintain it at this level. Stir for 7 minutes. Avoid grinding of the alumina.
3. Rinse the stirring bar and electrodes with deionized water. Allow the alumina to settle for 4 minutes, then discard the clear supernatant fluid.
4. Transfer the alumina quantitatively with deionized water to a glass column of 1.2 cm diameter. Wash with two 10-ml portions of deionized water. The water should flow through the column at a rate of 1 to 2 ml per minute.
5. Following the water wash, add 3 ml of 0.2*N* acetic acid to the column and discard the effluent; then add 9.4 ml of 0.2*N* acetic acid in two 4.7-ml portions. Collect the eluate in a calibrated centrifuge tube and dilute to 9.5 ml. This solution should be clear and colorless.
6. Add 0.5 ml of 0.2*M* EDTA and centrifuge to remove granules of alumina that may be present. Transfer to a test tube.
7. Number two series of test tubes from 1 to 8 and proceed as follows:

Tube No.	
1	Add 0.2 ml of working standard (0.2 μg NE)
2	Add 0.1 ml of working standard (0.1 μg NE)
3	Use as the reagent blank tube
4	Add 0.2 ml of eluate (sample tube)
5	Add 0.2 ml of eluate (sample blank tube)
6	Add 0.1 ml of eluate (sample tube)
7	Add 0.1 ml of working standard (0.1 μg NE) and 0.1 ml of eluate
8	Add 0.1 ml of eluate (sample blank tube)

8. Add to each tube 1 ml of 1*M* acetate buffer of pH 6.5.
9. Add 0.1 ml of 0.1*N* iodine solution to each tube. Allow to stand for 4 minutes. At this point prepare the 1% ascorbic acid and the sodium hydroxide-ascorbic acid solution.
10. Add 0.5 ml of 0.05*N* sodium thiosulfate to each tube. Add 1 ml of sodium hydroxide-ascorbic acid solution to each tube, except the two sample blanks, tubes 5 and 8.
11. Add 0.7 ml of 5*N* sodium hydroxide to tubes 5 and 8, allow to stand for 15 minutes, then add 0.3 ml of 1% ascorbic acid.
12. Dilute the contents of all tubes to 5 ml with deionized water and allow them to stand for 45 minutes.
13. Perform fluorometric measurements.
    (a) Set the spectrophotofluorometer at the peak wavelength for NE (activation peak at 395 mμ; fluorescence peak at 505 mμ).
    (b) Adjust the instrument so that the reading for the 0.2-μg NE standard is 80, then read the relative fluorescence of all tubes.
    (c) If a sample tube reads off the scale, dilute the eluate with deionized water and repeat the assay from step 7.

CALCULATION

1. Average the blank values and subtract from the appropriate tube readings.
2. Average the readings for 0.1 μg of the standards and for the 0.1-ml eluates.
3. Micrograms of catechol amines as NE equivalents per 24 hours equals

$$\frac{\text{reading of 0.1 ml eluate}}{\text{reading of 0.1 }\mu\text{g NE}} \times 10 \times \frac{\text{urine volume (ml)}}{\text{volume of urine aliquot (ml)}}$$

NOTES

1. Substances such as quinidine, quinine and tetracyclines may interfere with the determination.

REAGENTS

1. Hydrochloric acid (6*N*)

   Dilute 500 ml of concentrated hydrochloric acid to 1000 ml with distilled water.
2. Hydrochloric acid (2*N*)

   Dilute 167 ml of concentrated hydrochloric acid to 1000 ml with distilled water.
3. Alumina (aluminum oxide, acid-washed)

   Add 1000 ml of 2*N* hydrochloric acid to 300 g of alumina. Boil the mixture for 30 minutes in a reflux apparatus, then decant the supernatant fluid. Add 1000 ml of distilled water to the sediment and stir briefly. Allow the alumina to settle for 5 minutes, then pour off the supernatant fluid. Repeat the washing and decanting process with distilled water at least 10 times, until the wash water clears after 5 minutes of settling and has a pH of 4 to 5. Filter the alumina, using a suction funnel. Dry overnight at room temperature, then heat the alumina for 2 hours in an oven at 100°C. Store in a bottle.
4. Deionized water

   Deionize distilled water by passing it through a commercial deionizer.

5. Sodium hydroxide (5*N*)
   Dissolve 100 g of sodium hydroxide pellets in deionized water and dilute to 500 ml.
6. Sodium hydroxide (0.5*N*)
   Dilute 50 ml of 5*N* sodium hydroxide solution to 500 ml with deionized water.
7. Ascorbic acid (1%)
   Dissolve 100 mg of ascorbic acid in 10 ml of deionized water just before use.
8. Sodium hydroxide-ascorbic acid solution
   Mix 3 volumes of 1% ascorbic acid with 7 volumes of 5*N* sodium hydroxide just before use.
9. Hydrochloric acid (0.01*N*)
   Dilute 0.17 ml of 6*N* hydrochloric acid to 100 ml with deionized water.
10. Sodium thiosulfate (0.05*N*)
    Dissolve 2.5 g of sodium thiosulfate ($Na_2S_2O_3 \cdot 5H_2O$), reagent grade, in deionized water and dilute to 200 ml.
11. EDTA (0.2*M*)
    Dissolve 37.2 g of disodium ethylenediaminetetraacetate (reagent grade) in warm deionized water, cool, then dilute to 500 ml.
12. Acetic acid (0.2*N*)
    Dilute 5.8 ml of glacial acetic acid to 500 ml with deionized water.
13. Acetic acid (1*M*)
    Dilute 30 ml of glacial acetic acid to 500 ml with deionized water.
14. Sodium acetate (1*M*)
    Dissolve 41 g of sodium acetate (reagent grade) in deionized water and dilute to 500 ml.
15. Acetate buffer (1*M*, pH 6.5)
    Adjust the pH of 400 ml of 1*M* sodium acetate to 6.5 by the addition of 1*M* acetic acid, using a pH meter.
16. Acetate buffer (1*M*, pH 3.5)
    Adjust the pH of 400 ml of 1*M* acetic acid with 1*M* sodium acetate, using a constant-pH monitoring apparatus.
17. Iodine solution (0.1*N*)
    Dissolve 2.5 g of sodium iodide (reagent grade) and 0.635 g of reagent-grade iodine in 50 ml of deionized water. This reagent and all those above are stable at room temperature.
18. Norepinephrine stock standard (1000 μg/ml)
    Dissolve 18.2 mg of *l*-norepinephrine bitartrate monohydrate in 10 ml of 0.01*N* hydrochloric acid. Keep in a refrigerator, where it will be stable for at least 6 months.
19. Norepinephrine working standard (1 μg/ml)
    Dilute 0.1 ml of the stock standard with 0.01*N* hydrochloric acid to 100 ml. Keep in a refrigerator, where it will be stable for at least 6 months.

REFERENCES

Crout, R., Catechol Amines in Urine. Standard Methods of Clinical Chemistry, *3*, p. 62, Seligson, D., ed. Academic Press, New York, 1961.

Lund, A., Fluorometric Determination of Adrenaline in Blood. III. A New Sensitive and Specific Method. Acta Pharmacol. Toxicol., *5*, 231, 1949.

'Cortisol', Plasma

PRINCIPLE

The free (nonconjugated) 11-hydroxycorticosteroids are extracted from plasma with dichloromethane and then measured fluorometrically.

NORMAL VALUES

On samples drawn from adults between 8 and 9 a.m., the range is 8—24 μg/100 ml, with a mean of 17 μg/100 ml.

SPECIMEN

Heparinized plasma.

PROCEDURE

Run all samples in duplicates.

1. Mark four tubes as follows: "Blank", "Standard", "Control", "Specimen". Add 15 ml of dichloromethane to each.
2. Add to the blank tube 2 ml of water, to the standard tube 2 ml of working standard, to the control tube 2 ml of control serum, and to the specimen tube 2 ml of plasma.
3. Stopper the tubes and mix the contents for 20 minutes with a mechanical shaker.
4. Remove the aqueous supernate by aspiration.
5. Mark another set of tubes as above and transfer 10 ml of dichloromethane extract, respectively, from the first to the second set of extraction tubes.
6. Measure the fluorescence with an Aminco-Bowman spectrophotofluorometer or other precision instrument. Use an activating wavelength of 475 mμ and an emission wavelength of 530 mμ. Arrange up to twelve extracts in sequence for fluorometry. Number up to twelve cuvettes corresponding to the extracts.
7. At 45-second intervals, add 5 ml of fluorescence reagent to each tube, beginning with the blank. Stopper the tubes and shake for 20 seconds.
8. After the phases have separated, aspirate and discard the upper (dichloromethane) phase. Transfer the bottom phase to the marked cuvettes.
9. Measure the fluorescence, making readings consecutively at 45-second intervals, beginning at 15 minutes from the time of addition of fluorescence reagent to the first tube.

CALCULATION

$$\frac{A - B}{S - B} \times 30 = \mu g \text{ cortisol}/100 \text{ ml}$$

A, B, and S are the fluorometer values for specimen, blank, and standard respectively; 30 is the concentration of the working standard (μg/100 ml).

NOTES

1. Medications such as estrogens, corticosterone and cortisol will cause high values.

2. All glassware should be thoroughly cleaned. Sources of lint and dust should be eliminated as much as possible.

REAGENTS

1. Glass-distilled water
2. Dichloromethane (spectro grade)
3. Ethanol (95%, redistilled)
4. Fluorescence reagent
   Add 150 ml of 95% ethanol to a 1-liter beaker and place in an ice bath. With stirring, slowly add 350 ml of concentrated sulfuric acid (reagent grade). This solution is stable at room temperature if stored in a glass-stoppered bottle.
5. Cortisol stock solution I (1 mg/ml)
   Dissolve 10 mg of cortisol in redistilled 95% ethanol to make 10 ml of solution. Store in a refrigerator.
6. Cortisol stock solution II (0.01 mg/ml)
   Dilute 1 ml of stock solution I with distilled water to 100 ml. Store in a refrigerator.
7. Cortisol stock solution III (1 μg/ml)
   Dilute 5 ml of stock solution II with distilled water to 50 ml. Store in a refrigerator.
8. Cortisol working standard (30 μg/100 ml)
   Dilute 3 ml of stock solution III with distilled water to 10 ml. Prepare fresh daily.
9. Control serum
   Use pooled serum and keep it frozen.

REFERENCES

Gantt, C. L., Maynard, D. E., and Hamwi, G. G., Experience with a Simple Procedure for the Determination of Plasma and Urine Free 11-Hydroxycorticosteroids. Metabolism, *13*, 1327, 1964.

Mattingly, D., A Simple Fluorometric Method for the Estimation of Free 11-Hydroxycorticoids in Human Plasma. J. Clin. Pathol., *15*, 374, 1962.

Maynard, D. E., Folk, R. L., Riley, T. R., Wieland, R. G., Gwinup, G., and Hamwi, G. J., A Rapid Test for Adrenocortical Insufficiency. Ann. Internal Med., *64*, 552, 1966.

Cortisol Metabolites, Urine

PRINCIPLE

This technic has the advantage that it measures most of the cortisol metabolites, including cortols, allocortols, cortolones, and allocortolones, which are not measured by the Porter-Silber method. Furthermore, it is more specific than the Norymberski method. It consists of the conversion of all known cortisol metabolites, except the 17-ketosteroids, to a mixture of 11-beta-hydroxyetiocholanolone and, to a lesser extent, 11-beta-hydroxyandrosterone, both of which are then measured with the Zimmerman color reaction.

NORMAL VALUES

Adult males: 10.0—20.5 mg/24 hours
Adult females: 6.3—17.4 mg/24 hours

SPECIMEN

A 24-hour urine must be collected without preservative and analyzed while fresh or freshly frozen.

PROCEDURE

1. Place a 100-ml aliquot of a 24-hour urine collection in a 250-ml round-bottom flask. Add to this 30 ml of 1*M*, pH-5 sodium acetate buffer and 20 ml of Ketodase®.* Fit the flask with a ground-glass stopper.
2. Incubate for 20 hours at 38°C.
3. Add 50 g of sodium chloride, which results in a concentration of 30% with respect to the salt. Extract with three 70-ml portions of ethyl acetate, using a 250-ml separatory funnel.
4. Wash the extract 3 times with 3*N* sodium hydroxide. Backwash the sodium hydroxide extracts with 30 ml of ethyl acetate and combine the washings with the ethyl acetate extract.
5. Wash the combined ethyl acetate extracts with five 20-ml portions of water. Wash the water extracts with 30 ml of ethyl acetate and combine the washings with the ethyl acetate extracts.
6. Evaporate the combined ethyl acetate extracts to dryness with a flash evaporator. Dissolve the residue in 0.4 ml of absolute alcohol, then add 30 ml of benzene. Transfer to a 125-ml separatory funnel.
7. Extract gently with ten 30-ml portions of water and add 90 g of sodium chloride to the combined water extracts. Extract the saline water solution with three 40-ml portions of ethyl acetate. Evaporate the ethyl acetate extract to dryness, then transfer the residue quantitatively to a 100-ml round-bottom flask by adding 5 ml of absolute ethanol to the flask and drawing this up with a Pasteur pipette. Repeat with 3 ml, then with 2 ml of absolute ethanol. Add 1 ml of water to the flask.
8. Add 0.3 g of sodium borohydride to the above aqueous ethanolic solution. Allow it to stand at room temperature for 4 hours (the flask should be unstoppered,

*Warner-Chilcott Laboratories, Morris Plains, New Jersey, 07950.

to allow the hydrogen produced to escape), then reflux for 16 hours, using a heating mantle.

9. Evaporate the bulk of ethanol under a stream of nitrogen. Add 40 ml of water and then 10% acetic acid, drop by drop, until a pH of 5 is reached. Add 15 g of sodium chloride and extract with three 30-ml portions of ethyl acetate. Wash the extract with 10 ml of water, wash the aqueous washings with 20 ml of ethyl acetate, then combine the ethyl acetate wash with the ethyl acetate extract. Evaporate the ethyl acetate to dryness, then dissolve the residue in 10 ml of absolute ethanol.
10. Dissolve 100 mg of periodic acid in 10 ml of water and add it to the above ethanolic solution. Stopper the flask and allow it to stand in the dark at room temperature for 2 to $2\frac{1}{2}$ hours.
11. Add 40 ml of water to the flask and extract with three 40-ml portions of benzene. Wash the combined benzene extracts with 1*N* sodium hydroxide, followed by water until the washes are neutral. Evaporate the benzene solution to dryness, dissolve the residue in absolute ethanol, then transfer quantitatively to a 25-ml volumetric flask and adjust to the mark with ethanol rinses of the flask.
12. Color reaction.
    (a) Add 1 ml of the unknown ethanolic solution from step 11 to each of three test tubes having ground-glass stoppers. Add 1 ml (40 μg) of working standard solution to each of two other test tubes. Use two additional empty tubes as blanks.
    (b) Evaporate the contents of each tube to dryness under a gentle stream of nitrogen, then desiccate for at least 3 hours.
    (c) Place the desiccated tubes in ice, keeping them stoppered at all times. Add 0.2 ml of *m*-dinitrobenzene and 0.2 ml of alcoholic potassium hydroxide to each tube, including the blanks, and mix. Store the stoppered tubes in a refrigerator for 3 hours.
    (d) Add 7 ml of 80% ethanol to each tube immediately after the 3-hour period, then proceed to measure the absorbances of the tubes against an alcohol blank at wavelengths of 430 and 520 mμ.

CALCULATION

1. Subtract the reagent blank reading.
2. The ratio of the reading at 520 mμ to that at 430 mμ should be 2.1 or greater for the standard, and 1.7 or more for the unknown.
3. Carry out the following calculation:

$$\text{mg of 11-}\beta\text{-hydroxy etiocholanolone}/\text{tube} = \frac{0.040 \times (\text{average reading of unknown at 520 m}\mu - \text{blank})}{\text{average reading of standard at 520 m}\mu - \text{blank}}$$

4.

$$\frac{\left(\text{mg of 11-}\beta\text{-hydroxy-etiocholanolone}/\text{tube}\right) \times 25 \times \text{total urine volume} \times 1.2 \times 1.2}{100} = \text{mg of cortisol metabolites per 24 hours}$$

NOTES

1. Soak all glassware in soap detergent and rinse with tap water. After rinsing, soak in concentrated sulfuric acid, rinse with water, and then, finally, with distilled water. Dry in an oven or in air.

REAGENTS

1. Ammonium sulfate crystals (analytical reagent)
2. Sodium acetate buffer (pH 5, 1*M*)
   Add 11.55 ml of glacial acetic acid to 200 ml of water (solution A). Dissolve 32.8 g of sodium acetate in 400 ml of water (solution B). To obtain the 1*M* sodium acetate buffer, pH 5, mix 148 ml of solution A with 252 ml of solution B.
3. Sodium chloride crystals (analytical reagent)
4. Benzene (thiophene-free, purified by redistillation)
5. Ethyl acetate (reagent grade, redistilled)
6. Sodium borohydride (purity 98% or better)
7. Periodic acid (analytical reagent)
8. *m*-Dinitrobenzene
   Purify by recrystallization according to the method of Callow as follows:
   (a) dissolve 20 g of *m*-dinitrobenzene in 750 ml of warm 95% ethanol and place in a refrigerator overnight;
   (b) add 100 ml of 2*N* sodium hydroxide, wash the crystals to neutrality with distilled water in a Buchner funnel under low suction, then dry in a desiccator;
   (c) dissolve the crystals in 300 ml of absolute ethanol and recrystallize in the cold; separate the crystals and dry in a desiccator over Drierite ®*; repeat this step until the crystals are white, fine, and long.
9. Absolute ethanol
   Purify according to the method of Callow as follows: to commercial absolute ethanol add 4 g of *m*-phenylenediamine dihydrochloride per liter; allow to stand in the dark for 1 week; distill in an all-glass system; discard the head and tail fractions (about 100 ml each); keep sealed under nitrogen in a refrigerator.
10. Ethanolic potassium hydroxide
    Prepare and treat according to Wilson and Carter. Place 100 ml of absolute ethanol in a Pyrex glass-stoppered bottle and allow it to stand in an ice bath. Add 15 mg of ascorbic acid powder and shake. Add 25 g of potassium hydroxide pellets, bubble a stream of nitrogen gently through the mixture for 10 seconds, then stopper. Shake intermittently for 15 to 20 minutes, keeping the temperature near 0°C. Take an aliquot and determine the acidity by titrating with 1*N* sulfuric acid, using phenol red as the indicator. Each time the bottle is opened, flush out the air space before stoppering. Continue adding 1*N* sulfuric acid and shaking until the normality is approximately 2.6, then filter through a Buchner funnel, using vacuum and Whatman #50 filter paper. While filtering, direct a stream of nitrogen over the surface of the fluid. Transfer the solution to a graduated cylinder with a glass stopper. Flush out the air space with nitrogen. Adjust the normality to 2.5 ± 0.02 with absolute ethanol, flushing out the air space with nitrogen after each sampling. After the final adjustment, add 15 mg of powdered ascorbic acid. The presence of slight turbidity need cause no concern. Store in a freezer. Just before using, take the container from the freezer, pour a portion into a clean tube, flush out the airspace over the liquid in the bottle with nitrogen, then return the container to the freezer. Immediately pipette the cold

*W. A. Hammond Drierite Co., Xenia, Ohio 45385.

solution. If handled with care, this reagent can be stable for as long as 3 months.

11. Ketodase ®
    Brand of beta-glucuronidase derived from beef liver and containing 5,000 units/ml.
12. Distilled water
13. Sodium hydroxide (3*N*)
    Dissolve 360 g of sodium hydroxide pellets in 2950 ml of distilled water.
14. 11-β-Hydroxyetiocholanolone standard stock solution (0.2 mg/ml)
    Add 5 mg of 11-beta-hydroxyetiocholanolone to a 25-ml volumetric flask, dissolve with absolute ethanol, then adjust to the mark. Keep in a refrigerator.
15. 11-β-Hydroxyetiocholanolone working standard (40 μg/ml)
    Add 5 ml of the stock solution to 20 ml of absolute ethanol. Keep in a refrigerator when not in use.

REFERENCES

Callow, N. H., Callow, R. K., and Emmens, C. W., Colorimetric Determination of Substances Containing the Grouping $CH_2 \cdot CO$ in Urine Extracts as an Indication of Androgen Content. Biochem. J., *32*, 1312, 1938.

Jefferies, W., Michelakis, A. M., and Price, J. W., Urinary Cortisol Metabolites in Adrenocortical Hyperfunction. J. Clin. Endocrinol. Metab., *26*, 219, 1966.

Michelakis, A. M., A New Method for Measuring Cortisol Metabolites. J. Clin. Endocrinol. Metab., *22*, 1071, 1962.

Wilson, H., and Carter, P., Stabilization of the Alcoholic Potassium Hydroxide in Colorimetric 17-Ketosteroid Determinations. Endocrinology, *41*, 417, 1947.

17-Hydroxycorticosteroids, Urine (17-OHCST; Porter-Silber Chromogens)

PRINCIPLE

This technic measures urinary corticosteroids that have the C-17,C-21-dihydroxy-C-20-keto side chain. Therefore it measures only a fraction of the urinary cortisol metabolites. The urinary corticosteroid-glucuronide conjugates in an aliquot of a 24-hour urine specimen are hydrolized with beta-glucuronidase. The 17-hydroxy-corticosteroids are then extracted with an organic solvent and measured colorimetrically as the phenylhydrazine reaction products.

NORMAL VALUES

4—8 mg/g creatinine.

SPECIMEN

Urine collected over 24 hours in a bottle containing 10 ml of glacial acetic acid. Run the determination while the urine is fresh or freshly frozen.

PROCEDURE

1. Measure and record the urine volume.
2. Run the determination in groups of 10 specimens or less.
3. Filter about 10 ml of each urine and adjust the pH to 5.0 with concentrated acetic acid or 20% sodium hydroxide, using pH paper with the range of 3.0—5.5.
4. With each set of unknowns, set up two 50-ml glass-stoppered centrifuge tubes as blanks and pipette 1 ml of water into each.
5. Into each of three tubes pipette 1 ml of working standard (6 μg/ml).
6. For each unknown, pipette 1 ml of urine (see step 3) into a tube.
7. From this point on, all tubes are treated exactly in the same manner. Add 0.2 ml of Ketodase®* to each tube, and 3.8 ml of acetate buffer. Place all tubes in a 37°C water bath for 18 to 24 hours.
8. Remove the tubes from the bath and allow them to cool at room temperature. Add 25 ml of freshly distilled chloroform to each tube, stopper, then shake them for about 2 minutes. Centrifuge for 10 minutes, then remove the aqueous layer and interface by aspiration.
9. Add 2 ml of 0.1*N* sodium hydroxide to each tube and mix by inverting 8 to 10 times. Allow the layers to separate, then discard the aqueous phase by aspiration.
10. Filter the washed chloroform extract through Whatman #43 filter paper into a clean and dry 25-ml test tube.
11. Color reaction.
    (a) Pipette 10 ml of the chloroform extract into each of two 15-ml centrifuge tubes. Designate one tube as the test tube and the other as the control tube.

*Warner-Chilcott Laboratories, Morris Plains, New Jersey 07950.

(b) To each control tube add 0.5 ml of blank reagent. To the test tubes add 0.5 ml of phenylhydrazine reagent.
(c) Mix vigorously for about 1 minute, then centrifuge for 10 minutes at 2,000 rpm.

12. Measure the absorbance the next day in a high-resolution spectrophotometer such as the Beckman DU, Model 2400, at 410 mμ as follows:
    (a) read the blanks of the control group against water, then set the lowest-reading blank at zero and read the remainder of the controls;
    (b) repeat this for the test group.
13. Measure the creatinine excretion in the 24-hour urine.

CALCULATION

1. Subtract the readings of the controls from the readings of the corresponding tubes marked as test tubes to obtain the corrected readings.
2. Average the corrected standard readings.
3.

$$\text{mg of 17-OHCST/ml} = \frac{\text{reading of unknown (corrected)} \times \text{mg of standard}}{\text{reading of standard (corrected)}}$$

4.

$$\text{mg of 17-OHCST/24 hrs} = \text{(mg of 17-OHCST per ml of urine)} \times \text{(total volume, in ml, of 24-hr urine)}$$

5.

$$\text{mg of 17-OHCST/g of creatinine} = \frac{\text{mg of 17-OHCST per 24 hrs}}{\text{g of creatinine per 24 hrs}}$$

NOTES

1. Soak all glassware in soap detergent and rinse with tap water. After rinsing, soak the 15-ml centrifuge tubes and their stoppers in concentrated sulfuric acid, then rinse with water. Finally, rinse all glassware with distilled water, then dry in an oven or in air.

REAGENTS

All chemicals used should be reagent grade unless otherwise specified.

1. Distilled water
2. Glacial acetic acid
3. Sodium hydroxide (20% *W*/*V*)
   Dissolve 20 g of sodium hydroxide pellets in water and dilute to 100 ml.
4. Ketodase®
   Beta-glucuronidase, 5,000 units/ml. Available from Warner-Chilcott Laboratories, Morris Plains, New Jersey 07950.
5. Acetate buffer (0.2*N*, pH 5.0)
   Mix 30 ml of 0.2*N* acetic acid (11.8 ml of glacial acetic acid per liter) with 70 ml of 0.2*N* sodium acetate (27.22 g of sodium acetate per liter). Adjust to pH 5.0 with 0.2*N* acetic acid or with 0.2*N* sodium acetate.
6. Chloroform
   Place 4 g of 2,4-dinitrophenylhydrazine in 400 ml of chloroform and distill in the dark.

7. Sodium hydroxide (0.1*N*)
   Dissolve 4 g of sodium hydroxide in water and dilute to 1000 ml.
8. Sulfuric acid (63% *V/V*)
9. Ethyl alcohol
   Purify according to the method of Callow as follows: to commercial absolute ethanol add 4 g of *m*-phenylenediamine dihydrochloride per liter; allow to stand in the dark for 1 week; distill in an all-glass system; discard the head and tail fractions (about 100 ml each); keep sealed under nitrogen in a refrigerator.
10. Phenylhydrazine hydrochloride
    Purify in the manner described below.
    (a) Boil 95% ethanol, using a steam bath and reflux condenser. Dissolve 32 g of phenylhydrazine hydrochloride in 790 ml of boiling ethanol. Add 10 to 15 g of norite A and mix. Reflux for 10 minutes. While hot, quickly filter through Whatman #2 filter paper. Let the solution cool to room temperature, then place in a refrigerator overnight.
    (b) Filter the crystals and wash with cold ethanol, then dry and weigh. Recrystallize by repeating step (a), but use an amount of ethanol equal to the weight of the crystals × 790/32 ml.
    (c) Recrystallize two more times, following steps (a) and (b), but omit the norite. Dry the crystals thoroughly in a desiccator over Drierite®*, then store in a brown bottle in a vacuum desiccator.
11. Blank reagent
    Mix 2 volumes of dilute sulfuric acid with 1 volume of purified ethanol. This solution is stable indefinitely.
12. Phenylhydrazine reagent
    Dissolve 8.7 mg of phenylhydrazine hydrochloride in 20 ml of reagent blank. Make this up fresh each time.
13. Hydrocortisone standard stock solution
    Dissolve 20 mg of powdered hydrocortisone (free alcohol) in 1 liter of distilled water.
14. Hydrocortisone working standard (6 μg/ml)
    Dilute 3 ml of the stock standard with water to 10 ml. Keep refrigerated.

REFERENCES

Callow, N. H., Callow, R. K., and Emmens, C. W., Colorimetric Determination of Substances Containing the Grouping $CH_2 \cdot CO$ in Urine Extracts as an Indication of Androgen Content. Biochem. J., *32*, 1312, 1938.

Silber, R. H., and Busch, R. D., The Specificity of the Reaction of Phenylhydrazine with 17,21-Dihydroxy-20-Ketosteroids. J. Clin. Endocrinol., *15*, 505, 1955.

Silber, R. H., and Porter, C. C., The Determination of 17,21-Dihydroxy-20-Ketosteroids in Urine and Plasma. J. Biol. Chem., *210*, 923, 1954.

*W. A. Hammond Drierite Co., Xenia, Ohio 45385.

17-Ketosteroids, Urine

PRINCIPLE

Urinary conjugated 17-ketosteroids are hydrolyzed with acid and extracted with ethylene dichloride. The neutral 17-ketosteroids are then separated and measured by reacting them with *m*-dinitrobenzene (Zimmerman reaction)

NORMAL VALUES

Age (years)	<2	2—5	5—10	10—16	16—60	>60
Male (mg/24 hour)	<1.2	1.2—3	3—6	6—15	10—20	5—15
Female (mg/24 hours)	<1.2	1.2—3	3—6	5—12	5—15	3—14

SPECIMEN

A 24-hour urine specimen, collected without preservative, is analyzed while fresh or freshly frozen.

PROCEDURE

1. Perform all analyses in duplicate.
2. Add 0.1 ml of 8% formaldehyde to 5 ml of urine, then add to it 16 ml of 4.3*N* hydrochloric acid.
3. Set tubes in a boiling water bath for 10 minutes.
4. Cool to room temperature, then add exactly 20 ml of ethylene dichloric to each acid and shake mechanically for 5 minutes.
5. Centrifuge, if necessary, to separate the layers.
6. Aspirate and discard the aqueous phase, then add 5 ml of 1*N* hydrochloric acid; shake well. Allow to stand for 5 minutes.
7. Aspirate and discard the aqueous phase, then add 5 ml of water and shake well. Allow to stand for 5 minutes.
8. Aspirate and discard the aqueous phase, then add 5 ml of 3*N* sodium hydroxide and shake well. Allow to stand for 10 minutes.
9. Aspirate and discard the aqueous phase, then add 10 ml of water and shake well. Wait for 10 minutes.
10. Repeat step 9.
11. Aspirate and discard the aqueous phase, then add 5 ml of water and shake well. Allow to stand for 15 minutes.
12. Aspirate and discard the aqueous phase.
13. Filter the extract into test tubes through Whatman #43 filter paper.
14. Pipette exactly 10 ml of extract into 18 × 150 mm glass-stoppered centrifuge tubes. Pipette 0.5 ml (0 050 μg) of DHEA working standard into two tubes.
15. Dry all tubes with a stream of filtered air, then place them in an evacuated desiccator overnight.
16. Colorimetry (Zimmerman reaction).
    (a) Place all tubes (unknowns, standards, and two blank tubes) in ice.
    (b) Add 0.2 ml of *m*-dinitrobenzene reagent and 0.2 ml of alcoholic potassium hydroxide to each tube and shake well.

(c) Refrigerate for 3 hours.
(d) Add 7.5 ml of 80% alcohol to each.
(e) Measure the absorbances at 430 and 520 mμ.

CALCULATION

1. Average absorbances of the blanks at 430 and 520 mμ respectively.
2. Average absorbances of the standards at 430 and 520 mμ respectively.
3. Subtract blank absorbances at 430 and 520 mμ from the corresponding absorbances of the standards and the unknowns.
4. Calculate factor A:

$$A = 1 - \left[\frac{0.6 \times (\text{av. reading of standards at 430 m}\mu - \text{av. reading of blanks at 430 m}\mu)}{\text{av. reading of standards at 520 m}\mu - \text{av. reading of blanks at 520 m}\mu}\right]$$

5. Calculate factor B (correction for interfering chromogens):

$$B = \frac{(\text{520 reading of unknown} - \text{blank}) - 0.6\ (\text{430 reading of unknown} - \text{blank})}{\text{factor A}}$$

6.

$$\frac{\text{concentration of standard (0.05 mg)} \times B}{\text{average reading of standards at 520 m}\mu - \text{blank}} = \text{mg/2.5 ml of urine}$$

7.

$$\frac{(\text{mg/2.5 ml urine}) \times (\text{total urine volume/24 hours})}{2.5} = \text{mg 17-KS/24 hrs}$$

8. Average the results of the duplicate samples.

REAGENTS

Use distilled water in making all reagents.

1. Hydrochloric acid (4.3*N*)
   Dilute 360 ml of concentrated hydrochloric acid with distilled water to 1000 ml.
2. Hydrochloric acid (1*N*)
   Dilute 167 ml of concentrated hydrochloric acid with distilled water to 2000 ml.
3. Sodium hydroxide (3*N*)
   Dissolve 360 g of sodium hydroxide pellets in water. When cool, dilute to 3000 ml.
4. Ethylene dichloride (reagent grade)
   Can be used as such. If necessary to purify, shake with 5*N* sulfuric acid, let stand, discard the acid phase, then redistill in an all-glass apparatus.
5. Ethanol (80%)
   Dilute 1600 ml of 95% ethanol with distilled water to 1900 ml.
6. *m*-Dinitrobenzene reagent
   Purify by recrystallization according to the method of Callow as follows:
   (a) dissolve 20 g of *m*-dinitrobenzene in 750 ml of warm 95% ethanol and place in refrigerator overnight;
   (b) add 100 ml of 2*N* sodium hydroxide, wash the crystals with distilled water in a Buchner funnel under low suction until they are neutral, then dry in a desiccator;

(c) dissolve the crystals in 300 ml of absolute ethanol and recrystallize in the cold; separate the crystals and dry in a desiccator over Drierite®*; repeat this step until the crystals are white, fine, and long.

7. Formaldehyde (8%)
   Dilute 100 ml of AR formalin with water to 500 ml.

8. Absolute ethanol
   Purify according to the method of Callow as follows: to commercial absolute ethanol add 4 g of *m*-phenylenediamine dihydrochloride per liter; allow to stand in the dark for 1 week; distill in an all-glass system; discard the head and tail fractions (about 100 ml each); keep sealed under nitrogen in a refrigerator.

9. Ethanolic potassium hydroxide
   Prepare and treat according to Wilson and Carter. Place 100 ml of absolute ethanol in a Pyrex glass-stoppered bottle and allow it to stand in an ice bath. Add 15 mg of ascorbic acid powder and shake. Add 25 g of potassium hydroxide pellets, bubble a stream of nitrogen gently through the mixture for 10 seconds, then stopper. Shake intermittently for 15 to 20 minutes, keeping the temperature near 0°C. Take an aliquot and determine the acidity by titrating with 1*N* sulfuric acid, using phenol red as the indicator. Each time the bottle is opened, flush out the air space before stoppering. Continue adding 1*N* sulfuric acid and shaking until the normality is approximately 2.6, then filter through a Buchner funnel, using vacuum and Whatman #50 filter paper. While filtering, direct a stream of nitrogen over the surface of the fluid. Transfer the solution to a graduated cylinder with a glass stopper. Flush out the air space with nitrogen. Adjust the normality to 2.5 ±0.02 with absolute ethanol, flushing out the air space with nitrogen after each sampling. After the final adjustment, add 15 mg of powdered ascorbic acid.The presence of slight turbidity need cause no concern. Store in a freezer. Just before using, take the container from the freezer, pour a portion into a clean tube, flush out the air space over the liquid in the bottle with nitrogen, then return the container to the freezer. Immediately pipette the cold solution. If handled with care, this reagent can be stable for as long as 3 months.

10. Dehydroepiandosterone (DHEA)† standard stock solution
    Dissolve 100 mg of DHEA in 100 ml of ethanol.

11. Dehydroepiandosterone (DHEA) working standard (0.1 mg/ml)
    Dilute 2.5 ml of stock solution with absolute ethanol to 25 ml.

REFERENCES

Callow, N. H., Callow, R. K., and Emmens, C. W., Colorimetric Determination of Substances Containing the Grouping $CH_2 \cdot CO$ in Urine Extracts as an Indication of Androgen Content. Biochem. J., *32*, 1312, 1938.

Talbot, N. B., Berman, R. A., and MacLachlan, E. A., Elimination of Errors in the Colorimetric Assay of Neutral Urinary 17-Ketosteroids by Means of a Color Correction Equation. J. Biol. Chem., *143*, 211, 1942.

Wilson, H., and Carter, P., Stabilization of the Alcoholic Potassium Hydroxide in Colorimetric 17-Ketosteroid Determinations. Endocrinology, *41*, 417, 1947.

Zimmerman, W., Eine Farbreaktion der Sexualhormone und Ihre Anwendung zur Quantitativen Kolorimetrischen Bestimmung. Hoppe-Seyler's Z. Physiol. Chem., *233*, 257, 1935.

Zimmerman, W., Kolorimetrische Bestimmung der Keimdrüsenhormone. Hoppe-Seyler's Z. Physiol. Chem., *245*, 47, 1937.

*W. A. Hammond Drierite Co., Xenia, Ohio 45385.
†Available from Sigma Chemical Co., St. Louis, Missouri 63118.

Iodine, Protein-Bound (PBI), Serum

PRINCIPLE

This is a method for the quantitative estimation of protein-bound iodine (PBI), using the ceric-arsenite-iodide color reaction. The concentration of PBI is read directly from a semi-logarithmic plot of the color reaction data.

NORMAL VALUES

Range: 3.7—7.2 μg/100 ml serum
Mean: 5.0 μg/100 ml serum

SPECIMEN

Serum.

PROCEDURE

1. Perform all determinations in duplicate. In each series of unknown samples include a reagent blank without serum and a control serum of known PBI content.
2. Add 7 ml of water, 1 ml of 10% zinc sulfate, and 1 ml of 0.5*N* sodium hydroxide to 1 ml of serum in a 15 × 125 mm Pyrex test tube. Mix thoroughly, then centrifuge for 10 minutes. Decant the supernatant and add 10 ml of water. Break the precipitate into a fine suspension, using a glass stirring rod, then centrifuge for 5 minutes. Decant the supernatant and wash the precipitate once more.
3. Place the same stirring rod into the tube and add 1 ml of 4*N* sodium carbonate in two portions as follows: allow half of the volume to flow down the sides of the tube, then break the precipitate into a homogeneous suspension; use the rest of the carbonate to wash the sludge from the stirring rod.
4. Dry the tubes overnight in an oven at 80 to 90°C. Remove the tubes from the oven and place them in a slanting position in a cold muffle furnace. Heat the furnace gradually over a period of 1 hour until it reaches 610°C and maintain it at this temperature for 3 hours. Remove the tubes from the furnace and cover them with aluminum foil. Keep the furnace temperature at 900°C for 4 hours to remove any iodine contamination.
5. Add 2 ml of 2*N* hydrochloric acid to each tube. Allow the tubes to stand until there is no longer an odor of hydrogen sulfide (about 10 minutes).
6. To prepare the standards, add duplicate 1-ml portions of each working standard and sodium carbonate solution to 15 × 125 mm test tubes, then add 1 ml of 4*N* hydrochloric acid to each tube.
7. Cerate color production. Treat blanks, standards, controls, and unknowns the same way from this stage on.
   (a) Add 3 ml of 3*N* sulfuric acid to each tube by allowing it to flow down the sides. Mix thoroughly by the flicking technic. Centrifuge the tubes for 5 minutes.
   (b) Remove 4 ml of supernatant fluid from each tube and place it in 18 × 150 mm tubes. Add 0.5 ml of 0.1*N* sodium arsenite to each tube and mix by the flicking technic.

(c) With a blow-out pipette add 1 ml of ceric ammonium sulfate to each tube at 30-second intervals. Mix the contents of each tube immediately by the flicking technic. The room temperature should be 24°C. Allow the reaction to take place for 18 minutes; then, using a blow-out pipette, add 0.5 ml of brucine sulfate to each tube in the same time sequence in which the ceric reagent was added. Mix by the flicking technic.

(d) Read the samples within 24 hours in a Klett-Summerson photoelectric colorimeter, using a No. 42 blue filter and water as a reference solution.

CALCULATION

1. Make a graph on semi-logarithmic paper, with the serum PBI equivalents of the standards on the horizontal axis and the colorimeter readings on the vertical axis.
2. By using this graph, convert the colorimeter readings of the unknown samples directly to μg PBI/100 ml serum.

NOTES

1. The incinerated reagent blank should check within 0.2 μg/100 ml with the tube containing 1 ml of sodium carbonate solution.
2. Avoid room and glassware contamination with iodine.
3. Use incineration tubes only once.
4. Clean glassware by soaking overnight in a sulfuric acid-dichromate solution, then rinsing thoroughly with deionized water.

REAGENTS

Use deionized water for the preparation of all solutions. Test reagent-grade chemicals for their iodine concentration; use lots containing minimum concentrations of iodine.

1. Zinc sulfate (10%)

    Dissolve 100 g of zinc sulfate ($ZnSO_4 \cdot 7H_2O$) in water and dilute to 1 liter.

2. Sodium hydroxide (0.5*N*)

    Dissolve 20 g of sodium hydroxide in water and dilute to 1 liter. A permanent pink color should be produced when titrating 10.8 to 11.2 ml of this solution with 10 ml of the 10% zinc sulfate in 50 ml of water, using phenolphthalein as the indicator.

3. Sodium carbonate (4*N*)

    Dissolve 212 g of anhydrous sodium carbonate (Na_2CO_3) in water and dilute to 1 liter.

4. Hydrochloric acid (2*N*)

    Dilute 167 ml of hydrochloric acid, sp. gr. 1.19, with water to 1 liter.

5. Hydrochloric acid (4*N*)

    Dilute 334 ml of hydrochloric acid, sp. gr. 1.19, with water to 1 liter.

6. Sulfuric acid (3*N*)

    Add 84 ml of sulfuric acid, sp. gr. 1.84, to water and dilute to 1 liter.

7. Ceric ammonium sulfate solution

    Dissolve 5 g of ceric ammonium sulfate ($Ce(SO_4)_2 \cdot 2\,(NH_4)_2SO_4 \cdot 4H_2O$) in a mixture of 400 ml of water and 500 ml of 3*N* sulfuric acid, then dilute to 1 liter. Since different brands of ceric ammonium sulfate have different moisture contents, an adjustment can be made as follows: place 1.0 ml of

$4N$ sodium carbonate in a tube; place 1.0 ml of the standard containing 0.12 μg iodide per ml in another tube; treat both tubes as standards; the colorimeter (Klett-Summerson) reading of the standard should be between 200 and 250, and that of the blank should be between 850 and 900; if the readings are below the prescribed range, more ceric sulfate is added; if the readings exceed these ranges, the ceric sulfate solution is diluted with $3N$ sulfuric acid.

8. Brucine sulfate (1%)
   Dissolve 10 g of brucine sulfate in water by warming, then dilute to 1 liter.
9. Sodium arsenite ($0.1N$)
   Dissolve 4.95 g of arsenic trioxide (As_2O_3) in 25 ml of 4% sodium hydroxide by warming, then dilute with 300 ml of water. To the resultant solution add $7N$ sulfuric acid until the solution is acid to litmus paper. Dilute this solution to 1 liter.
10. Iodide standard reference solution (100 μg/ml)
    Dissolve 130.8 mg of well-dried potassium iodide in water and dilute to 1 liter.
11. Iodide standard stock solution
    Dilute 2 ml of the reference solution with $4N$ sodium carbonate to 1 liter.
12. Iodide working standards
    Dilute 20, 40, and 60 ml of the stock solution with $4N$ sodium carbonate solution to 100 ml in order to obtain standards containing 0.04, 0.08, and 0.12 μg of iodide per ml respectively.

REFERENCE

Faulkner, L. W., Levy, R. P., and Leonards, J. R., Simplified Technique for the Determination of Serum Protein-Bound Iodine. Clin. Chem., *7*, 637, 1961.

Vanilmandelic Acid (VMA), Urine

PRINCIPLE

Vanilmandelic acid (VMA) is oxidized to vanillin with potassium ferricyanide. The vanillin is extracted, then treated with an indolephosphoric acid reagent to produce a salmon-colored complex, which is measured colorimetrically and is proportional to the concentration of VMA.

NORMAL VALUES

0.7—6.8 mg/24 hours.

SPECIMEN

Collect urine over 24 hours. Instruct the patient to abstain from medication and from bananas, chocolate, tea, and coffee for 2 days prior to collection of urine. Collect urine specimen in a brown glass bottle containing 25 ml of 6*N* hydrochloric acid. Store the urine in a refrigerator.

PROCEDURE

1. Transfer 50 ml of urine into an Erlenmeyer flask (capacity 100 to 150 ml) containing 5 ml of concentrated hydrochloric acid. Add 5 g of Florisil®*. Mix for 10 minutes by swirling, then filter through Whatman #1 filter paper.
2. Transfer 10 ml of the urinary filtrate into each of two 50-ml glass-stoppered centrifuge tubes. Transfer 1 ml of vanilmandelic acid working standard and 1 ml of concentrated hydrochloric acid into another centrifuge tube and dilute with distilled water to 10 ml to provide a "standard". To another centrifuge tube add 1 ml of concentrated hydrochloric acid and dilute with distilled water to 10 ml to serve as a "reagent blank".
3. Add 45 ml of ethyl acetate to each tube and stopper. Shake each vigorously for 2 minutes, then centrifuge for 5 minutes. Remove the aqueous infranatant fluid by aspiration and discard it. Recentrifuge the tubes briefly, then remove the small amount of aqueous infranatant fluid by aspiration.
4. Add 5 ml of potassium carbonate to each tube and stopper. Shake vigorously for 2 minutes, then centrifuge. Without delay, aspirate the supernatant organic phase and discard it. Immediately add 2.5 ml of concentrated hydrochloric acid to each carbonate extract, shake the tubes, then allow them to stand for 5 minutes.
5. Add 1 ml of potassium ferricyanide solution to the reagent blank, to the standard, and to one of the urine extract tubes. Do not add ferricyanide to the duplicate urine extract, which serves as "urine blank". Add 1 ml of zinc sulfate solution to all of the centrifuge tubes and shake them. Place all tubes in a 37°C water bath in the dark for 2 hours, except the urine blank tube, which is stored in a refrigerator. Protect the tubes from direct light throughout step 5.
6. Add 45 ml of toluene to each centrifuge tube and stopper. Shake vigorously for 2 minutes, then centrifuge. Remove the aqueous infranatant fluid by aspiration and discard it. Recentrifuge briefly, then remove the small amount of aqueous infranatant fluid that usually collects at the tip of each tube by aspiration.
7. Decant the toluene extract into another 50-ml centrifuge tube, taking care to avoid dislodging the precipitate present. Add 3.4 ml of potassium carbonate

*Floridin Co., 2 Gateway Center, Pittsburgh, Pennsylvania 15222.

reagent to each toluene extract. Stopper the tubes, shake vigorously for 2 minutes, then centrifuge.

8. Insert a 3-ml volumetric pipette through the toluene layer into each infranatant carbonate extract. Expel the drop of toluene from the pipette by gently blowing through the pipette. Without delay, transfer 3 ml of each carbonate extract into 19 × 105 mm Coleman colorimeter cuvettes.
9. Place the colorimeter cuvettes in an ice bath. Very slowly add 0.5 ml of concentrated sulfuric acid to each. Agitate the cuvette during addition of sulfuric acid to avoid excessive heating or foaming.
10. Add 4 ml of cold indole-phosphoric acid reagent to each cuvette. Stopper the cuvettes and mix by inversion, then place them in an ice bath.
11. Precisely 5 minutes after the addition of the indole-phosphoric acid reagent, measure the absorbance at 495 mμ in a Coleman Junior spectrophotometer. If the measurements of absorbance are greater than 0.8, repeat the procedure on smaller urine samples.
12. Prepare a calibration curve by treating standard samples containing 0, 10, 20, 30, 40, 50, 60, 70, and 80 μg of vanilmandelic acid according to the procedure as outlined. Plot the concentrations of vanilmandelic acid versus the absorbances on rectangular coordinate paper to obtain a calibration curve. The curve should approach linearity in the range of absorbance less than 0.7 mμ.

CALCULATION

$$\text{mg VMA/100 ml} = \frac{A_{\text{urine sample}} - A_{\text{blank}}}{A_{\text{standard}} - A_{\text{reagent blank}}} \times 0.55$$

$$\text{mg VMA/24 hrs} = \frac{\text{VMA (mg/100 ml)} \times \text{urine volume (ml)}}{100}$$

REAGENTS

1. Vanilmandelic acid stock standard (1 mg/ml)
   Add 50 mg of vanilmandelic acid to a 50-ml volumetric flask and dissolve in 0.01*N* hydrochloric acid. Dilute to the mark with 0.01*N* hydrochloric acid and store in a refrigerator. This solution is stable for at least 1 month.
2. Vanilmandelic acid working standard (50 μg/ml)
   Transfer 5 ml of the stock standard into a 100-ml volumetric flask and dilute to the mark with distilled water. Store in a refrigerator. Prepare fresh each week.
3. Potassium carbonate (0.4*M*)
   Transfer 55.3 g of potassium carbonate (anhydrous, reagent grade) into a 1-liter volumetric flask and dissolve in distilled water, then dilute to the mark.
4. Potassium ferricyanide (0.6% *W/V*)
   Dissolve 0.6 g of potassium ferricyanide (reagent grade) in 100 ml of distilled water and store in a brown glass bottle in a refrigerator. This solution is stable for 3 days.
5. Zinc sulfate (1.2% *W/V*)
   Dissolve 1.2 g of anhydrous zinc sulfate in distilled water to make 100 ml of solution.
6. Ethanolic indole reagent
   Dissolve 500 mg of indole (reagent grade) in absolute ethanol and dilute with the absolute ethanol to 100 ml. Store in a refrigerator.

7. Phosphoric acid (85%, reagent grade)
   Store in a refrigerator.
8. Mixed indole-phosphoric acid reagent
   Dilute 1 ml of ethanolic indole reagent to 40 ml with cold 85% phosphoric acid in a 50-ml glass-stoppered mixing cylinder. Prepare this reagent immediately before use and keep chilled in an ice bath.
9. Concentrated hydrochloric acid (reagent grade)
10. Concentrated sulfuric acid (reagent grade)
11. Ethyl acetate (reagent grade)
12. Toluene (reagent grade)
13. Activated magnesium silicate (60/100 mesh Florisil®)

REFERENCE

Sunderman, F. W., Jr., Cleveland, P. D., Law, N. C., and Sunderman, F. W., A Method for the Determination of 3-Methoxy-4-Hydroxymandelic Acid (Vanilmandelic Acid) for the Diagnosis of Pheochromocytoma. Am. J. Clin. Pathol., *34*, 293, 1960.

BLOOD BANK

Sectional Directory

Introduction

Any compilation of laboratory procedures referring to the field of blood banking runs into several difficulties. More than any other branch of the clinical laboratory, the blood bank deals with commercially produced agents of highly variable quality. Each manufacturer produces a special product, which works best when used as he prescribes. The compiler cannot specify particular incubator times and temperatures for a particular test, because these conditions will vary widely with the type of serum used. A procedure manual can at best impress upon the worker that, in order to ensure optimal results in the immunohematology laboratory, the most important thing to do is to read the label. In our laboratory we keep a loose-leaf notebook, and all package literature or other directions from typing sera and other reagents are filed and referred to whenever there is any question about procedure. Each manufacturer of typing sera has prepared manuals of immunohematology that cover the subject admirably. They are available on request and serve as free competition to any procedure manual in this field. Also, the official manual of the American Association of Blood Banks is a complete and authoritative compilation of many technics used in the blood banks.

Considering these factors, the reason we believe that our contribution to blood bank literature might be useful is because we have attempted to present the work in a concise fashion that avoids being bookish only by assuming that its readers know something about the field and can intelligently interpret their results. It is also hoped that the format used to present the procedures is easier to follow than that of other manuals. Finally, the inclusion of several useful procedures not commonly found elsewhere should make this compilation more valuable to the reader.

John W. King, M.D., Ph.D.

Red-Cell Suspensions

PRINCIPLE

Many of the procedures in the blood bank require the use of red-cell suspensions ranging from 2 to 5%. There are wide tolerances allowed in the strength of these suspensions, but it is desirable that some uniformity be followed. One way to ensure this is to ascertain that the blood bank technicians know what a cell suspension of the more commonly used concentrations looks like. It is good practice in training technicians to have them prepare suspensions of red cells of known concentration in order to make them familiar with the appearance of these suspensions.

PROCEDURE

1. Prepare a suspension of red blood cells in physiological saline by mixing whole blood or macerated clot in saline. Shake vigorously. Allow larger clots to settle.
2. Decant cell suspension into another test tube. Centrifuge to pack cells.
3. Pipette 1 ml of packed cells into a container holding 49 ml of saline. This represents a 2% suspension of cells.
4. Pipette 1 ml of cells into 19 ml of saline. This represents a 5% suspension.
5. Mix these suspensions by shaking vigorously. Pipette aliquots of each preparation into test tubes commonly used for most blood bank tests and observe.

NOTES

1. While it is not practical, nor necessary, for this procedure to be carried out daily, it is a desirable exercise to require of all technicians in training as an aid in teaching the proper application appearance of these cell suspensions.

REAGENTS

1. Whole blood (oxalated, versenated, or clotted).
2. Physiological saline

sodium chloride	9.0 g
distilled water	1000.0 ml

Blood Grouping—ABO System

Tube Method

PRINCIPLE

Blood groups can be determined by the use of anti-A and anti-B grouping sera to demonstrate the presence of the antigen (A or B) on the red cells. In the first stage of the reaction the antigenic sites on the red cells are coated with antibody globulin of the same specificity. In the second stage the coated cells become sufficiently linked to one another to produce agglutination.

SPECIMEN

Venous or capillary blood.

PROCEDURE

1. Puncture the patient's fingertip and transfer 2 drops of blood to a 10 × 75 mm tube partially filled with saline. Blood obtained by venipuncture may also be used.
2. Mix by shaking, fill the tube with saline, centrifuge, discard supernatant, and refill with fresh saline. Repeat the washing.
3. Make a 2% suspension of cells.
4. Place 2 drops of the cell suspension in each of two tubes.
5. Label the tubes with patient's name and "Anti-A" or "Anti-B".
6. Add 1 drop of anti-A grouping serum to the tube labeled "Anti-A".
7. Add 1 drop of anti-B grouping serum to the tube labeled "Anti-B".
8. Spin for 30 seconds in a Serofuge or similar type of centrifuge.
9. Tap the tubes gently. If there is no agglutination, the cells will resuspend evenly. Examine all apparently negative reactions under a low-power microscope.

INTERPRETATION

1. Agglutination in "Anti-A" tube: group A.
2. Agglutination in "Anti-B" tube: group B.
3. No agglutination in either "Anti-A" or "Anti-B": group O.
4. Agglutination in both "Anti-A" and "Anti-B": group AB.

NOTES

1. As weak subgroups of A may be missed, cells testing as group O should be rechecked by routinely testing in the same manner with anti-A,B serum.
2. For any but the most casual screening procedures, reverse grouping using the patient's serum against known A and B cells should be performed.

REAGENTS

1. Anti-A grouping serum
2. Anti-B grouping serum
3. Anti-A,B grouping serum.

Blood Grouping—ABO System

Slide Method

PRINCIPLE

Blood groups can be determined by the use of anti-A and anti-B grouping sera to demonstrate the presence of the antigens (A or B) on the red cell. In the first stage of the reaction the antigenic sites on the red cells are coated with antibody globulin of the same specificity. In the second stage the coated cells become sufficiently linked to one another to produce agglutination. The tube method is considered slightly more sensitive than the slide method, but the slide method has its proponents and is a useful screening test.

SPECIMEN

Whole blood, oxalated or clotted.

PROCEDURE

1. Draw a vertical line through the center of a glass slide held horizontally, or use ceramic slides suitably divided.
2. Label the upper portion of the slide to the left "Anti-A"; label the upper portion of the right side "Anti-B".
3. Mix the blood sample well by inversion or, if clotted, by macerating the clot in its serum. With a glass dropper or two wooden applicator sticks place a drop of blood on the side labeled "Anti-A" and a drop on the side labeled "Anti-B".
4. Add 1 drop of anti-A grouping serum to the side labeled "Anti-A".
5. Add 1 drop of anti-B grouping serum to the side labeled "Anti-B".
6. With a clean wooden applicator stick mix the blood sample and anti-A serum. Spread the mixture so that it covers an oval area about the size of a quarter.
7. With a clean wooden applicator stick mix the blood sample and anti-B serum. Spread the mixture as above.
8. Hold the slide over a light source, such as a view box. (Do not place the slide on the view box; heat from the light may decrease the strength of the reactions.)
9. Hold the slide in your hands and tilt it back and forth. Observe for agglutination for exactly 2 minutes.

INTERPRETATION

1. Agglutination with anti-A: group A.
2. Agglutination with anti-B: group B.
3. Agglutination with neither anti-A nor anti-B: group O.
4. Agglutination with both anti-A and anti-B: group AB.

NOTES

1. As weak subgroups of A may be missed, cells testing as group O should be rechecked by routinely testing with anti-A,B serum.

2. For any but the most casual screening procedures, reverse grouping using the patient's serum against known A and B cells is required.
3. Subgrouping of group A or AB bloods may be desirable. This can be carried out in the same manner as described above for determining A and B, using absorbed B (anti-A_1) serum or the appropriate lectin.

REAGENTS

1. Anti-A grouping serum
2. Anti-B grouping serum
3. Anti-A,B grouping serum

Serum Grouping—ABO System

PRINCIPLE

Depending on which blood group antigen is on the red cell, the opposite antibody will normally be found in the serum, provided that the patient is not less than one year old. When the A antigen is present on the red cell, anti-B will be present in the serum. When the B antigen is present on the red cell, anti-A will be present in the serum. By adding cells of known groups to the patient's serum, the blood group of the patient can be found. This should be used as a check of the regular grouping method.

Antibodies to A are sometimes found in the serum of individuals who are A_2, A_2B, or weaker subgroups of A. About 25% of A_2B individuals have anti-A in their serum, while the corresponding value for anti-A in A_2 individuals is less than 5%. People who have suppressor genes (Bombay type) will have cells that fail to agglutinate with any grouping serum (anti-A, anti-B, anti-H), but they will have antibodies that will agglutinate group A, B, and O cells.

SPECIMEN

Serum.

PROCEDURE

1. Obtain 1 ml of patient's serum.
2. Make a 2% suspension of known A cells in normal saline. Label the tube "A Cells".
3. Make a 2% suspension of known B cells in normal saline. Label the tube "B Cells".
4. Label two other small test tubes "A" and "B".
5. Place 2 drops of serum into each tube.
6. To the tube marked "A" add 1 drop of the 2% suspension of A cells.
7. To the tube marked "B" add 1 drop of the 2% suspension of B cells.
8. Mix the contents in both tubes by shaking, then centrifuge for 1 minute.
9. Hold the tubes up to a light source and observe for agglutination.

INTERPRETATION

1. Agglutination in "A" tube only: group B.
2. Agglutination in "B" tube only: group A.
3. Agglutination in both "A" and "B": group O.
4. Agglutination in neither "A" nor "B": group AB.
5. If serum grouping does not agree with cell grouping, recheck both procedures to reconcile your results.

REAGENTS

1. Selected red blood cells known to be group A
2. Selected red blood cells known to be group B

Secretion of Blood Group Antigens

PRINCIPLE

About 80% of Caucasians secrete blood group substances in their saliva. Determination of secretion may be useful in diagnosing some of the weaker subgroups of A, in studying paternity exclusions, and in studying the possibilities of erythroblastosis developing in an unborn child whose mother is group O and whose father is group A. Individuals of groups A, B, and AB secrete the corresponding antigens. Group O individuals secrete H substances, which can be detected by anti-H sera and by anti-H lectins. People other than group O also secrete H substances, but in lesser amounts than found in the saliva of group O people.

These substances are detected by agglutinin absorption technics. The saliva is allowed to react with the appropriate reagent; after a suitable incubation period, residual activity of the reagent is measured, using appropriate reagent red blood cells. In secretors the salivary antigens inactivate the antisera or lectins, so that the reagent test cells are not agglutinated. In nonsecretors the antisera continue to be active, and the reagent cells are agglutinated.

Individuals who secrete antigens in their saliva also secrete these same substances in their tears, cerebrospinal fluid, urine, and other body fluids.

SPECIMEN

Collect 3 ml of saliva from the patient by having him expectorate directly into a clean test tube. (Be sure that he rinses his mouth several times with water before collecting the specimen; food residues, dentifrices, chewing gum, or blood from bleeding gums may invalidate the result.) Specimens from children may be collected by using a cotton swab and rinsing the swab in a few drops of saline or by aspirating the saliva directly from the mouth with a medicine dropper.

The specimen should be inactivated promptly by placing the test tube in boiling water for 10 minutes. Most specimens become cloudy with heating and must be clarified by centrifugation. Remove and save the supernatant. If the test is to be delayed, the specimen can be preserved by freezing.

PROCEDURE

1. If the patient's blood group is group O, the test must be set up against anti-H. If the patient is of any other blood group, anti-A or anti-B serum, as appropriate, may also be used.
2. Set up a five-tube serial dilution of saliva as follows:

Tube	1	2	3	4	5
Saliva	0.2 ml	—	—	—	—
Saline	0.2 ml	0.2 ml	0.2 ml	0.2 ml	0.2 ml
Dilution	1:2	1:4	1:8	1:16	1:32

   Make serial dilutions by transferring 0.2 ml of the saline-saliva mixture from tube 1 to tube 2, then from tube 2 to tube 3, etc.
3. Add 1 drop of anti-H lectin to each tube.
4. Incubate at room temperature for 10 minutes, then add 0.2 ml of the red-cell suspension. Centrifuge, then read for agglutination.
5. Compare titers against proper positive and negative controls.

NOTES

1. It may not be necessary to set up a quantitative procedure. Because the strength of the antisera and lectins does vary, the quality of the specimen to be tested may vary enough to cause either false positives or negatives.
2. Suitable positive and negative control saliva should be included to ascertain that the system is working properly. It is a simple matter to screen random volunteers to pick out appropriate control material.
3. The use of group A_2 cells rather than A_1 cells is not mandatory; it is considered better in that the A_2 cells are a more sensitive indicator of reduction of titer of the absorbed serum than A_1 cells.

REAGENTS

1. Anti-H lectin

   This is available commercially. Anti-H sera are rarely available, but the lectin is an effective substitute.
2. Group O cells (5% suspension)

REFERENCES

Anonymous, Hyland Reference Manual of Immunohematology. A Concise Review of Principles and Procedures, 3rd ed. Hyland Laboratories, Los Angeles, California, 1965.

Krant, M. J., Martin, Margaret S., and Bandruj, Cynthia S., Salivary Secretion of Blood Group Factors in Cancer. J. Am. Med. Assoc., *204*, 153, 1968.

Screening for Dangerous Universal Donors

PRINCIPLE

The use of group O donors as donors for patients of other blood groups is a practice that should be discouraged. Unfortunately there are situations in which this cannot be avoided. The objection to the use of group O blood as universal donor blood, aside from the fact that the supply of such blood for group O patients is used up, is that some group O people develop immune-type antibodies for A and B cells. These antibodies are hemolysins and, as such, are capable of producing serious and sometimes fatal reactions in group A and B recipients. In the past, group O bloods have been titered for agglutinins to screen the high-titer donors. While this is a useful procedure, a more realistic approach is the screening of group O bloods for hemolysins and eliminating as universal donor blood any that show evidence of hemolytic activity. Rejected bloods can be conserved and used in transfusions for group O subjects.

SPECIMENS

1. Serum from the blood samples to be screened.
2. Reagent group A and B cells, 5% suspensions.
3. Complement, fresh or lyophilized, made daily in a dilution of 1:15 and kept refrigerated when not in use.

PROCEDURE

1. For each specimen to be tested, set up a serial dilution of serum from 1:5 to 1:80. Make dilutions in duplicate, so that you can test with both group A and group B cells.

Tube	1	2	3	4	5
Serum	0.1 ml	—	—	—	—
Saline	0.4 ml	0.25	0.25	0.25	0.25
Dilution	1:5	1:10	1:20	1:40	1:80

2. Transfer 0.25 ml from tube 1 to tube 2, mix, and transfer 0.25 ml from tube 2 to tube 3, etc. Discard 0.25 ml from tube 5 to keep the volume in each tube uniform.
3. Add 0.1 ml of 1:15 dilution of complement to each tube.
4. Add 0.2 ml of 5% suspension of group A cells to each tube.
5. Incubate at 37°C for 30 minutes, centrifuge, and read for hemolysis and agglutination.

INTERPRETATION

Any hemolysis beyond 1:5 disqualifies a blood as safe universal donor blood.

NOTES

1. No attempt is made to titer the complement, as it is used in excess. However, appropriate controls should be run, using serum from a person who is known to have hemolysins. This serum may be stored indefinitely, as it is reactivated by the addition of complement each time it is used.

2. No attempt is made to balance the complement in this reaction, as this is not the same type of reaction as the Kolmer-Wasserman, in which the concentration of complement must be carefully balanced in respect to antigen and antibody concentration.
3. A recent report pointing out a further complication of universal-donor transfusions is that of Barnes and Allen concerning the increased difficulties in cross-matching and transfusing patients transfused with universal-donor blood as compared with those who received group-specific blood.

REFERENCES

Barnes, A., and Allen, T. E., Transfusions Subsequent to Administration of Univeral Donor Blood in Vietnam. J. Am. Med. Assoc., *204*, 147, 1968.

Grove-Rasmussen, M., Shaw, R. S., and Marceau, E., Hemolytic Transfusion Reactions in Group A Patient Receiving Group O Blood. Am. J. Clin. Pathol., *23*, 828, 1953.

Rh Typing—The D (Rh_o) Factor

Saline Tube Method

PRINCIPLE

The original method for determining Rh factors was the saline agglutinin test, which was carried out in tubes and required incubation at 37°C for 30 minutes. This procedure is still an accepted method, and in many instances is still the best method. Care must be taken to use typing serum marked for saline tube test.

SPECIMEN

Clotted or oxalated blood.

PROCEDURE

1. Prepare a 2% suspension of red blood cells in saline. Wash once if blood is fresh, several times if blood is hemolyzed.
2. Place 2 drops of cell suspension in a test tube (10 × 75 mm). Add 1 drop of typing serum. Mix cells and serum by shaking vigorously for a few moments.
3. Incubate at 37°C for 30 minutes.
4. Centrifuge. Shake or roll gently to break up sedimented cells. Read macroscopically for agglutination.
5. If no agglutination is present, proceed to test for D^u (see p. 129).
6. The test may be modified to test for any of the other Rh antigens (C, D, E, c, and e), if appropriate sera are used.

NOTES

1. Saline tube tests are probably the best method of determining Rh antigens. Saline-reacting serum is rarely available for the c (hr′) antigen; when it is available, our own experience indicates that it usually does not give clear-cut reactions. It is, therefore, preferred that this test be done as a modified (high-protein) tube test or as a slide test.
2. Saline sera for the other Rh antigens are available and give excellent reactions when used as indicated by the manufacturer.

REAGENTS

1. Anti-D (Rh_o) saline tube test serum

Rh Typing—The D (Rh_o) Factor

Slide Method

PRINCIPLE

The Rh factor D (Rh_o) was the first of the Rh factors to be described and is by far the most important clinically. It is present in the cells of about 85% of Caucasians and 95% of Negroes. With appropriate serum, this antigen can be demonstrated by using the slide technic originally described by Diamond. The slide test described here is faster than test tube methods, and suitable for small-scale work. One disadvantage of this method is that apparent Rh-negative bloods cannot be studied further for D^u without making a new preparation.

SPECIMEN

Clotted or oxalated blood.

PROCEDURE

1. Turn on a view box and place a slide directly on it to warm. The slide should reach a temperature of about 40 to 45°C.
2. When the slide is warm, mix the blood by inversion or by macerating the clot in its own serum. Using a wooden applicator, a soda straw or a glass dropper, place 1 drop of blood in each of two divisions of a slide. Mark "Test" and "Control".
3. Add 1 drop of anti-D (Rh_o) typing serum specifically prepared for the slide or rapid tube method to the test drop of blood.
4. Add 2 drops of 22% bovine albumin to the control drop.
5. Mix the blood and typing serum or albumin with a clean applicator stick.
6. Set a timer and for 2 minutes slowly rock the view box back and forth.
7. Observe for agglutination.

INTERPRETATION

1. No agglutination in anti-D slide division or control division: Rh_o negative.
2. Agglutination in anti-D slide division, no agglutination in control division: Rh_o positive.
3. Agglutination in both slide divisions indicates an auto-antibody, and the proper Rh reaction cannot be determined by this technic.

NOTES

1. Saline suspensions of cells should not be used, because slide anti-D (Rh_o) serum will sensitize Rh_o-positive cells, but will not agglutinate them in this medium.
2. The common view boxes on the market permit the use of ordinary microscope slides or of larger ceramically marked slides. The author's own preference is for the larger slide, which can be rinsed off and reused rather than discarded.

REAGENTS

1. Anti-D (Rh_o) slide typing serum
2. Bovine albumin (22%)

The D^u (Rh_o Variant) Problem

PRINCIPLE

Red blood cells not agglutinated by potent anti-D (Rh_o) serum can sometimes be shown to have combined with the antibody in the typing serum, although no visible reaction has occurred. The presence of the antibody on the surface of the red cells can be demonstrated by carrying out a direct Coombs test on the cells to show the presence of the globulin. Such sensitized cells are agglutinated by the Coombs serum, which has no effect on unsensitized cells. These cells are known as D^u (Rh_o variant) cells.

Because such antigens are known to cause sensitization of the patient and to be responsible for transfusion reactions and hemolytic diseases of the newborn, it is essential that all donors be tested for D^u before they are used in Rh-negative transfusions. Blood positive for D^u should be used as Rh-positive donor blood or reserved for other D^u patients.

Recipients who are D^u positive must be treated in a somewhat different manner. The D^u phenomenon can be produced either by the inheritance of a weakly reacting D, or the genetically normal D may be suppressed by the presence of the C (rh′) gene in a double dose. Individuals with the genotypes CDe/Cde, CDE/Cde, etc., can develop antibodies to c (hr′), which is present in a double dose in Rh-negative blood. Consequently they are in at least as much danger when transfused with Rh-negative as with Rh-positive blood. Because it seems somewhat safer to use Rh-positive blood for the suppression-type D^u patients, it is necessary to determine the status of the C (rh′) and c (hr′) genes in these patients before transfusing them.

SPECIMEN

Clotted, versenated, or fingertip blood.

PROCEDURE

1. This procedure is a continuation of the saline tube method of D (Rh_o) typing (see p. 127).
2. After determining with the anti-D (Rh_o) antiserum that a blood is negative, wash the cell-antiserum mixture 3 times with saline.
3. It is well to use the patient's cells without the anti-D (Rh_o) serum as a negative control and to use Rh-positive cells sensitized with incomplete anti-D (Rh_o) as a positive control (see p. 128).
4. Completely decant the final washing and add 2 drops of the anti-human globulin serum.
5. Resuspend the cells by shaking vigorously. Centrifuge the resulting suspension for 30 seconds. Read both macroscopically and microscopically.
6. Test any blood determined to be D^u positive for reaction to anti-C and anti-c sera (see pp. 127, 128).
7. Bloods that react with both of these sera or with the anti-c alone are considered genetic D^u and are transfused as Rh-negative recipients.
8. Bloods that fail to react to the anti-c serum, but do react with anti-C, are considered homozygous for C; hence they are suppressed-type D^u and should be transfused as Rh-positive recipients. This latter type of D^u is often referred to as a "high-grade D^u".

NOTES

1. It is not completely clear how the D^u fits into Weiner's studies of subtypes of Rh_o. Yet it is necessary for blood banks to take cognizance of the differences in D (Rh_o), if they wish to avoid potentially dangerous reactions.
2. A new aspect of the importance of D^u is the possibility of reactions in D^u-positive women who are treated with Rhogam® to prevent sensitization by a Rh-positive pregnancy. Therefore all women to be treated with this reagent must be typed for D^u prior to administration of the serum.

REAGENTS

1. Anti-human globulin serum
2. Rh-negative cells, as a negative control
3. Rh-positive cells sensitized anti-D (Rh_o), as a positive control

   These may be prepared by mixing one drop of anti-D (Rh_0) serum prepared for the slide test with 5 ml of a 5% suspension of Rh-positive cells. Such cells should give a strong reaction when tested with anti-human globulin serum.

Determination of Rh Genotypes

PRINCIPLE

When a family is faced with the problem of Rh incompatibilities between the husband's blood and the wife's blood, the physician often turns to the laboratory for help. Information about the husband's Rh genotype can help the physician advise the family whether they should have further pregnancies or whether they must be reconciled to being unable to have more children and plan for an adoption. If the father is heterozygous for the Rh factor responsible for erythroblastosis of an infant, he still has an even chance of fathering a child compatible with its mother's blood and hence unafflicted. If he is homozygous, then all his offspring will have the incompatible antigen, and all future pregnancies can be expected to produce erythroblastotic children.

In over 90% of the cases of hemolytic disease of the newborn, the offending antigen is the D (Rh_0) antigen. While antisera are available to detect antigens determined by the genes C and E and by their alleles c and e, an antiserum for d is not available, and only antigen D can be defined by an antiserum. Because antiserum for d has not been satisfactorily demonstrated, we have no laboratory procedure to determine homozygosity or heterozygosity for D. (The situation is somewhat similar to that existing in group A, where we are unable to distinguish individuals who are homozygous for A from those who are heterozygous and carry a gene for O as well as for A.)

To get around this problem, use is made of the fact that individuals who are heterozygous for C are most often also heterozygous for the D locus. Thus a Rh-genotype determination is carried out by allowing the patient's cells to react with antisera for C, c, D, E, and e, and sometimes with antisera for C^w. The resulting data can be used to evaluate the possible presence of a gene for d.

PROCEDURE

1. Determine the reaction of the father's cells to appropriate antisera for D, C, c, E, and e, using technics outlined elsewhere.
2. Determine the same antigen reactions on any other family members available, especially the paternal grandparents, uncles and aunts, and the siblings of the affected child.
3. Review the data. If any of the siblings of the affected child or its paternal grandparents are negative for D, then the father must be heterozygous and carry the gene for d.
4. If no Rh-negative family members are found, use the father's data and refer to the chart on the next page. The reactions given in the five left-hand columns refer to cell reactions with the antisera. To the right are the possible genotypes and the frequency of each.

Example:

The father's blood reacts D + C + E − c + e +. This indicates a phenotype of CDe (Rh_1) that may be produced by the following genotypes: CDe/cde, CDe/CDe, and cDe/Cde. Of these, only the second one constitutes a homozygote for D, and the frequency of this genotype is much lower than that of the first and most likely choice. Therefore the family should be advised that there is an excellent chance of future normal pregnancies and be encouraged to try again.

FREQUENCY OF Rh TYPES AND GENOTYPES

Reaction with Antisera to					Types		Genotypes		Frequency Percent
D (Rh_o)	**C (rh′)**	**E (rh″)**	**c (hr′)**	**e (hr″)**	**Race-Sanger**	**Wiener**	**Race-Sanger**	**Wiener**	**Race-Sanger**
Rh_o Negative (15%)									
0	0	0	+	+	cde	rh	cde/cde	rr	15.10
0	+	0	+	+	Cde	rh′rh	Cde/cde	r′r	0.76
0	+	0	0	+		rh′rh′	Cde/Cde	r′r′	0.01
0	0	+	+	+	cdE	rh″rh	cdE/cde	r″r	0.92
0	0	+	+	0		rh″rh″	cdE/cdE	r″r″	0.01
0	+	+	+	+	CdE	rh′rh″ rh_yrh	Cde/cdE CdE/cde	r′r″ r^yr	0.02 0.00
0	+	+	0	+		rh_yrh'	CdE/Cde	r^yr'	0.00
0	+	+	+	0		rh_yrh''	CdE/cdE	r^yr''	0.00
0	+	+	0	0		rh_yrh_y	CdE/CdE	r^yr^y	0.00
Rh_o Positive (85%)									
+	0	0	+	+	cDe	Rh_o	cDe/cde cDe/cDe	R^0r R^0R^0	2.00 0.06
+	+	0	+	+	CDe	Rh_1rh	CDe/cde CDe/cDe cDe/Cde	R^1r R^1R^0 R^0r'	31.68 2.09 0.05
+	+	0	0	+		Rh_1Rh_1	CDe/CDe CDe/Cde	R^1R^1 R^1r'	16.61 0.80
+	0	+	+	+	cDE	Rh_2Rh	cDE/cde cDE/cDe cDe/cdE	R^2r R^2R^0 R^0r''	10.96 0.72 0.06
+	0	+	+	0		Rh_2Rh_2	cDE/cDE cDE/cdE	R^2R^2 R^2r''	1.99 0.34
+	+	+	+	+	CDE	Rh_1Rh_2	CDe/cDE CDe/cdE cDE/Cde	R^1R^2 R^1r'' R^2r'	11.50 0.97 0.28
						Rh_zRh	CDE/cde CDE/cDe cDe/CdE	R^zr R^zR^0 R^0R^y	0.19 0.01 0.00
+	+	+	0	+		Rh_zRh_1	CDE/CDe CDE/Cde CDe/CdE	R^zR^1 R^zr' R^1R^y	0.20 0.00 0.00
+	+	+	+	0		Rh_zRh_2	CDE/cDE CDE/cdE cDE/CdE	R^zR^2 R^zr'' R^2r^y	0.07 0.01 0.00
+	+	+	0	0		Rh_zRh_z	CDE/CDE CDE/CdE	R^zR^z R^zR^y	0.000 0.000

NOTES

1. The application of family data to this problem has been neglected in the past. A recent example in our own laboratory of a CDe (Rh_1) father who was positive for c (hr′) ended unhappily when it was shown that an older sibling of the affected baby was cDe/cde. This indicated that the father had contributed a gene for cDe to this child and was, in fact, homozygous with the probable genotype CDe/cDe.

REFERENCE

King, J. W., Determination of Genotypes by Family Studies. Cleveland Clinic Quarterly, *33*, 119, 1966.

Direct Antiglobulin (Coombs) Test

PRINCIPLE

This procedure is designed to demonstrate the presence of an antibody (globulin) coating on erythrocytes. The addition of an antiglobulin serum to a saline suspension of red cells will produce agglutination of coated cells and will not agglutinate uncoated cells. Such sera may be prepared in the laboratory; they are also available commercially. They are produced by injecting human globulins into a rabbit or other suitable animal. Absorption of such sera with washed normal red cells will remove any antibodies for erythrocytes and leave the antiglobulin antibodies.

PROCEDURE

Washing Cells

In washing cells in preparation for a direct Coombs test or similar technic, it should be remembered that, for each washing to be successful, the cells must be resuspended after each centrifugation. The usual test tubes are 10 × 75 mm and are too small to allow mixing by inversion of the tube. The best way to accomplish the mixing is to decant the supernatant by inverting the tubes over a sink or pan, then placing the tubes back in the rack to allow the residual saline to collect on top of the sedimented cells. These cells can then be resuspended in this residual saline by vigorously shaking the tubes and by tapping them on the bottom to dislodge the button of cells. This suspension can be further mixed with saline by squirting the saline directly into the suspension as the tube is filled.

Test Procedure

1. Prepare a suspension of red cells in saline by mixing 2 or 3 drops of a thick suspension of cells with saline in a test tube (13 × 75 mm).
2. Centrifuge, then decant the supernatant fluid.
3. Resuspend the cells in a few drops of saline and add saline to fill the tube. Centrifuge and decant as in step 2.
4. Repeat step 3.
5. Make a 2—5% suspension of these cells in saline.
6. Transfer 2 drops of this suspension to each of two small test tubes (10 × 75 mm).
7. Fill both small tubes with saline and centrifuge for 30 seconds.
8. Decant completely the saline from each tube.
9. Add 2 drops of anti-human globulin serum to one tube, and 2 drops of saline to the other. Resuspend the cells.
10. Centrifuge for 30 seconds.
11. Roll the tubes to resuspend the cells.
12. Observe both macroscopically and microscopically for agglutination. Compare the two tubes to avoid misinterpretation of unbroken packed cells.

NOTES

1. When washing the cells, care should be taken not to allow the saline to stand on the cells longer than necessary, as some antibodies may be eluted more easily

than others. The routine use of cold saline for washing will serve to help avoid this problem.

2. Washing of the cells must be done thoroughly, as any protein remaining on the cells will react with the Coombs serum and may produce false negative reactions.

INTERPRETATION

1. Agglutination: positive direct Coombs.
2. No agglutination: negative direct Coombs.

REAGENTS

1. Patient's red blood cells as clotted or versenated blood
2. Anti-human globulin serum

Indirect Antiglobulin (Coombs) Test

PRINCIPLE

This test is designed to detect incomplete antibodies in a patient's serum. These antibodies are globulins that are capable of coating red cells, but do not agglutinate the red cells. It is carried out in two steps. First, selected red blood cells of known antigen content are exposed to the suspected serum. After the red cells have been washed with saline to remove excess globulin, they are tested for sensitization by mixing them with the antiglobulin serum.

SPECIMEN

Fresh serum.

PROCEDURE

1. Place 2 drops of the serum to be tested in a properly labeled test tube.
2. Add 2 drops of a 2—4% saline suspension of the selected red blood cells.*
3. Incubate for 1 hour at 37°C. A similarly prepared tube may also be incubated at 4°C to test for cold-reacting antibodies, including anti-H, anti-P, anti-Le^a, and anti-Ti^a.
4. Centrifuge, then examine for agglutination. If none is present, continue with step 5.
5. Rapidly wash the cells 3 times in normal saline.
6. Add broad-spectrum anti-human globulin (Coombs) serum according to the manufacturer's directions.
7. Centrifuge only enough to pack the cells.
8. Resuspend lightly, then examine macroscopically for agglutination. If negative, recentrifuge and read microscopically.

INTERPRETATION

1. If the cells agglutinate when treated with anti-human globulin serum, it may be assumed that an incomplete antibody is present in the serum. The indirect Coombs test is also used in typing blood cells with antibodies of known specificity that are only reactive by the antiglobulin method (anti-Fy^a, etc.), or in cases where the antigen is not detectable by ordinary methods.
2. The specificity of the antibody may be determined by using a panel of cells of known antigen content. These are most easily obtained commercially.

NOTES

1. Antibodies tend to elute from cells if the washing time is unduly prolonged. When developing cold antibodies, be careful to keep the cells cold during washing.

*The erythrocytes chosen must contain the antigenic group against which the antibody is directed. For isoantibodies, a small pool of group O cells containing D, C, E, c, e, K, Le^a, and Ky^a is suggested. These reagent cells are available commercially.

This can be done by using cold saline and a refrigerated centrifuge or ice water in the centrifuge cups.

REAGENTS

1. Selected red blood cells
2. Anti-human globulin serum

Screening Technic for Atypical Antibodies, Donors and/or Patients

PRINCIPLE

The term "atypical antibody" was introduced to describe any antibodies that react with red blood cells, except the isoantibodies of the ABO system.

The presence of atypical antibodies is detected by adding pooled group O red cells to the serum of the donor or patient. It is usually impractical for the individual bank to prepare its own pool of cells, as it requires a considerable reserve of donors to provide an adequate spectrum of antigens in the donor pool. Several excellent commercial products, meeting rigid standards, are available.

SPECIMEN

Serum.

PROCEDURE

1. Obtain clotted blood and centrifuge at high speed for 5 minutes.
2. With a glass dropper, remove the serum and put it into a labeled tube.
3. Label one tube "S" (for saline) and one tube "Alb" (for albumin).
4. Add 2 drops of serum to each tube.
5. Add 1 drop of pooled red cells to each of the above tubes.
6. Add 2 drops of 22% bovine albumin to the tube labeled "Alb".
7. Centrifuge both tubes for 1 minute, then read macroscopically for agglutination and/or hemolysis.
8. Resuspend the mixtures in both tubes and place them in a 37°C incubator for 30 minutes.
9. Remove the tubes from the incubator and centrifuge them for 1 minute at 3,400 rpm. Examine with the naked eye for agglutination.
10. If there is no agglutination or hemolysis in the tube marked "S", the tube may be discarded.
11. Fill the tube marked "Alb" with normal saline and centrifuge it. Decant the saline.
12 Continue washing 3 times. Decant the saline as completely as possible after the last washing.
13. Add 2 drops of anti-human globulin serum to the cells and mix well.
14. Centrifuge for 1 minute at 3,400 rpm, then examine macroscopically as well as microscopically for agglutination.

INTERPRETATION

1. No agglutination or hemolysis: negative for atypical antibodies.
2. Agglutination: see Antibody Identification (p. 140).
3. In the event of a transfusion problem unexplained by the screening studies done at 37°C, it is sometimes helpful to repeat the above procedure, using refrigerator temperatures. Ordinarily, cold antibodies are of much less significance than warm-acting antibodies, but on rare occasions they may be of interest.

4. Agglutination after incubation at 37°C is characteristic of the antibodies for the Rh factors.
5. Agglutination by the Coombs technic is characteristic of some anti-Rh, Kell, Duffy, Kidd, Xg, and other antibodies.

REAGENTS

1. Bovine albumin (22%)
2. Antiglobulin serum
3. Pooled red cells

Antibody Identification

PRINCIPLE

Detection of an antibody in the serum of a patient or donor must be followed by the identification of the antibody, if possible. Some information about the nature of the antibody is available from the screening test, and the conduct of the identification tests should be guided by this information. If the serum appears to react most strongly in saline at room temperature or lower, it should be tested against the panel of cells in this way. If the antibody reacts best at 37°C, the tests should be incubated at this temperature. If the screening examination reveals an antibody demonstrable by the Coombs technic, the test can be confined to this method. If a number of antibodies are present, absorption technics may have to be used to identify the individual antibodies.

SPECIMEN

Serum and cells.

PROCEDURE

1. Label test tubes for each panel cell specimen available and another for the patient's cells.
2. Place 1 drop of each of the panel cells into the corresponding tubes.
3. Place 1 drop of the patient's cells into the corresponding tube.
4. Fill each tube with saline, centrifuge, then decant the saline.
5. Add 2 drops of the serum to be tested to each tube.
6. Add 2 drops of 22% bovine albumin to each tube.
7. Centrifuge for 1 minute, then examine for agglutination.
8. Incubate all tubes for 15 minutes at 37°C.
9. Centrifuge for 1 minute, then examine for agglutination.
10. Wash 3 times with large volumes of normal saline. Completely decant the saline after the last washing.
11. Add 2 drops of anti-human globulin serum to the washed cells and mix well.
12. Centrifuge for 1 minute at 3,400 rpm, then examine microscopically for agglutination.
13. Incubate negative tubes for 15 minutes at 37°C, recentrifuge, and read for agglutination both macroscopically and microscopically.

INTERPRETATION

1. If a specific antibody or antibodies are present, a regular pattern should be observed that can be interpreted from consideration of the antigen content of the various cells making up the panel.
2. If a mixture of antibodies is present, agglutinin absorption studies may be required.

NOTES

1. If the panel cells are very fresh, it may not be necessary to wash the cells as in step 3. However, it is a good rule to always wash reagent cells before use.

2. Commercial panels are made up of selected cells and, except for the largest and most active blood banks, are more practical than maintaining one's own donors. It is advisable to alternate one's standing orders for panels, so that panels from two different companies are available as needed in the blood bank.

REAGENTS

1. Panel of known cells
2. Bovine albumin (22%)
3. Anti-human globulin serum

Elution of Antibodies

PRINCIPLE

Antibodies bound to red cells can often be identified only if they are released from the red cell and tested against a known panel. Conversely, this technic can be used to identify antigens, the best example of which is the identification of some of the weaker subgroups of A. Although elution technics may be carried out by heating the cells-antibody mixtures to 56°C, the method presented here has worked better for the authors. It consists of lysis of the cells with ether and recovery of the antibody in the saline layer. The presence of hemolysis does not seem to interfere with the subsequent antigen–antibody reaction.

SPECIMEN

Clotted, or EDTA-treated, or oxalated blood.

PROCEDURE

1. Prepare a 25% suspension of red cells in saline (keep saline bottle in the refrigerator).
2. Wash 3 times in large volumes of saline, then pack the cells.
3. Add 1 volume of saline and 2 volumes of ether to the packed cells.
4. Shake the mixture by hand for at least 2 minutes.
5. Centrifuge for 10 minutes at 3,000 rpm.
6. Remove the ether layer with a Pasteur pipette and discard it.
7. Remove the eluate from underneath the stroma, then discard the stroma.

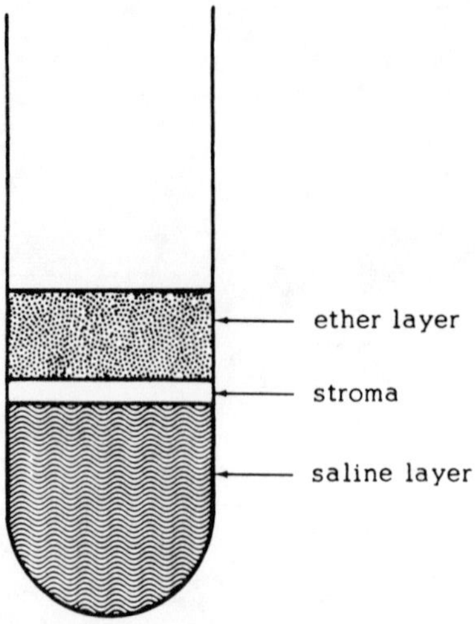

8. Allow the eluate to stand for 30 minutes in a water bath at 37°C to eliminate traces of ether; shake occasionally. Do not leave the eluate in the water bath overnight.
9. Test the eluate against the panel in a manner comparable with testing serum for antibodies.

REFERENCE

Rubin, H., Antibody Elution from Red Blood Cells, J. Clin. Pathol., *16*, 70, 1963.

ABO Titers

PRINCIPLE

Titers of anti-A and anti-B agglutinins usually do not exceed 1:256 in normal blood. Elevations in titers occur in ABO-incompatible pregnancies or following incompatible transfusion. The test is often ordered in pregnancies in which the wife is group O and the husband another group as a measure of the prognosis of such pregnancy. The test may be less significant than chemical examination of the amniotic fluid; nevertheless, the test is frequently ordered and seems to have some usefulness.

SPECIMEN

Serum.

PROCEDURE

1. Set up twelve tubes for each titer as shown in the table below:

Tube No.	Normal Saline (ml)	Patient's Serum (ml)	Titer
1		0.1	
2	0.1	0.1	1:2
3	0.1		1:4
4	0.1		1:8
5	0.1		1:16
6	0.1		1:32
7	0.1		1:64
8	0.1		1:128
9	0.1		1:256
10	0.1		1:512
11	0.1		1:1024
12	0.1		1:2048

2. Mix the contents of tube 2 and transfer 0.1 ml to tube 3. Continue dilution through tube 12. Discard 0.1 ml from tube 12.
3. Add 2 drops of A cells to each of the tubes for the anti-A titer. Add 2 drops of B cells to each of the tubes for the anti-B titer.
4. Centrifuge for 30 seconds, then check for agglutination. Record the results.
5. Add 2 drops of 22% bovine albumin to each of the tubes that appear negative.
6. Incubate for 1 hour at 37°C.
7. Wash the contents of each tube 3 times with cold normal saline. Completely decant the saline after the last washing.
8. Add 2 drops of Coombs serum and resuspend the cells.
9. Centrifuge for 30 seconds. Resuspend the cells gently, then read both macroscopically and microscopically. Record the results. If the test is still positive in tube 12, record the result as greater than 1:2048.

NOTES

1. Most procedure manuals do not carry this titration beyond the saline agglutination phase. However, developing the Coombs serum will enhance the titer and, in some instances, detect immune antibodies not demonstrated by agglutination.

REAGENTS

1. Suspension of group A and group B cells (5%)

Rh Titer

PRINCIPLE

Any antibodies to the Rh factors are evidence of pathology. It is sometimes important to estimate the increase in such antibodies, expecially in pregnancy. Although there is a trend toward relying more and more on chemical tests on amniotic fluid, the Rh titer is still an important test.

SPECIMEN

Serum.

PROCEDURE

Screening Test

Before an Rh titer is performed on a serum, check the serum to determine if there is an Rh antibody present. This is done as follows.

1. Set up four tubes.
   Tube 1: 2 drops of patient's serum plus 2 drops of 5% suspension of group O Rh-positive cells in saline.
   Tube 2: 2 drops of patient's serum plus 2 drops of 5% suspension of group O Rh-negative cells in saline.
   Tube 3: 2 drops of patient's serum plus 1 drop of 5% suspension of group O Rh-positive cells in 22% bovine albumin.
   Tube 4: 2 drops of patient's serum plus 1 drop of 5% suspension of group O Rh-negative cells in 22% bovine albumin.
2. Incubate all four tubes for 1 hour at 37°C.
3. At the end of the hour, centrifuge for 30 seconds in a clinical centrifuge and record the results.
4. Wash the contents of all four tubes 3 times, add two drops of commercial antihuman globulin serum, shake thoroughly, and centrifuge for 30 seconds. Record the results.
5. Tubes 2 and 4 are negative controls and, therefore, should not exhibit agglutination.

Rh Titer

If the patient has saline agglutinins, use saline as a diluent for the titration and test with cells suspended in saline. (It is also advisable to titer with bovine albumin, since albumin antibodies of higher titer often exist along with the saline agglutinins.) If the patient's serum reacted with cells suspended in bovine albumin or exhibited a positive indirect-Coombs reaction, use bovine albumin as a diluent and test with cells suspended in bovine albumin. In those cases where the indirect Coombs was the only positive test, the titration should reveal a prozone containing a high-protein-reacting antibody. In rare instances, however, specific antibodies may be present that do not clump cells suspended in albumin, even on titration. In these instances it is necessary to perform a saline titration of such sera and to follow with an indirect Coombs test on each tube.
The test is performed as follows:

1. Dilutions are made by using a series of twelve 10 × 75 mm test tubes.

2. Each tube, except the first, receives 0.1 ml of diluent (saline or bovine albumin).
3. With a 0.2-ml pipette deliver 0.1 ml of patient's serum to the first tube and 0.1 ml to the second tube. Mix the contents of tube 2 and deliver 0.1 ml of the mixture to tube 3.
4. Continue serial dilutions through tube 12. The 0.1 ml remaining after tube 12 is discarded.
5. Each tube receives 2 drops of the suitable test cell suspension (group O Rh-positive cells suspended in saline or in bovine albumin).
6. Incubate the test tubes for 1 hour at 37°C.
7. Centrifuge, then record the results.
8. The titration values will run from undiluted (tube 1), 1:2 (tube 2), etc., to 1:2048 (tube 12).
9. Perform the Coombs test as indicated.
10. Wash the contents of each tube 3 times with normal saline. Completely decant the saline after the last washing.
11. Add 2 drops of Coombs serum and resuspend the cells.
12. Centrifuge for 30 seconds. Resuspend the cells gently, then check for agglutination both macroscopically and microscopically. Record the results.

NOTES

1. With the Rh titer procedure it is advisable to use a separate pipette for each transfer of diluted serum.
2. The patient's serum should be frozen and preserved to serve as a baseline for subsequent titers.

REAGENTS

1. Known group O Rh-positive cells
   Two types are required; if available, one CDe and one cDE are preferred.
2. Known group O Rh-negative cells
   Cells must be negative for CDE and for D^u.
3. Anti-human globulin serum.

Cross-Matching

PRINCIPLE

The purpose of the cross-match procedure is to ensure compatibility between the donor blood selected and the patient. Ideally, the processing of the donor's and patient's blood specimens prior to the actual cross-matching should be so thorough that an incompatible cross-match does not occur. It must be remembered that the cross-match will detect actual incompatibilities, and not potential ones. Errors in ABO grouping will usually be detected, because such errors are usually associated with the presence of antibodies that can be observed in either the major or minor cross-matching procedure. The procedure does not detect incorrect Rh typing, because Rh antibodies are not normally present in blood.

Since the cross-match is expected to detect incompatible antibodies, and because the various blood group antibodies react optimally in a variety of ways, there is no single cross-match procedure that is uniformly reliable for routine use. To circumvent this problem, it is necessary to plan the routine cross-match test to detect the maximum possible number of antibodies.

The fate of the donor's cells in the recipient's circulation is of major significance, while the possible incompatibility between donor's serum and patient's cells is minor because of the dilution of donor's serum into the patient's blood volume during transfusion and also because of the large mass of the patient's red cells. If a careful antibody search of the donor's serum fails to detect any unusual antibodies, the minor cross-match may be eliminated at the discretion of the pathologist in charge. The cross-match technic described below includes both major and minor sides, however, and is designed to detect both complete and incomplete antibodies. In addition, the immediate spin will often detect prozoned incomplete antibodies together with antibodies of the cold-acting type, such as Lewis, M, or N, along with ABO incompatabilities, whether of the hemolytic type or not.

PROCEDURE

1. Prepare a 2% suspension of the recipient and donor cells in saline, and a 5% suspension of cells in serum. The serum suspension can be easily made by aspirating cells and serum from the macerated clot of the pilot tube.
2. Label four test tubes (13 × 120 mm) as follows.

Tube 1: "Major Saline"	Tube 3: "Major Albumin"
Tube 2: "Minor Saline"	Tube 4: "Minor Albumin"

3. Place 2 drops of recipient serum and 2 drops of a 2% suspension of donor cells in saline into tube 1.
4. Place 2 drops of donor serum and 2 drops of a 2% suspension of recipient cells in saline into tube 2.
5. Centrifuge both tubes for 30 seconds, then read microscopically (low-power objective).
6. Incubate both tube 1 and tube 2 for 15 minutes at 37°C. Centrifuge for 30 seconds, then read microscopically. Discard tube 2. Save tube 1 for step 11.
7. Place 2 drops of recipient serum and 1 drop of a 5% suspension of donor cells suspended in their own serum into tube 3.
8. Place 2 drops of donor serum and 1 drop of a 5% suspension of recipient cells suspended in their own serum into tube 4.
9. Add 2 drops of 22% albumin to both tube 3 and tube 4.

10. Incubate for 15 minutes at 37°C. Centrifuge for 30 seconds, then read microscopically.
11. Wash tubes 1, 3, and 4 three times with saline, completely decanting the supernatant saline from each tube at the conclusion of the last washing.
12. Add 2 drops of Coombs serum to each of these tubes. Resuspend the cells by vigorous shaking. Centrifuge for 30 minutes, then read both microscopically and macroscopically.

INTERPRETATION

1. No agglutination or hemolysis denotes compatibility.
2. If in any phase agglutination or hemolysis occurs, the cross-match is considered incompatible, and another donor is selected. Later the cause of the original incompatibility should be ascertained, and this information inserted into the patient's chart and the blood bank record for future reference.

NOTES

1. Many blood banks have eliminated the minor cross-match, contending that they have had no incidents in which significant reactions have been prevented by using this technic. Similarly, some technics have eliminated the immediate spin in the saline cross-match. Our own experience indicates that both these technics have value, as we feel that significant incompatibilities have been avoided by the use of these procedures.

REAGENTS

1. Bovine albumin (22%)
2. Anti-human globulin serum (Coombs serum)
3. Suspension of donor and recipient cells in saline (2%)
4. Suspension of donor and recipient cells in their own serum (5%)

REFERENCE

Rosenfield, R. E., Compatibility Tests: An Appraisal. Med. Clin. N. Am., *50*, 1643, 1966.

Investigation of Transfusion Reactions

PRINCIPLE

All transfusion reactions should be investigated in an attempt to determine their causes. This requires a thorough recheck of every aspect of the transfusion, including clerical records and procedures as well as the serologic aspects of blood banking. The identification of both the recipient and the donor or donors should be checked along with the specimens used for testing and the actual container of blood employed, if it is available.

The procedure below should be followed when the blood bank is notified of a transfusion reaction.

PROCEDURE

1. Recall the bottle of blood. If the blood has already been given to the patient, the emptied container, along with the administration set or other tubing, should be retrieved.
2. Culture the blood left in the bottle, using thioglycollate medium or another medium. Incubate both at room temperature and at 37°C.
3. Obtain a post-transfusion specimen from the patient. It is best to collect both versenated and clotted blood.
4. Find the pilot tubes of the unit given to the patient and also the patient's pre-transfusion specimen.
5. Observe the post-transfusion specimens for evidence of hemolysis in the serum or plasma. If indicated, a serum hemoglobin determination may be done by the chemistry laboratory.
6. Regroup and do Rh typing on donor pilot tube, blood from the transfusion bottle, and patient's pre- and post-transfusion specimens. Screen patient and donor sera for atypical antibodies, using commercial screening cells.
7. Repeat the cross-matches, using blood from the bottle and the patient's pre-transfusion specimen.
8. Do a direct Coombs test on the patient's post-transfusion specimen. If positive, do the test on the pre-transfusion specimen.
9. Have all urine specimens sent to the blood bank to be tested for hemoglobinuria.
10. If the transfusion has been with group O blood to a group A or B recipient, check the donor blood for hemolysins (see p. 125).
11. Report all findings to the pathologist in charge of the blood bank.

NOTES

1. It is worthwhile to require that the nursing service routinely retain all blood containers on the patient's ward for possible return to the blood bank. The small amount of blood left in such containers and in the tubing is usually adequate for transfusion-reaction follow-ups.
2. Pilot tubes from both patient and donor should be held in the blood bank for 7 days after a transfusion to allow rechecking of a blood group or cross-match, if necessary.
3. Many transfusion reactions never demonstrate antibodies, and many occur without hemolysis.

Preparation of AHG Cryoprecipitate

PRINCIPLE

For many years blood bank supervisors have been cautioning physicians to be sure to thaw completely the fresh-frozen plasma used in treating hemophilic patients. It was generally believed that the major part of the antihemophilic activity of the plasma was concentrated in the precipitate and did not go into solution until a unit of fresh-frozen plasma was completely liquefied. This casual observation has been exploited to give us a method of concentrating the AHG to the point where most of the activity of a unit of plasma can be concentrated in a volume of less than 5.0 ml. This technic will produce products of reasonable uniformity with the facilities available in most blood banks.

PROCEDURE

1. Donors are selected and bled according to AABB and NIH regulations. Only donors with good veins should be used, as it is important to draw the blood rapidly in order to avoid holding the blood at room temperature for any extended period. Plastic double packs should be used.
2. When the program can be set up to have repeat donors for AHG production, it is desirable to titer the donors' blood and select those with the highest titers of AHG.
3. After phlebotomy is completed, centrifuge the unit of blood in a precooled refrigerated centrifuge (4°C) for 15 minutes at maximum speed.
4. Express plasma into the side pocket, using a plasma expressor. It is essential that the bag into which the plasma is collected be only two-thirds full, to permit expansion during freezing.
5. Clamp the tubing between the blood bag and the side pocket bag containing the plasma, then place the sedimented red cells into a bath of ice water at 0°C.
6. Place the plasma bag into a bath of alcohol containing dry ice. (Some banks prefer not to use alcohol and merely pack the plasma bag in crushed dry ice, as they feel that there is some danger—admittedly remote—of the alcohol getting into the plasma through the plastic. Another alternative is to place the plasma bags directly into the freezer; this entails separating the two bags and using the red cells as packed cells and the plasma as single-unit plasma. Some banks produce AHG concentrates by plasmaphoresis of their donors. This requires that the red cells be returned to the donor.)
7. Once the plasma bag is frozen, which will usually take about 15 minutes in the mixture of alcohol and dry ice (−70°C), the frozen plasma and cells are placed in the regular blood bank refrigerator to thaw overnight.
8. The next day, centrifuge the two bags again for 20 to 30 minutes in a refrigerated centrifuge. The AHG precipitate will adhere to the bottom of the plasma bag as a soft white mass.
9. Remove the bag from the centrifuge and return the supernatant plasma to the red-cell bag, retaining the precipitate in the plasma bag.
10. Replace the reconstituted unit in the blood bank, marking it "AHG-Poor Blood".
11. When thawing the units of AHG for use, place the bags in a water bath at 37°C with constant agitation and keep them under observation, so that the units are not in the bath for a longer time than necessary.

12. When the original volume of the concentrate is 5.0 ml or less, it may be necessary to add 5.0 ml of sterile saline to the material to bring the precipitate into solution. If the volume of the concentrate is 10 ml, it is usually possible to reconstitute the material without adding saline. When properly prepared, the precipitate should go into complete solution, so that a clear, smooth liquid results.
13. As the usual dose is at least 5 units, it is usually best to pool the entire prescribed dose and administer it in one syringe.

NOTES

1. Care should be taken in handling the plastic bags after they have been subjected to the low temperature of the dry ice. These bags are very brittle and can easily break. Attempts to use liquid nitrogen instead of dry ice in our blood bank ended in disaster, as the plastic became too brittle under these conditions to tolerate handling.
2. The procedure should not be undertaken unless a refrigerated centrifuge capable of centrifuging four units of blood at a time is available. The centrifuge should be powerful enough to separate the cells and plasma in a maximum of 15 minutes.

REFERENCES

Pool, Judith G., Hershgold, E. J., and Pappenhagen, A. R., High-Potency Antihaemophilic Factor Concentrate Prepared from Cryoglobulin Precipitate. Nature, *203*, 312, 1964.

Pool, Judith G., and Shannon, A. E., Production of High-Potency Concentrates of Antihemophelic Globulin in a Closed Bag System, Assay *in vitro* and *in vivo*. New Engl. J. Med., *273*, 1443, 1965.

HEMATOLOGY

Sectional Directory

Introduction

Any collection of tests used in the average hematology laboratory can usually be divided into two groups. In the first group are those tests that have been in use for many years and, having withstood the test of time, are of proven value. These procedures most often measure variations in number and appearance of the formed elements of the blood and employ mechanical rather than chemical principles. In the second group of procedures one finds the more recently developed and possibly more esoteric tests, which are often chemical in nature and are used to investigate hemolytic and hemorrhagic problems.

In this brief hematology section, tests have been selected for their practical value and reliability on the basis of our personal experience with them. The format has been selected with a view to brevity without loss of clarity.

George C. Hoffman, M.B., B.Chir., M.C.Path.

Hemoglobin

PRINCIPLE

The red cells in a specimen of blood are hemolyzed, and the hemoglobin is converted into either oxy- or cyanmethemoglobin. Cyanmethemoglobin is most commonly used. The optical density or percent transmittance of a dilute solution is measured, and the hemoglobin concentration of the original sample is computed from a reference curve.

NORMAL VALUES

Men: 13.5—18.0 g/100 ml
Women: 11.5—16.5 g/100 ml

SPECIMEN

Freshly drawn blood collected into a tube containing a solid anticoagulant, such as sodium EDTA.

PROCEDURE

A. Cyanmethemoglobin Method

1. Place exactly 5 ml of Drabkin's solution in a clean, dry test tube.
2. Add 0.02 ml of well-mixed blood. In order to make this measurement as accurate as possible, draw blood into the pipette just beyond the 0.02-ml mark, wipe the outside of the pipette clean, and withdraw the slight excess of blood by touching the end of the pipette against a cloth. Rinse the pipette several times in Drabkin's solution to ensure complete removal of blood from the pipette.
3. Mix thoroughly, then allow to stand at room temperature for 2 minutes.
4. Switch on the photometer; allow to warm up, if necessary, and set the wavelength scale to 540 mμ (or insert an appropriate filter).
5. Measure optical density or percent transmittance of the unknown and compute hemoglobin concentration from the reference curve. It is preferable to measure two samples and average the results.

B. Oxyhemoglobin Method

1. Add 0.02 ml of well-mixed blood to 5 ml of 0.04% (V/V) ammonium hydroxide in distilled water, using the technic described in steps 2 to 4 for the cyanmethemoglobin method.
2. Measure the optical density or percent transmittance in a suitable filter photometer or spectrophotometer.
3. Read hemoglobin concentration from the reference curve.

REFERENCE CURVE

A. Cyanmethemoglobin Method

Highly accurate cyanmethemoglobin standards that meet the requirements of the College of American Pathologists are commercially available. These standards are labeled according to the concentration of cyanmethemoglobin in the solution. The equivalent hemoglobin content of whole blood will depend on the dilution of whole blood used; in the present case this is 0.02 ml in 5 ml of Drabkin's solution, or a dilution of 1:251. If the standard contains, for example, 55 mg of cyanmethemoglobin per 100 ml, then the reading obtained with it will be equivalent to $\frac{55 \times 251}{1000}$ or 13.80 g hemoglobin per 100 ml whole blood. The standard curve is made by plotting the optical density (ordinate) against hemoglobin concentration in g/100 ml on arithmetic graph paper, or by plotting the percent transmittance (ordinate) against hemoglobin concentration in g/100 ml on single-cycle semi-logarithmic graph paper. In either case, at least three points should be plotted. These points should lie on a straight line that passes through the zero point if optical density is used, and through the 100% point if percent transmittance is used.

B. Oxyhemoglobin Method

1. Calibrate the instrument with dilutions of a standard cyanmethemoglobin solution as described in the cyanmethemoglobin method.
2. Prepare 4 or 5 dilutions of a specimen of normal blood, using the donor's plasma as diluent.
3. Measure the hemoglobin content of these specimens, using the cyanmethemoglobin method.
4. Determine the optical density or percent transmittance of these samples, using the oxyhemoglobin method, and construct the oxyhemoglobin reference curve. These secondary standards may not be stable in diluted form; however, the original blood samples may be stored for several days.

NOTES

1. The cyanmethemoglobin method of measuring hemoglobin is popular because of the stability of cyanmethemoglobin solutions and hence the reliability of standards. Furthermore, cyanmethemoglobin has a wide absorbancy band and hence is well suited to filter photometers as well as spectrophotometers. The oxyhemoglobin method can be performed with an accuracy comparable to the cyanmethemoglobin method and may be standardized indirectly with a cyanmethemoglobin standard.
2. Automatic diluting apparatus is available and is very useful when many measurements have to be made. These instruments require very careful calibration and are a more likely source of error than the photometer.
3. Ready availability of photometers has rendered other instruments outdated for the measurement of hemoglobin. Instruments that read hemoglobin directly in g/100 ml are available. Although a standard curve is not required with these instruments, they must be calibrated with primary or secondary standards.
4. The time required for the hemoglobin in a sample of blood to be converted to cyanmethemoglobin depends more on the time taken to lyse the red cells than on the speed of the chemical reaction.

REAGENTS

1. Drabkin's solution

sodium bicarbonate	1.00 g
potassium cyanide	0.05 g
potassium ferricyanide	0.29 g

Combine the above ingredients with sufficient distilled water to make 1000 ml. Store in a brown bottle. The solution should be a clear yellow and may be stored for a month or more. It is advisable to make a fresh solution at monthly intervals. The small amount of potassium cyanide in this solution is unlikely to be a source of danger; nevertheless, the container should be clearly labeled as poisonous.

Hematocrit

Microhematocrit Method

PRINCIPLE

Whole blood is centrifuged at high speed until the red cells have been reduced to a constant packed-cell volume. This volume is reported as a percentage of the whole-blood volume.

NORMAL VALUES

Men: 40—54%
Women: 37—47%

SPECIMEN

1. Venous blood anticoagulated with sodium EDTA.
2. Capillary blood collected directly into heparin-coated microhematocrit tubes can be used as an alternative.

PROCEDURE

1. Fill a capillary tube (75 × 1.5 mm) to approximately three fourths of its length with well-mixed blood. Alternatively, draw capillary blood collected from a finger puncture directly into a heparin-coated capillary tube.
2. Seal the colored end of the capillary tube with molding clay or by heat fusion.
3. Place the capillary tube into a slot in a microhematocrit centrifuge head, with the unsealed end near the hub. Tighten the head cover and close the centrifuge lid. There are several commercially available microhematocrit centrifuges of comparable reliability.
4. Turn the centrifuge on and operate for the desired length of time. This is usually 2 minutes, but see the note below.
5. The hematocrit value is most simply calculated by the use of a "hematocrit reader", several types of which are commercially available.

NOTES

1. The macrohematocrit technic of Wintrobe involves the use of calibrated hematocrit tubes with a 110 × 2.5 mm internal diameter. These are filled with blood to the 100 mark and centrifuged for 30 minutes at about 2,260 *g*. The hematocrit obtained by this method is higher than that obtained by maximal packing in the microhematocrit method. Since the normal values for the red-cell indices (MCV and MCHC) were based on the Wintrobe method, it is theoretically necessary either to ascertain the speed of centrifugation that gives similar results in the microhematocrit method, or to establish new normals. In practice, the difference between a hematocrit value read after 2 minutes of centrifugation is usually less than 1% greater than the value obtained after 5 minutes of centrifugation.

Red Blood Cell Count

PRINCIPLE

Blood is diluted with an isotonic solution, and the number of cells in a known volume is counted in a hemocytometer.

NORMAL VALUES

Men: 4.5—6.5 × $10^6/mm^3$
Women: 4.0—5.5 × $10^6/mm^3$

SPECIMEN

Venous blood collected in a dry anticoagulant; versenate (sodium EDTA) is most commonly used. Alternatively, blood obtained from a fingertip may be drawn directly into a diluting pipette.

PROCEDURE

1. Prepare a 1:200 dilution of blood, using a red-cell diluting pipette.
   (a) Draw well-mixed blood to the 0.5 mark.
   (b) Wipe the outside of the pipette.
   (c) Draw diluting fluid to the 101 mark.
2. Fill a second pipette in the same manner.
3. Shake the pipettes for 3 minutes immediately before filling the hemocytometer.
4. Expel the first 4 to 6 drops from the pipettes and fill one side of the counting chamber from each pipette.
5. Allow the cells to settle for a few minutes.
6. Under high-power magnification, count the cells in the center and in the four corner squares (each containing 16 small squares) of the central ruled area. When cells touch or overlap the edges of the squares, count only those touching the left and upper lines, disregarding those cells touching the right or lower lines.

CALCULATION

1. Average the counts obtained in the two chambers.
2. Red blood cells per mm^3 in the original blood =

$$\frac{\text{cells counted} \times \text{dilution factor}}{\text{volume counted in mm}^3} = \frac{\text{cells counted} \times 200}{0.02\ \text{mm}^3} = \text{cells counted} \times 10^4$$

NOTES

1. The results obtained by good technologists using the most accurate equipment may vary within ±10% when counting the same specimen. The variations associated with diurnal changes, posture of the patient when the blood is drawn, and the method of drawing must all be added to this figure.

REAGENTS

The following diluting solutions may be used.

1. Saline (0.85%)
2. Hayem's solution

sodium sulfate	2.5 g
sodium chloride	0.5 g
mercuric chloride	0.25 g
distilled water	100 ml

3. Gower's solution

sodium sulfate	12.5 g
glacial acetic acid	33.3 ml
distilled water	100 ml

SPECIAL EQUIPMENT

1. Hemocytometer with improved Neubauer ruling.
2. Red-cell diluting pipettes.

REFERENCE

Biggs, R., and MacMillan, R. L., The Error of the Red Cell Count. J. Clin. Pathol., *1*, 288, 1948.

Red Cell Indices

PRINCIPLE

If the red-cell count, hematocrit and hemoglobin content of a blood specimen are known, it is possible to calculate the average volume and the average hemoglobin content of the individual red cells as well as the concentration of hemoglobin in the red cells.

NORMAL VALUES

Mean cell volume (MCV): 82—92 μ^3
Mean cell hemoglobin (MCH): 27—32 pg
Mean cell hemoglobin concentration (MCHC): 32—36% (g/100 ml)

CALCULATION

A. Mean Cell Volume (MCV)

If the total volume of red cells in a given volume of blood (hematocrit) and the total number of red cells in that volume are known, then the volume of an average single red cell can be calculated.

Example

Hematocrit	45%
Red-cell count	5,000,000/mm^3

Thus, each mm^3 of whole blood contains 5 million red cells, which occupy 0.45 mm^3. Hence, one red cell occupies $\frac{0.45}{5{,}000{,}000}$ mm^3. This is most conveniently reported in terms of cubic micra (1 mm^3 = 1 × 10$^9\mu^3$). Hence, one red cell occupies

$$\frac{0.45 \times 10^9}{5 \times 10^6}\,\mu^3 = \frac{450}{5}\,\mu^3 = 90\,\mu^3.$$

In practice, the following formula is used:

$$\text{MCV} = \frac{\text{Hematocrit } \% \times 10}{\text{RBC/mm}^3 \text{ in millions}}\,\mu^3,$$

or, as applied to the stated example,

$$\text{MCV} = \frac{45 \times 10}{5}\,\mu^3 = 90\,\mu^3.$$

B. Mean Cell Hemoglobin (MCH)

If the hemoglobin content in a given volume of blood and the number of red cells in that volume are known, then the weight of hemoglobin in an average red cell can be calculated.

Example

Hemoglobin	15 g/100 ml
Red-cell count	5,000,000/mm^3

Thus, each mm^3 of blood contains 5 million red cells and 15×10^{-5} g of hemoglobin. Hence, one red cell contains $\frac{15 \times 10^{-5}}{5 \times 10^5}$ g of hemoglobin. This is more conveniently reported in terms of picograms (micro-micrograms) of hemoglobin. Hence, one red cell contains

$$\frac{15 \times 10^{-5} \times 10^{12}}{5 \times 10^6} = 30 \text{ pg of hemoglobin.}$$

In practice, the MCH is most simply calculated from the following formula:

$$\text{MCH} = \frac{\text{Hb g/100 ml} \times 10}{\text{RBC/mm}^3 \text{ in millions}} \text{ pg hemoglobin,}$$

or, as applied to the stated example,

$$\text{MCH} = \frac{15 \times 10}{5} = 30 \text{ pg hemoglobin.}$$

C. Mean Cell Hemoglobin Concentration (MCHC)

If the hemoglobin concentration and the hematocrit of a given volume of blood are known, the concentration of hemoglobin in the same volume of red cells (as distinct from whole blood) can be calculated.

Example

Hemoglobin	15 g/100 ml
Hematocrit	45%

Thus, 45 ml of red cells contain 15 g of hemoglobin, and hence 100 ml of red cells contain

$$\frac{15 \times 100}{45} \text{ g hemoglobin} = 33\% \text{ (g/100 ml).}$$

In practice, the MCHC is most simply calculated from the following formula:

$$\text{MCHC} = \frac{\text{Hb in grams} \times 100}{\text{Hematocrit}} = \% \text{ (g/100 ml),}$$

or, as applied to the stated example,

$$\text{MCHC} = \frac{15 \times 100}{45} = 33\% \text{ (g/100 ml).}$$

NOTES

1. The changes seen in the three major morphologic types of anemia are outlined in the following table:

Type of Anemia	MCV	MCH	MCHC
Microcytic, hypochromic	↓	↓	↓
Macrocytic, normochromic	↑	↑	N
Normocytic, normochromic	N	N	N

2. The spherocyte is the only type of red cell exhibiting an increased MCHC. A decreased MCHC is almost invariably the result of iron deficiency.

3. The term "mean cell hemoglobin concentration" is a misnomer in that the MCHC is not directly related to the number and size of red cells.
4. The validity of reported results should always be checked by examining a well-stained blood film.

Reticulocyte Count

PRINCIPLE

Reticulocytes contain remnants of RNA, which are precipitated as filaments and granules when the cells are vitally stained. The stained reticulocytes are counted in a blood film and may be reported either in absolute numbers or as a percentage of the number of red cells.

NORMAL VALUES

0.5—2.0/100 red cells, or 25,000—75,000/mm^3.

SPECIMEN

Venous blood collected in a dry anticoagulant; versenate (sodium EDTA) is most commonly used. Alternatively, blood obtained from a fingertip may be mixed directly into the stain.

PROCEDURE

1. Place 2 drops of brilliant cresyl blue solution into the well of a porcelain spot plate and allow to evaporate. These plates may be stored for several days.
2. Mix 2 drops of blood with the stain.
3. Allow the mixture to stand for 2 or 3 minutes, with the well covered by a cover slip to prevent drying.
4. Prepare two or more smears on cover slips or slides and air-dry.
5. Counterstain with Wright's stain.
6. Mount the preparation.
7. The reticulocyte count is determined by counting, under oil immersion, the number of reticulated cells seen per 1000 red cells. The procedure is simplified if the size of the field is reduced. This can be accomplished by placing a diaphragm of cardboard or paper, with a small hole cut into its center, into the ocular of the microscope.
8. The number of reticulocytes may be reported as a percentage (the number of reticulocytes per 100 red cells), or as the number per mm^3 of blood, using the following formula:

$$\text{reticulocytes/mm}^3 = \frac{\text{reticulocytes/100 rbc} \times \text{rbc/mm}^3}{100}$$

NOTES

1. The precision of the reticulocyte count increases with the number of reticulocytes counted. When 1% reticulocytes are present, the precision is approximately $\pm 50\%$. When 10% reticulocytes are present, the precision is increased to approximately $\pm 20\%$.
2. The area of the smear that is counted must be thin, with no rouleaux formation or overlapping of red cells.

3. Precipitation of the RNA may be incomplete if the blood sample contains an excess of anticoagulant. The ratio of stain to blood may vary widely without affecting the result.
4. Stain precipitated on the red cells may be confused with reticulation. This can best be avoided by refiltering the stain.

SOLUTIONS

1. Saturated alcoholic solution of brilliant cresyl blue

   Dissolve 1 g of brilliant cresyl blue in 100 ml of 95% alcohol. Shake intermittently for 48 hours. Filter small amounts of this stock solution into a dropping bottle for use as required.

White Blood Cell Count

PRINCIPLE

Blood is diluted in a solution that lyses red blood cells, and the remaining nucleated cells in a known volume are counted in a hemocytometer.

SPECIMEN

Venous blood collected in a dry anticoagulant; versenate (sodium EDTA) is most commonly used. Alternatively, blood obtained from a fingertip may be drawn directly into a diluting pipette.

PROCEDURE

1. Prepare a 1:20 dilution of blood, using a white-cell diluting pipette.
   (a) Draw well-mixed blood to the 0.5 mark.
   (b) Wipe the outside of the pipette.
   (c) Draw diluting fluid to the 11 mark.
2. Repeat step 1 with a second pipette.
3. Shake the pipettes for 3 minutes immediately before filling the hemocytometer.
4. Expel the first 4 to 6 drops from the pipettes and fill one side of the counting chamber from each pipette.
5. Allow the cells to settle for a few minutes.
6. Under high-power magnification, count the cells in the four large corner squares of the ruled area (each containing 16 small squares). When cells touch or overlap the edges of squares, count only those touching the left and upper lines, disregarding those cells touching the right or lower lines.

CALCULATION

1. Average the counts obtained in the two chambers.

2. $$\text{WBC/mm}^3 = \frac{\text{cells counted} \times \text{dilution factor}}{\text{volume counted in mm}^3} =$$

$$\frac{\text{cells counted} \times 20}{0.1 \times \text{number of large squares counted}} = \text{cells counted} \times 50$$

NOTES

1. The results obtained by a good technologist using the most accurate equipment may vary within $\pm 12\%$ when counting the same specimen. The variations associated with diurnal changes, posture of the patient when blood is drawn, and the method of its drawing must all be added to this figure. When all variables are taken into account, results may vary $\pm 20\%$ when the white-cell count is 10,000/mm^3.
2. Since nucleated red cells (NRBC) are also counted in this method, it is sometimes necessary to correct the white-cell count. The correction factor is obtained by counting the number of NRBC per 100 WBC in the blood smear; then

$$\frac{\text{number of cells counted/mm}^3}{(100 + \text{number of NRBC})} \times 100 = \text{WBC/mm}^3.$$

REAGENTS

The following diluting solutions may be used.

1. Glacial acetic acid (1%)
2. Türk's solution

 Add 3 ml of glacial acetic acid and 1 ml of 1% aqueous solution of gentian violet to enough distilled water to make 100 ml.

SPECIAL EQUIPMENT

1. Hemocytometer with improved Neubauer ruling.
2. White-cell diluting pipettes.

REFERENCE

Berg, W. N., Blood Cell Counts: Their Statistical Interpretation. Am. Rev. Tuberc., *52*, 179, 1945.

Absolute Eosinophil Count

PRINCIPLE

Blood is diluted in a fluid that stains eosinophil granules red, lyses other white blood cells, and renders red cells invisible.

NORMAL VALUES

50—500/mm^3, with $\pm 30\%$ diurnal variation.

SPECIMEN

Venous blood collected in a dry anticoagulant; versenate (sodium EDTA) is most commonly used. Alternatively, blood obtained from a fingertip may be drawn directly into a diluting pipette.

PROCEDURE

1. Draw well-mixed blood to the 0.5 mark of a white-cell diluting pipette.
2. Wipe the outside of the pipette.
3. Draw Pilot's diluting fluid to the 11 mark.
4. Repeat step 1 with a second pipette.
5. Shake the pipettes for 3 minutes.
6. Expel and discard the first 4 to 6 drops from each pipette.
7. Fill both sides of a hemocytometer from each pipette.
8. Allow the hemocytometer to stand for 15 minutes, covering it with an inverted petri dish to avoid evaporation.
9. Count all eosinophils in the entire ruled area in both chambers.

CALCULATION

1. Average the counts from both chambers.
2. $$\text{Eosinophils/mm}^3 = \frac{\text{eosinophils counted} \times \text{dilution factor}}{\text{volume counted}}$$

   (a) For improved Neubauer ruling:

   $$\text{eosinophils/mm}^3 = \frac{\text{eosinophils counted} \times 20}{0.9}$$

   (b) For Fuchs-Rosenthal ruling:

   $$\text{eosinophils/mm}^3 = \frac{\text{eosinophils counted} \times 20}{3.2}$$

   (c) For Speirs-Levy ruling:

   $$\text{eosinophils/mm}^3 = \frac{\text{eosinophils counted} \times 20}{2}$$

REAGENTS

1. Pilot's solution

propylene glycol	50 ml
distilled water	40 ml
phloxine (1% aqueous solution)	10 ml
sodium carbonate (10% aqueous solution)	1 ml
heparin sodium	100 units

SPECIAL EQUIPMENT

1. White-cell diluting pipettes.
2. Hemocytometers with improved Neubauer, Fuchs-Rosenthal, or Speirs-Levy rulings.

REFERENCE

MacFarlane, J. C. W., and Cecil, G. W., Eosinophil Counting: A Modification of Pilot's Method. Brit. Med. J., *2*, 1187, 1951.

Platelet Count

PRINCIPLE

The platelets in a diluted sample of blood are counted in a hemocytometer. Several methods are available for rendering the platelets easily visible.

NORMAL VALUES

200,000—450,000/mm^3

PROCEDURE

1. Draw blood into a red-cell diluting pipette, wipe the outside of the pipette, and adjust the volume exactly to the 0.5 mark.
2. Draw either 1% ammonium oxalate or cresyl blue solution exactly to the 101 mark.
3. Shake for 3 minutes.
4. Discard the first few drops from the pipette.
5. Fill both sides of a hemocytometer having improved Neubauer ruling.
6. Allow the cells to settle for about 15 minutes. (Place the hemocytometer under a petri dish lid with moist blotting paper to prevent drying.)
7. If the cresyl blue solution is used, the platelets will stain a lilac color; if the ammonium oxalate is used, they will appear as bright refractile bodies. With the latter diluent, platelets may be counted either by phase contrast or by simple light microscopy. When cresyl blue is used, the platelets are most easily seen under light microscopy. Whichever method is employed, the platelets lying within the four corner squares and the central square of the large central ruled area are counted. Those platelets touching the upper and left borders of the squares are counted; those touching the lower and right borders are not counted.

CALCULATION

1. Average the counts obtained in the two chambers.
2. $$\text{platelets/mm}^3 \text{ in original blood} = \frac{\text{platelets counted} \times \text{dilution factor}}{\text{volume counted as mm}^3}$$

$$= \frac{\text{platelets counted} \times 200}{0.02 \times \text{mm}^3} = \text{platelets counted} \times 10^4$$

NOTES

1. When two pipettes are used to fill two counting chambers and the true platelet count is 250,000/mm^3, then the confidence limits are 195,000—350,000/mm^3. At a true platelet count of 50,000, the limits are 39,000—61,000/mm^3.
2. The disposable blood-diluting system available from Becton-Dickinson is well suited to platelet counting. Ammonium oxalate is used, but the dilution is 1:100, and the final formula is therefore

$$\text{platelets/mm}^3 = \text{platelets counted} \times 5{,}000.$$

REAGENTS

1. Ammonium oxalate (1%)

   Dissolve 1 g of ammonium oxalate in 100 ml of distilled water.

2. Cresyl blue solution (Rees-Ecker)

sodium citrate	3.80 g
brilliant cresyl blue	0.05 g
neutral formaldehyde	0.22 ml

   Combine the above ingredients and add distilled water to make 100 ml. Filter before use.

REFERENCE

Brecher, G., and Cronkite, E. P., Morphology and Enumeration of Blood Platelets. J. Appl. Physiol., *3*, 365, 1950.

Leukocyte Alkaline Phosphatase Stain

PRINCIPLE

Leukocyte alkaline phosphatase (LAP) hydrolyzes a substrate of alpha-naphthol phosphate. The liberated naphthol is coupled with a diazotized amine and precipitates as colored granules in the cell cytoplasm. The nuclei are counterstained with aqueous neutral red. The quantity of precipitate gives a rough measure of the LAP content of the cell.

NORMAL VALUES

The normal "score" ranges from 7 to 100.

SPECIMEN

Fresh, air-dried blood smears on chemically clean (acid-washed) slides.

PROCEDURE

1. Place slides in cold (0—4°C) fixative for 30 seconds.
2. Rinse briefly in tap or distilled water and dry thoroughly.
3. Filter the incubation mixture directly onto the slides and allow to stand at room temperature for 15 minutes.
4. Rinse the slides thoroughly in distilled water and air-dry.
5. Counterstain the smears with 0.1% aqueous solution of neutral red for 3 minutes.
6. Rinse the smears very briefly in running distilled water and air-dry.
7. Examine the unmounted preparation under oil immersion and quantitate the blue granular cytoplasmic precipitate in mature neutrophils by the scoring method of Kaplow. The staining is scored as 0 to 4 in each of 100 mature neutrophils.

   Grade 0: no visible granules.
   Grade 1: very few granules.
   Grade 2: a few granules obviously present.
   Grade 3: a moderate number of granules.
   Grade 4: cytoplasm densely packed with granules.

   The scores for each of 100 neutrophils are added and reported. For instance:

		Score
35	neutrophils scored 0	0
39	neutrophils scored 1	39
24	ncutrophils scored 2	48
2	neutrophils scored 3	6
0	neutrophils scored 4	0
100	Total Score	93

   The possible range of scores is 0 to 400.

NOTES

1. The staining characteristics of this method are somewhat more vivid and easier to score than the methods of Kaplow or of Hoffman and Lucich; however, the

stain fades more rapidly, and the scoring must be performed as soon as the slide is prepared. The use of mounting material and cover slip often results in even more rapid fading of the stain.

2. We have been unable to find a simple mounting method that does not result in rapid fading of the LAP stain and prefer to proceed with unmounted preparations. However, the authors of this method state that Permount®* is a satisfactory mounting medium.
3. Since scoring involves subjective interpretation, each laboratory should establish its own normal range.
4. The LAP score is mainly of value in distinguishing chronic granulocytic leukemia (LAP absent or markedly reduced) from other myeloproliferative disorders and leukemoid reactions (LAP increased).

REAGENTS

1. Fixative

   Mix 9 parts absolute methanol with 1 part 10% formalin. This solution is stored at −20°C and may be kept for 1 to 2 weeks.
2. Stock substrate solution

   Dissolve 30 mg of naphthol AS phosphate† in 0.5 ml of N,N-dimethylformamide‡. Add 100 ml of 0.2*M* tris buffer, pH 9.1. This solutions is stable for several months when stored at 1—5°C.
3. Incubation mixture.

   Dissolve fast-blue BBN§ in the stock substrate solution in the proportion of 1 mg per 1 ml. The mixture is stirred and filtered directly onto the slides. This mixture must be freshly prepared before each use.
4. Neutral red counterstain (0.1%)

   Dissolve 100 mg of neutral red in 100 ml of distilled water.

REFERENCES

Hoffman, G. C., and Lucich, V. J., The Clinical Application of a Modified Azo Dye Technic for the Determination of Alkaline Phosphatase Activity in Neutrophils. Cleveland Clin. Quart., *27*, 146, 1960.

Kaplow, L. S., Histochemical Procedure for Localizing and Evaluating the Leukocyte Alkaline Phosphatase Activity in Smears of Blood and Marrow. Blood, *10*, 1023, 1955.

Rutenberg, A. M., Rosales, C. L., and Bennett, J. M., An Improved Histochemical Method for the Demonstration of Leukocyte Alkaline Phosphatase Activity: Clinical Application. J. Lab. Clin. Med., *65*, 698, 1965.

*Fisher Scientific Co.
†Cyclo Chemical Corporation, Los Angeles, California.
‡Fisher Scientific Co.
§General Analine and Film Corporation, New York, New York.

Peroxidase Stain

PRINCIPLE

Benzidine is oxidized by peroxide in the presence of peroxidase. The oxidized benzidine forms a dark-blue compound in the presence of sodium nitroprusside.

PROCEDURE

1. Place 10 drops of solution A on a freshly prepared air-dried blood smear and allow to stand for $1\frac{1}{2}$ minutes.
2. Add 5 drops of solution B and allow the mixture to stand for 3 to 4 minutes.
3. Rinse the slide with tap water for 3 minutes.
4. Counterstain with either Wright's or Giemsa's stain.

NOTES

1. Granulocytes maturing beyond the promyelocyte stage and immature and mature monocytes are peroxidase-positive, whereas lymphocytes and plasma cells are peroxidase-negative.
2. The use of the stain to distinguish leukemia cell types is limited by the fact that all blasts are peroxidase-negative.

REAGENTS

1. Solution A

   Dissolve 0.3 g of benzidine in 99 ml of 95% ethanol. Add 1 ml of saturated aqueous solution of sodium nitroprusside. This solution is stable for 6 to 12 months at room temperature.
2. Solution B

   Add 0.3 ml of 3% hydrogen peroxide to 15 ml of distilled water. This solution must be freshly prepared before each use.

Iron Stain (Siderocyte Stain)

PRINCIPLE

The presence of iron granules in the cells of the bone marrow or peripheral blood can be detected by the Prussian blue reaction. A siderocyte is a red cell containing iron granules. A sideroblast is a nucleated red cell containing iron granules. The siderotic granules also stain with Romanowsky dyes, in which case they are called "Pappenheimer bodies".

Siderocytes are not normally found in the peripheral blood. They appear following splenectomy and in some instances of altered hemoglobin synthesis. Sideroblasts are normally found in the bone marrow. Iron granules are also found in some histiocytes, as well as free in the bone marrow fragments. An iron stain of the bone marrow is a useful aid in the diagnosis of iron deficiency.

PROCEDURE

1. Prepare air-dried films of peripheral blood or bone marrow on slides or cover slips.
2. Fix in absolute methanol for 10 to 15 minutes.
3. Air-dry the films.
4. Stain with Prussian blue reagent for 10 minutes.
5. Wash thoroughly in distilled water.
6. Counterstain for a few seconds in aqueous solution of eosin (0.1%) or safranin (0.1%). Alternatively, the films may be counterstained with Wright's stain.

NOTES

1. This method may be used for demonstrating iron in films previously stained with Wright's stain. Films several months old may be used. The slight disadvantage of Wright's stain as a counterstain is that it may be difficult to detect small siderotic granules in basophilic erythroid precursors.

REAGENTS

1. Potassium ferrocyanide solution (2%)

potassium ferrocyanide	2 g
distilled water	to 100 ml

2. Prussian blue reagent

   Mix equal volumes of 2% potassium ferrocyanide and 0.2*N* hydrochloric acid immediately before use.

REFERENCE

Sundberg, R. D., and Broman, H., The Application of the Prussian Blue Stain to Previously Stained Films of Blood and Bone Marrow. Blood, *10*, 160, 1955.

The Lupus Erythematosus (L.E.) Cell Test

PRINCIPLE

The L.E. cell test is a means of demonstrating the presence of antinuclear factor in the serum of patients with disseminated lupus erythematosus. When the patient's clotted blood is vigorously stirred, some nuclear material is released from the damaged leukocytes. Antinuclear factor reacts with this nuclear material, which is then phagocytized by a neutrophil to form an L.E. cell. When a group of neutrophils collect around the nuclear material, the result is a "rosette".

SPECIMEN

5 ml of clotted whole blood.

PROCEDURE

1. Break up the clot by vigorously mixing with an applicator stick or similar implement.
2. Strain the blood through a layer of gauze into a clean test tube.
3. Centrifuge the blood and prepare several smears of the buffy coat on slide or cover slip.
4. Stain with Wright's stain and examine for L.E. cells and rosettes.

INTERPRETATION

The presence of even one L.E. cell should be reported as a positive result. Increasing numbers of L.E. cells may be reported semiquantitatively as 1+, 2+, 3+, or 4+ positive. The presence of definite rosettes, but no L.E. cells, should be reported as 1+.

NOTES

1. Since the L.E. factor or antinuclear factor that is being tested for is in the patient's serum, it is possible to use normal bone marrow or dog bone marrow as the source of nuclear material and neutrophils. Except in the rare instance of the patient having marked neutropenia, there is no advantage in using these alternative sources, since they do not increase the sensitivity of the test.
2. There are many variations of the L.E. cell test, but we have found the clot method most simple and at least as sensitive as other methods.
3. When the fluorescent-antibody technic is used to demonstrate the antinuclear factor, a positive result is found in many "autoimmune" disorders, including disseminated L.E. The L.E. cell test appears to be more specific for disseminated L.E.
4. The L.E. cell must be distinguished from a "tart" cell. The latter contains a phagocytized whole nucleus or cell and does not exhibit the smooth "frosted glass" appearance of the engulfed nuclear material of the L.E. cell.

Osmotic Fragility of Red Cells

Quantitative Test

PRINCIPLE

Red cells are placed in a series of sodium chloride solutions of decreasing strength, and the percentage of cells hemolyzed is calculated from the amount of hemoglobin released into the supernate.

Any change in the shape of red cells may alter their ability to withstand reduction in the osmotic pressure of the medium in which they are suspended. Red cells whose shape varies from the normal biconcave disc toward a spherocytic shape have increased sensitivity to reduced osmotic pressure. Flat, thin red cells, such as target cells, are able to withstand a greater reduction in osmotic pressure than normal red cells.

NORMAL VALUES

Lysis of normal red cells begins between 0.50 and 0.45% sodium chloride and is complete between 0.35 and 0.30%.

SPECIMEN

Heparinized or defibrinated blood. Blood collected in oxalate or citrate is unsuitable because of the added salt.

PROCEDURE

1. Number a series of test tubes from 1 to 17.
2. Place 5 ml of buffered sodium chloride ranging from 0.1 to 0.85% into tubes 1 through 16.
3. Place 5 ml of distilled water into tube 17.
4. Add 0.1 ml of blood to each tube.
5. Mix gently, then incubate the tubes at room temperature for 1 hour.
6. Centrifuge the tubes at approximately 700 *g* to sediment any intact red cells.
7. Measure the hemoglobin content of the supernatant, using the 0.85%-saline tube as a blank and the distilled-water tube as the 100%-hemolysis standard. Any convenient colorimeter may be used, but the 100%-hemolysis standard should register an optical density (OD) of 0.5 or less.

CALCULATION

1. Calculate the percent lysis for tubes 1 through 15 from the following formula:

$$\frac{\text{OD of test}}{\text{OD of standard}} \times 100 = \text{hemolysis } \%$$

2. Report the results in graph form, with the percent hemolysis plotted against percent sodium chloride concentration. The normal range should be indicated on the graph. The median corpuscular fragility, which is the concentration of sodium chloride producing 50% lysis, may also be recorded.

NOTES

1. The method described here utilizes a 1:50 dilution of blood. Depending on the colorimeter used, it may be necessary to use a 1:100 or 1:200 dilution to produce a 100%-lysis tube with an OD of about 0.5 without further dilution of the supernate.
2. The results are affected by the relative volume of sodium chloride to blood (which should be greater than 20:1), the pH of the blood-sodium chloride mixture (hence the necessity for buffered sodium chloride), and the temperature during incubation.
3. If the osmotic fragility of a sample of normal blood is measured at the same time as the test sample, then not only can a comparison be made, but also a gradual change in the normal curve may indicate the necessity for preparing fresh sodium chloride solutions.

REAGENTS

1. Stock buffered sodium chloride (equivalent to 10% NaCl)

NaCl	90 g
Na_2HPO_4	13.66 g
$NaH_2PO_4 \cdot 2H_2O$	2.43 g

   Dissolve in distilled water and dilute to 1 liter. If necessary, adjust pH to 7.4 with sodium hydroxide.

2. Dilutions

   Prepare a series of dilutions of the stock solution by adding distilled water in the quantities given in the table below. These solutions should be kept in well-stoppered bottles, preferably at refrigerator temperature.

Stock Solution (ml)	Distilled Water (ml)	Sodium Chloride (%)
0.50	49.50	0.10
0.75	49.25	0.15
1.00	49.00	0.20
1.25	48.75	0.25
1.50	48.50	0.30
1.75	48.25	0.35
2.00	48.00	0.40
2.25	47.75	0.45
2.50	47.50	0.50
2.75	47.25	0.55
3.00	47.00	0.60
3.25	46.75	0.65
3.50	46.50	0.70
3.75	46.25	0.75
4.00	46.00	0.80
4.25	45.75	0.85

REFERENCES

Guest, G. M., Osmometric Behavior of Normal and Abnormal Human Erythrocytes. Blood, *3*, 541, 1948.

Parpart, A. K., Lorenz, P. B., Parpart, E. R., Gregg, J. R., and Chase, A. M., The Osmotic Resistance (Fragility) of Human Red Cells. J. Clin. Invest., *26*, 636, 1947.

Osmotic Fragility of Red Cells

Incubation Method

PRINCIPLE

The sensitivity of the osmotic-fragility test is increased if the red cells are incubated at 37°C for 24 hours before the test is performed. This incubation increases the osmotic fragility of red cells of patients with spherocytosis, hereditary or acquired, and of some with hereditary nonspherocytic hemolytic anemia, to a greater extent than normal cells.

NORMAL VALUES

Hemolysis begins between 0.70 and 0.60% sodium chloride and is complete at 0.45 to 0.35%.

SPECIMEN

Sterile defibrinated blood is preferable; however, sterile heparinized blood may be used.

PROCEDURE

1. Incubate the sterile blood at 37°C for 24 hours.
2. Measure the osmotic fragility of the red cells as described in the quantitative osmotic-fragility test.

NOTES

1. When many spherocytes are present, the incubation alone may cause hemolysis, or hemolysis may occur in 0.85% sodium chloride. This makes it difficult to obtain a blank. If necessary, a saline blank may be used with only slight loss of accuracy. However, if the incubated osmotic fragility is that abnormal, the unincubated osmotic fragility will usually also be abnormal.

REFERENCES

Guest, G. M., Osmometric Behavior of Normal and Abnormal Human Erythrocytes. Blood, *3*, 541, 1948.

Parpart, A. K., Lorenz, P. B., Parpart, E. R., Gregg, J. R., and Chase, A. M., The Osmotic Resistance (Fragility) of Human Red Cells. J. Clin. Invest., *26*, 636, 1947.

The Autohemolysis Test

PRINCIPLE

When normal blood is incubated under sterile conditions at 37°C for 48 hours, less than 5% hemolysis occurs. However, blood containing spherocytes or red cells deficient in certain glycolytic enzymes exhibit much greater hemolysis. The effect of glucose or adenosine triphosphate (ATP) on the degree of hemolysis may be used as an aid in distinguishing some of the abnormalities.

The autohemolysis test is closely related to the incubated osmotic-fragility test, and the two tests are conveniently performed together.

NORMAL VALUES

0.1—5.0% hemolysis at 48 hours. With added glucose, the range is reduced to 0—0.7%.

SPECIMEN

15 ml of sterile defibrinated blood from the patient and from a normal individual.

PROCEDURE

1. Measure the hematocrits of both the patient's and the normal blood. Retain some preincubation serum for use as a blank, and samples of whole blood for use as a 100%-hemolysis standard.
2. Place 1 ml of the patient's blood into each of six sterile glass test tubes. Into each of another set of six test tubes place 1 ml of normal blood.
3. Add 0.05 ml of glucose to two of the normal and two of the patient's tubes.
4. Add 0.05 ml of ATP to another set of two normal and two patient's tubes. The remaining two pairs of tubes are carried through the procedure without an additive.
5. Gently mix each tube and place it in a 37°C incubator for 48 hours.
6. Pool the contents of each pair of tubes and mix, then measure the hematocrit.
7. Centrifuge each pool to obtain serum.
8. Make a dilution of each serum with 0.04% ammonia in water. A 1:10 dilution is satisfactory unless hemolysis is marked, in which case a 1:50 or even a 1:100 dilution may be more suitable. Make a similar dilution of the preincubation serum from the patient and from the normal control.
9. Make a 1:100 or a 1:200 dilution of normal and of the patient's whole blood in the remaining tubes with 0.04% ammonium hydroxide in water.
10. Using the diluted preincubation serum as a blank and the diluted whole blood as a 100% standard, measure the optical density (OD) of the test sera with a photocolorimeter.

CALCULATION

The percent hemolysis is obtained from the following formula:

$$\%\ \text{hemolysis} = \frac{R_{48} \times \left(\frac{100 - CV_{48}}{100}\right) \times 100}{R_0 \times \frac{\text{dilution of standard}}{\text{dilution of test}}},$$

or, assuming dilution of the standard as 1:100 and dilution of the test as 1:10,

$$\%\ \text{hemolysis} = \frac{R_{48}(100 - CV_{48})}{R_{10} \times 10},$$

where R_0 = colorimeter reading of diluted whole blood;
R_{48} = colorimeter reading of diluted serum, obtained after 48 hours of incubation; and
CV_{48} = hematocrit as a percent of the blood after 48 hours of incubation.

The correction is made for hematocrit so that the degree of hemolysis is related to the whole blood rather than to the serum compartment alone.

INTERPRETATION

Autohemolysis is increased when spherocytes, hereditary or acquired, are present, and in most instances of hereditary nonspherocytic hemolytic anemia. The latter is usually associated with red-cell enzyme deficiencies, the most common being glucose-6-phosphate dehydrogenase (G6PD) deficiency and pyruvate kinase (PK) deficiency.

The hereditary nonspherocytic hemolytic anemias were divided into Types I and II by Dacie. Type I is a heterogeneous group of enzyme deficiencies, of which G6PD deficiency is an example. Typically, the autohemolysis test shows normal to moderately increased hemolysis that is reduced by the addition of glucose or ATP. Type II appears to consist almost exclusively of cases of pyruvate kinase deficiency. These show a marked increase in autohemolysis, which is affected little by the addition of glucose, but is much reduced by the addition of ATP. All forms of spherocytes show increased autohemolysis, which is reduced to normal or near-normal levels by the addition of glucose.

NOTES

1. The multiplicity of red-cell enzyme defects now known to exist have reduced the diagnostic value of this test, but it is a useful screening test.
2. Other additives, such as adenosine, have been suggested to further refine the test.
3. On occasion the 100% standard and the blank may be slightly turbid, despite the use of dilute ammonium hydroxide. The addition of a drop of concentrated ammonium hydroxide will usually clear the solution.

REAGENTS

1. Glucose solution
   10% glucose in sterile 0.85% sodium chloride.
2. Adenosine triphosphate
   0.4*M* solution in sterile 0.85% sodium chloride (to give a final concentration in the blood of 0.02*M*).

REFERENCES

De Gruchy, G. C., Santamaria, J. N., Parsons, I. C., and Crawford, H., Nonspherocytic Congenital Hemolytic Anemia. Blood, *16*, 1371, 1960.

Selwyn, J. G., and Dacie, J. V., Autohemolysis and Other Changes Resulting from the Incubation *in vitro* of Red Cells from Patients with Congenital Hemolytic Anemia. Blood, *9*, 414, 1954.

Acid-Serum Hemolysis Test (Paroxysmal Nocturnal Hemoglobinuria)

PRINCIPLE

The red cells of patients with paroxysmal nocturnal hemoglobinuria (PNH) are lysed when placed in acidified serum (pH 6.5—7.0). Normal red blood cells do not lyse in acidified serum.

SPECIMEN

15 ml of defibrinated blood is obtained from the patient and from a normal individual of the same ABO blood group. The patient's red cells may be obtained from blood collected in any anticoagulant; red cells stored in ACD solution for several weeks may be used. However, the patient's serum is best obtained from defibrinated blood, since hemolysis may occur in blood allowed to clot. Defibrinated blood is prepared by gently shaking 15 ml of freshly drawn blood with glass beads. Fibrin formation around the beads is usually complete in 10 to 15 minutes.

PROCEDURE

1. Separate red cells and serum from both the patient's and the normal blood by centrifugation.
2. Decant the serum and inactivate a small amount of normal and patient's serum by heating in a 56°C water bath for 20 minutes.
3. Wash the red cells in at least 3 changes of 0.85% saline. Prepare an approximately 50% suspension of patient's and of normal red cells in 0.85% saline.
4. Place seven numbered test tubes in a 37°C water bath and make the mixtures listed in the following table (N = normal, P = patient, and 0.05 ml = 1 large drop).

Tube No.	Serum (0.5 ml)	Inactivated Serum (0.5 ml)	Red Cells (0.05 ml)	0.2*N* HCl (0.05 ml)	Hemolysis (in a positive test)
1	N	—	P	—	—
2	P	—	P	+	+
3	—	N	P	+	—
4	N	—	P	—	—
5	N	—	P	+	+
6	P	—	N	—	—
7	P	—	N	+	—

5. Incubate all tubes at 37°C for 1 hour.
6. Centrifuge all tubes and examine the supernate for hemolysis.

INTERPRETATION

PNH cells lyse in either normal or patient's acidified serum (tubes 2 and 5). Only a trace of lysis, if any, is seen in unacidified or inactivated serum (tubes 1, 3, and 4). Spherocytes may be lysed by acidified serum (tubes 2 and 5), but they will also be lysed by inactivated acidified serum (tube 3). If the patient's serum contains a lysin active at 37°C, then lysis will be visible in tubes 1, 2, 6, and 7.

NOTES

1. The proportion of cells lysed may be quantitated by comparing the hemoglobin in the suitably diluted supernate photometrically with a 100% lysis control.
2. PNH red cells are more sensitive to red-cell antibodies than normal red cells and thus are very useful for detecting low-titer antibodies in the blood bank.

Donath-Landsteiner Antibody (Paroxysmal Cold Hemoglobinuria)

PRINCIPLE

The Donath-Landsteiner (D-L) antibody acts optimally in the cold, but differs from the cold agglutinins in being a lysin. At temperatures from 0 to 18°C the D-L antibody is adsorbed onto red cells, and lysis occurs (in the presence of complement) when the temperature is raised to 30—37°C.

The D-L antibody may be found in the serum of patients suffering from paroxysmal cold hemoglobinuria and is not present in blood from normal individuals. It has an anti-T_j^a specificity that further differentiates it from the more common cold agglutinins, which have an anti-I specificity.

SPECIMEN

Freshly drawn whole blood collected in a syringe previously warmed to 37°C, or blood clotted at 37°C (see Note 2).

PROCEDURE

1. Place 3 to 5 ml of freshly drawn blood into two test tubes previously warmed to 37°C.
2. Allow one tube to clot at 37°C. Place the other tube immediately in a refrigerator (0—5°C), or in crushed ice, for 30 minutes.
3. Place the chilled tube in a 37°C water bath. After 1 hour, examine both tubes. If the D-L antibody is present, lysis will have occurred in the tube that was cooled and then warmed; as a result, the serum expressed during clot retraction will be heavily tinged with hemoglobin. The tube left at 37°C will show no evidence of lysis.

NOTES

1. It must be emphasized that the D-L antibody produces easily visible lysis, and not agglutination, in this test. Lysis should not occur during the cold-incubation phase.
2. An "indirect" D-L test may be performed by mixing 9 volumes of the patient's serum, obtained from blood clotted at 37°C, with 1 volume of a 50% suspension of washed group O red cells and then performing the test as described above. This indirect test may be used to titrate the D-L antibody by using varying dilutions of the patient's serum.
3. If the patient's blood is drawn soon after an attack of paroxysmal cold hemoglobinuria, it may be deficient in complement. Since complement is necessary for lysis to take place, the deficit may be made up by mixing the patient's serum with an equal volume of normal serum.

REFERENCE

Ham, T. H., Studies on Destruction of Red Blood Cells. I. Chronic Hemolytic Anemia with Paroxysmal Nocturnal Hemoglobinuria: An Investigation of the Mechanism of Hemolysis, with Observations on Five Cases. Arch. Internal Med., *64*, 1271, 1939.

Heinz Body Stain and Heinz Body Test for G6PD Deficiency

PRINCIPLE

Heinz bodies are small precipitates of denatured hemoglobin within the red cell. They may be stained with crystal violet, but are not visible in films treated with Wright's stain.

Heinz bodies may be produced both *in vivo* and *in vitro* by oxidant drugs. Red cells from patients with glucose-6-phosphate dehydrogenase deficiency are particularly sensitive to the action of oxidant drugs, and their effect may be used to distinguish enzyme-deficient from normal red cells. Heinz bodies are commonly seen following splenectomy, and this test may be positive in the presence of various unstable abnormal hemoglobins.

NORMAL VALUES

Fewer than 33% of normal red cells develop more than 5 Heinz bodies each when exposed to acetylphenylhydrazine. More than 45% of G6PD-deficient red cells develop more than 5 Heinz bodies.

SPECIMEN

Defibrinated blood may be used, or blood collected in heparin, sodium EDTA or sodium oxalate.

PROCEDURE

1. Add 0.1 ml of patient's blood to 2 ml of acetylphenylhydrazine solution. Prepare a control tube by adding 0.1 ml of normal blood to 2 ml of acetylphenylhydrazine solution.
2. Mix, then aerate both tubes by drawing the contents into and out of a pipette several times.
3. Incubate at 37°C for 2 hours.
4. Aerate both tubes again.
5. Incubate at 37°C for 2 hours.
6. Place 1 drop of the mixture onto a slide. Add 2 drops of crystal violet solution and mix.
7. Cover with a cover glass and allow the cells to settle for 5 minutes.
8. Examine 100 red cells microscopically under high power and note the percentage that contains 5 or more Heinz bodies.
9. If a permanent preparation is required, a film of the mixture of cells and stain may be made on a slide or cover slip, air-dried, and then mounted.

NOTES

1. If Heinz bodies are to be looked for without reacting the cells with acetylphenylhydrazine, 1 drop of blood is mixed with 2 drops of stain, and steps 6, 7, 8, and 9 are carried out.

2. Heinz bodies are visible as refractile bodies in a wet preparation of red cells suspended in saline.

REAGENTS

1. Buffer solution

   Dissolve 9.08 g of potassium dihydrogen phosphate in 1 liter of distilled water (0.066*M*). Dissolve 9.47 g of disodium hydrogen phosphate in 1 liter of distilled water (0.066*M*). Mix 13 ml of the first solution with 87 ml of the second solution and add 2 g of glucose. Store this solution at 4°C.

2. Acetylphenylhydrazine solution

   Dissolve 100 mg of acetylphenylhydrazine in 100 ml of buffer solution. Use within 1 hour of preparation.

3. Crystal violet

   Add 2 g of crystal violet to 100 ml of 0.73% sodium chloride in water. Shake for 5 minutes, then filter. Add another 100 ml of 0.73% sodium chloride solution. Store at room temperature.

REFERENCE

Beutler, E., Dern, R. J., and Alving, A. S., The Hemolytic Effect of Primaquine. VI. J. Lab. Clin. Med., *45*, 40, 1955.

Sickle Cell Preparation

PRINCIPLE

The structurally abnormal sickle hemoglobin (HbS) is relatively insoluble in the reduced form. When a red cell containing HbS is exposed to a reducing agent, the hemoglobin forms tactoids, which are in essence end-to-end polymers, and the membrane of the red cell is distorted. The sickle, holly-leaf, and other bizarre pointed shapes are readily seen under a microscope.

SPECIMEN

1 or 2 ml of blood collected in an anticoagulant, or red cells dislodged from a clot.

PROCEDURE

1. Mix together equal portions of an approximately 5% suspension of red cells and 2% sodium *m*-bisulfite solution.
2. Place a drop or two of this mixture on a slide and cover it with a cover slip.
3. Keep the preparation moist under an inverted petri dish.
4. After 30 minutes examine the slide for the presence of sickle cells. These cells should have at least two sharp points to distinguish them from other poikilocytes.

NOTES

1. Although the sickling phenomenon is not unique to HbS, other causes are so rare that a positive sickling test can be taken to indicate the presence of HbS in the red cells.
2. A positive sickling test will be found in the red cells of persons heterozygous or homozygous for HbS.
3. False negative results occasionally occur and usually result from the use of a sodium *m*-bisulfite solution that has not been freshly or correctly prepared. Stored blood may on occasion give a false negative result; hence the necessity for using fresh blood.

REAGENTS

1. Sodium *meta*-bisulfite solution

sodium *meta*-bisulfite	0.5 g
distilled water	25.0 ml

This solution should be freshly prepared immediately before each test. An exact 2% concentration is not essential, however, and it may be convenient to score a small test tube at the level that 0.5 g occupies and use it as a measure.

The Investigation of Hemorrhagic Disorders

The multiplicity of tests available for the study of hemostasis is a reflection of the complicated nature of the process and the lack of exact knowledge of its chemistry. In order to make the best use of the tests, it is necessary to keep in mind an outline of the various phases of hemostasis that they are designed to elucidate. Such an outline is presented below and will be referred to in each of the tests.

PHASES OF HEMOSTASIS

When a small blood vessel is punctured, the following series of events takes place, with considerable overlap. A defect in any one or more phases may cause a hemorrhagic diathesis.

Phase I

Platelets adhere to the damaged vessel wall and to each other, forming a loose plug. Local vascular contraction may also occur.

Phase II

Blood coagulation with the formation of a fibrin plug occurs and can be divided into three stages (see diagram).

Stage 1: the formation of prothrombin-converting factor.
Stage 2: the conversion of prothrombin to thrombin.
Stage 3: the conversion of fibrinogen to fibrin.

Stage 1 may proceed down the intrinsic pathway involving factors available in plasma and platelets, or down an extrinsic pathway when tissue thromboplastin is present. Although the intrinsic and extrinsic pathways may be studied separately *in vitro*, they act simultaneously *in vivo*, and both are necessary for effective hemostasis.

Phase III

The platelets enmeshed among the fibrin strands now contract, forming a firm plug. Clot retraction is dependent upon a retractile protein present in normal platelets.

Phase IV

The process of fibrinolysis prevents spread of the clot beyond the area in which it is required and aids in the early steps of repair and recanalization.

Phase V

Repair of the vessel wall and relining it with endothelium occurs. This phase is not usually considered part of the hemostatic process, but there is evidence that it cannot be completely separated. For example, wound healing is delayed and abnormal in patients who lack factor XIII (fibrin-stabilizing factor).

The Blood Coagulation Mechanism

DIAGRAMMATIC PRESENTATION OF THE BLOOD CLOTTING MECHANISM

Stage 1: formation of prothrombin activator; this may be formed either extrinsically when tissue thromboplastin is involved, or intrinsically from plasma constituents alone.

Stage 2: the conversion of prothrombin to thrombin.

Stage 3: the conversion of fibrinogen to fibrin by the proteolytic action of thrombin.

Calcium is required in all stages.

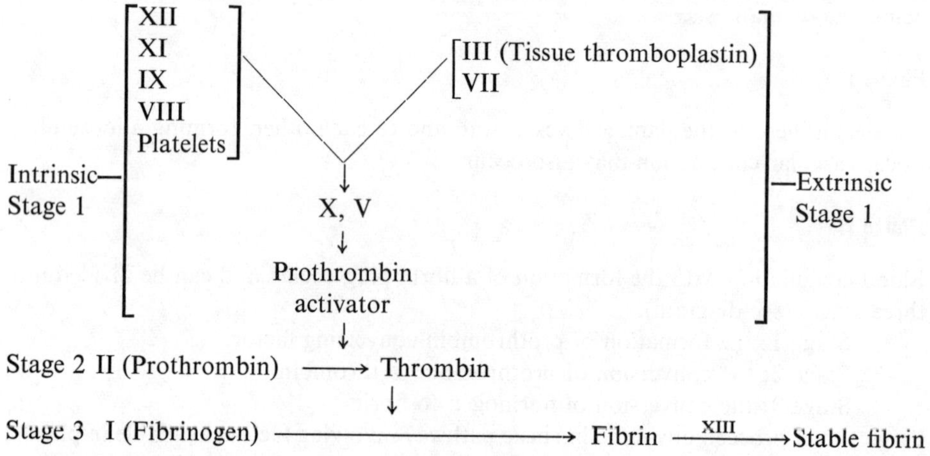

INTERNATIONAL NOMENCLATURE FOR BLOOD COAGULATION FACTORS AND THEIR MORE COMMON SYNONYMS

Factor	Synonym
I	Fibrinogen
II	Prothrombin
III	Tissue Thromboplastin
IV	Calcium
V	Labile Factor, Proaccelerin, Accelerin, Ac Globulin
VII	Stable Factor, Proconvertin, Serum Prothrombin Conversion Accelerator (SPCA)
VIII	Antihemophilic Globulin (AHG), Antihemophilic Factor (AHF)
IX	Plasma Thromboplastin Component (PTC), Christmas Factor
X	Stuart-Prower Factor
XI	Plasma Thromboplastin Antecedent (PTA)
XII	Hageman Factor
XIII	Fibrin-Stabilizing Factor

Whole-Blood Clotting Time

Ground-Glass Method

PRINCIPLE

The time it takes for whole blood to clot is a measure of the efficiency of all three stages of the intrinsic clotting pathway (see diagram). One of the major factors affecting the speed of clotting is the amount of contact with a foreign surface to which the blood is exposed. The method described here involves the addition of glass particles to the blood. This not only shortens the clotting time, but provides a clear-cut end point and greater sensitivity than the commonly used Lee-White method.

NORMAL VALUES

90 to 130 seconds. Significantly prolonged clotting times are obtained when, for instance, the plasma level of factor VIII (AHG) is less than 20%.

PROCEDURE

1. Place three 10 × 75 mm test tubes, each containing approximately 70 mg of ground glass (enough to fill the concavity of the bottom of the tube), in a 37°C water bath.
2. Draw approximately 4.0 ml venous blood into a glass or plastic syringe and immediately transfer 1.0 ml into each test tube.
3. Start a stopwatch.
4. Cork or cap the tubes as quickly as possible and mix each tube in turn by complete inversion.
5. Invert each tube in rapid succession until the blood forms a solid clot. Note the time to the nearest 5 seconds.
6. Report the average of the three clotting times.

NOTES

1. The quantity of ground glass is not critical. Doubling the amount shortens the normal clotting time by 5 to 10 seconds.
2. The stopwatch is started when the blood is added to the ground glass rather than when the blood enters the syringe, because the "contact" resulting during the variable time the blood is in the syringe is small compared to that resulting from the mixing with glass particles.
3. The test may be performed at room temperature with slight loss of sensitivity. The normal range extends to 150 seconds.
4. Each laboratory should establish a normal range.

MATERIALS

1. Glass particles

   The glass particles can be prepared by grinding discarded glassware with a pestle and mortar. The size varies from a fine dust to particles 1 to 2 mm in diameter. The size is not critical; however, commercially available powdered glass is so fine that it tends to cake and may fail to mix with the blood.

2. Heating block

   A portable electric heating block that can be plugged in at the patient's bedside or in the bleeding booth is convenient.

REFERENCE

Hoffman, G. C., and Snyder, A., The Ground-Glass Clotting Time. Cleveland Clin. Quart., *33*, 107, 1966.

One-Stage Prothrombin Time

PRINCIPLE

The clotting time of a mixture consisting of plasma, tissue thromboplastin (factor III) and calcium is a measure of the efficiency of the extrinsic blood coagulation pathway (see diagram). A prolonged clotting time may result from a deficiency of one or more of the following: factor V, factor VII, factor X, prothrombin (factor II), or fibrinogen (factor I). Alternatively, a circulating coagulant inhibiting one of these factors may be present. This test is most commonly used to monitor anticoagulant therapy with coumadin drugs and as a test of liver function.

NORMAL VALUES

11 to 14 seconds, depending on the tissue thromboplastin used. In the normal range the test is reproducible within 1 second.

SPECIMEN

4.5 ml of freshly drawn blood, collected either in 0.5 ml of 0.1*M* sodium oxalate solution or in 0.5 ml of 0.13*M* sodium citrate solution.

PROCEDURE

1. Centrifuge the blood to obtain plasma.
2. Place 0.2 ml of thromboplastin-calcium mixture (add 0.1 ml of thromboplastin to 0.1 ml of calcium chloride, if not already mixed) into each of two 10 × 75 mm test tubes.
3. Allow the tubes to warm for about 30 seconds.
4. Taking one tube at a time, blow 0.1 ml of plasma quickly into the thromboplastin mixture. Start a stopwatch.
5. Mix continuously and gently in a water bath for 10 seconds.
6. Remove the tube from the water bath, hold it in front of a bright light, and tilt it slightly every second until a clot appears. If the clotting time is prolonged, the tube should be dipped into the water bath between tiltings to keep its temperature near 37°C.
7. Each sample should be run in duplicate, and the results averaged.
8. A normal control must be included with each batch of tests.
9. Report the results in seconds. The result obtained with normal plasma should also be reported.

NOTES

1. The blood should be added to the anticoagulant immediately upon collection.
2. The one-stage prothrombin time is shorter when citrated plasma is used in place of oxalated plasma.
3. The venipuncture should be clean, since any tissue fluid mixed with the blood may alter the results.
4. The blood should be tested immediately, or refrigerated and run within 4 hours.

5. There are many ways of reporting the results of this test. The use of a reference dilution curve is particularly common, and the results are reported as percent of normal. Although this should theoretically lead to easy comparison of results obtained in different laboratories, there are variations in preparing the curve that may negate this apparent advantage. Thus it makes a considerable difference whether the reference curve is constructed on the basis of saline dilutions of normal plasma or of dilutions made with barium sulfate ($BaSO_4$) adsorbed plasma. Furthermore, percentages obtained from reference curves have little meaning in terms of individual clotting factors. Various ratios relating the patients to normal one-stage prothrombin times are also of little value, since all reference curves are hyperbolic.

REAGENTS

1. Thromboplastin

   Available from many commercial sources, usually in the form of a suspension of acetone-dried extract of brain tissue.

2. Calcium chloride (0.02*M*)

   Dissolve 2.22 g of anhydrous calcium chloride in 1 liter of distilled water. Many preparations are available in which thromboplastin and calcium are mixed ready for use.

3. Plasma control

   A pool of freshly drawn plasma, obtained from normal individuals. This also is available in lyophilized form from several commercial sources.

Partial-Thromboplastin Time (PTT)

PRINCIPLE

The PTT is a test of all stages of the intrinsic clotting pathway (see diagram) except platelet factor 3. In essence, a platelet substitute in the form of a phospholipid suspension, or "partial thromboplastin", is added to the plasma to be tested, and the clotting time following the addition of calcium is measured. The "activated" PTT is a variation in which Celite*, kaolin, or a similar substance provides added surface activation. By the addition of platelet substitute and surface activation, the two variables that exist when plasma alone is recalcified are minimized.

NORMAL VALUES

These must be determined for each laboratory; however, normal results for the unactivated test usually lie between 60 and 90 seconds, whereas those for the activated test lie between 40 and 60 seconds. In the normal range results are usually reproducible within a 2-second range. The sensitivity of the test is such that results are abnormal when, for instance, the test plasma contains 20% factor VIII.

SPECIMEN

4.5 ml blood added to 0.5 ml of a 0.13*M* solution of sodium citrate. (Blood collected in sodium oxalate may be used for the unactivated test, but is not suitable for the activated test.)

PROCEDURE

The procedure recommended for this test varies with the partial thromboplastin used and whether or not the test is "activated". The following method is employed when Thrombofax† is used as the phospholipid platelet substitute with Celite as the activator.

1. Centrifuge plasma to obtain platelet-poor plasma.
2. Place 0.1 ml of plasma into a 10 × 75 mm test tube in a 37°C water bath.
3. Add 0.1 ml of Celite suspension.
4. Mix gently for 15 seconds.
5. Add rapidly 0.2 ml of an equal mixture of calcium chloride and partial thromboplastin warmed to 37°C. Start a stopwatch.
6. Mix and allow to stand for approximately 30 second in a water bath.
7. Roll the tube gently between thumb and fingers over a black background until a fine thread-like fibrin clot forms around the edge of the solution. Record the time.

RESULTS

The average of duplicate results is reported in seconds. The results obtained using normal plasma and the same reagents are also reported.

*Johns-Manville Products Corporation, Celite Division, 22 East 40th Street, New York, New York 10016.
†Ortho Diagnostics, Raritan, New Jersey.

NOTES

1. Variations in technics may have considerable effect on the result; hence it is essential for each laboratory to determine its own normal values.
2. The test may be performed without the use of Celite as an activator.
3. The PTT is an excellent screening test for hemorrhagic disorders involving the intrinsic pathway of coagulation. It is much more sensitive than the Lee-White clotting test, and about equally as sensitive as the whole-blood clotting test with added glass particles.
4. The test may be used as the basis for the assay of many factors involved in the intrinsic coagulation pathway (see Assay of Factor VIII, p. 203).

REAGENTS

1. Partial thromboplastin

   Available from various commerical sources; may be obtained in liquid or dried form, with or without added calcium chloride, and with or without activator.
2. Calcium chloride

   Dissolve 2.22 g of anhydrous calcium chloride in 1 liter of distilled water.
3. Celite

   0.7% suspension in 0.85% sodium chloride.

REFERENCE

Rodman, N. F., Jr., Barrow, E. M., and Graham, J. B., Diagnosis and Control of the Hemophiloid States with the Partial-Thromboplastin Test. Am. J. Clin. Pathol., *29*, 525, 1958.

Prothrombin Consumption Test

PRINCIPLE

When blood clots via the intrinsic pathway (see diagram), prothrombin is converted to thrombin, and only small amounts of prothrombin are found in the serum. The amount of prothrombin remaining is a reflection of the efficiency of stage 1 of the intrinsic pathway. Thus a deficiency of factors XII, XI, VIII, IX, X, V, or platelet factor 3, or an inhibitor acting in this stage, will result in impaired prothrombin consumption, and hence greater than normal quantities of prothrombin remain in the serum. The residual prothrombin is estimated by performing, in essence, a one-stage prothrombin test on the serum, to which fibrinogen has been added.

In the method described here, the test is performed with and without addition of a platelet substitute. If an abnormal result is obtained that is corrected by platelet substitute, then platelet factor 3 is deficient or is not being released.

SPECIMEN

See procedure.

PROCEDURE

1. Place 0.1 ml of platelet substitute into one glass test tube, and 0.1 ml of saline into another.
2. Add 1.0 ml freshly drawn blood to each tube.
3. Observe at intervals until a clot has formed.
4. One hour after a clot has formed, remove the serum and refrigerate it until tested.
5. Add 0.1 ml of fibrinogen solution to 0.1 ml of serum.
6. To this mixture add 0.1 ml of thromboplastin and 0.1 ml of calcium chloride (or 0.2 ml of a commercially prepared mixture) and measure the clotting time in seconds.

INTERPRETATION

Serum Prothrombin Time		Interpretation
Without Platelet Substitute	With Platelet Substitute	
>25 secs	>25 secs	Normal
>25 secs	<20 secs	Platelet factor 3 deficient or not released
<20 secs	<20 secs	Defect in intrinsic stage 1 other than platelet factor 3.

REAGENTS

1. Tissue thromboplastin
   As used in the one-stage prothrombin test.
2. Calcium chloride (0.02*M*)
   Dissolve 2.22 g of anhydrous calcium chloride in 1 liter of distilled water (required only if not incorporated in the tissue thromboplastin preparation).

3. Fibrinogen (200 mg/100 ml distilled water)
   Commercially available bovine fibrinogen is adequate.
4. Platelet substitute
   Commercially available substitutes are used in the concentrate recommended for the partial-thromboplastin time determination.

REFERENCE

Owen, C. A., Jr., and Thompson, J. H. Jr., Soybean Phosphatides in Prothrombin-Consumption and Thromboplastin-Generation Tests: Their Use in Recognizing "Thrombasthenic Hemophilia". Am. J. Clin. Pathol., *33*, 197, 1960.

Thrombin Time

PRINCIPLE

The addition of thrombin to plasma causes the conversion of fibrinogen to fibrin, with the formation of a clot. A prolonged thrombin clotting time results from a deficiency of fibrinogen, the presence of an abnormal fibrinogen, or the presence of an inhibitor of fibrinogen–fibrin conversion.

SPECIMEN

Citrated blood from patient and from a control subject (4.5 ml blood with 0.5 ml of 3.2% trisodium citrate in water).

PROCEDURE

1. Place 0.1 ml of normal plasma and 0.1 ml of 0.85% sodium chloride into a test tube at 37°C.
2. Add 0.1 ml of thrombin solution, then start a stopwatch and measure the clotting time in seconds.
3. Repeat steps 1 and 2, using the patient's plasma.
4. If the patient's thrombin time is longer than that of the control, repeat steps 1 and 2, using 0.1 ml of an equal mixture of patient's and control subject's plasma.

INTERPRETATION

If the patient's thrombin time is more than 1.3 times longer than that of the control, the difference is probably significant. If the mixture of normal and patient's plasma has a thrombin time close to that of the control, a deficiency of fibrinogen probably exists (or, very rarely, a defective fibrinogen). If the thrombin time of the mixture is close to that of the patient, then an inhibitor is probably present.

NOTES

1. The use of calcified thrombin is not essential, but since the fibrinogen–fibrin conversion requires calcium, it seems a reasonable precaution.
2. The thrombin time is a better test for the detection of inhibitors than for the detection of fibrinogen deficiency, since there are more reliable quantitative tests for the latter. However, in emergency situations, such as may occur in obstetric wards, it is wise to maintain a stock of tubes containing dilute thrombin close at hand. Then, if afibrinogenemia is suspected, a small amount of whole blood may be added to the tube, and if no clot forms, then the suspicion is rapidly confirmed.
3. The inhibitors most likely to prolong the thrombin time are heparin and fragments of fibrinogen that result from fibrinolysis. Fibrinolysis leads to reduction in fibrinogen content and to the appearance of fibrinogen fragments; since this process may take time, it may be detected by performing serial thrombin time tests at 15-minute intervals after the blood is drawn. If the patient's thrombin time increases to a greater extent than the normal, increased fibrinolytic activity is present in the patient's plasma.

REAGENTS

1. Thrombin solution

   Many commercial preparations are available; human thrombin is preferable to bovine. A stock solution of approximately 50 units per ml, made according to the manufacturer's instructions, may be stored at −20°C for 3 to 4 months. From this solution a dilution with 0.025*M* calcium chloride is made that will give a clotting time of about 15 seconds with normal plasma.

The Thromboplastin Generation Test (TGT)

PRINCIPLE

The thromboplastin generation test is a test of stage 1 of the intrinsic clotting pathway (see diagram). The term "thromboplastin" refers to blood thromboplastin, more properly called "prothrombin-converting principle" to distinguish it from tissue thromboplastin. The TGT is a two-stage test. In the first stage a mixture of serum (factors XII, XI, IX, and X), adsorbed plasma (factors XII, XI, VIII, and V) and a suspension of platelets or platelet substitute is recalcified. In the second stage aliquots of this incubation mixture are tested at intervals for their ability to shorten the clotting time of recalcified normal plasma, which supplies stages 2 and 3 of the clotting system. By replacing the normal ingredients one at a time with those from the patient, it is possible to infer a missing factor or the presence of a circulating anticoagulant. The TGT may be used as an assay system for the various factors involved.

SPECIMENS

1. 5.0 ml of clotted blood from both the patient and a normal subject.
2. 5.0 ml of citrated blood (4.5 ml of blood added to 0.5 ml of 0.13*M* sodium citrate) from the patient and from 4 or 5 normal subjects.

PROCEDURE

1. Place 0.1 ml of normal platelet-poor plasma into each of eight to ten 10 × 75 mm test tubes in a 37°C water bath. These are the substrate tubes.
2. Place 0.3 ml each of diluted normal serum, diluted normal adsorbed plasma, and normal platelet suspension or substitute in a 13 × 100 mm test tube in a 37°C water bath. Add 0.3 ml of 0.025*M* calcium chloride, mix, and immediately start a stopwatch.
3. After approximately 50 seconds add 0.1 ml of calcium chloride to one of the substrate tubes and then, at 60 seconds, add 0.1 ml of the incubation mixture, mix, and start a second stopwatch. Tip the tube back and forth in the water bath and measure the time it takes for the clot to form.
4. Repeat step 3 at 1-minute intervals until the shortest clotting time is obtained. This is usually at the fourth to sixth minute of incubation. Record each clotting time to the nearest second.
5. Repeat steps 2, 3, and 4, utilizing each of the following incubation mixtures:
   (a) patient's serum, normal adsorbed plasma, normal platelet suspension or substitute;
   (b) normal serum, patient's adsorbed plasma, normal platelet suspension or substitute;
   (c) patient's serum, patient's adsorbed plasma, normal platelet suspension or substitute;
   (d) normal serum, normal adsorbed plasma, patient's platelet suspension.

INTERPRETATION

If all mixtures produce a substrate clotting time within 2 seconds of the normal, it can be assumed that the patient's intrinsic stage 1 is normal. If one or more of the combinations is abnormal, then the following possibilities exist (assuming a *single* deficiency or inhibitor):

Source of			If Abnormal, There Is a Deficiency of
Platelets	Serum	Adsorbed Plasma	
Normal	Normal	Patient	Factor V* or factor VIII
Normal	Patient	Normal	Factor IX or factor X*
Normal	Patient	Patient	Factor XI or factor XII†

*If factor V or factor X is deficient, then the patient will also have an abnormal one-stage prothrombin time.

†Factors XI and XII are present in both serum and adsorbed plasma.

NOTES

1. If a deficiency of, for instance, factor VIII is indicated from the results of the TGT and the one-stage prothrombin time, it is advisable to confirm the finding by:
   (a) demonstrating that the patient's plasma is unable to correct the defect in plasma from a known hemophiliac;
   (b) assaying the patient's plasma for factor VIII.
2. The TGT may be used to assay, for instance, factor VIII. First a TGT is run, using adsorbed plasma from a patient known to be deficient in factor VIII, but with no evidence of any anti-factor VIII activity; then the ability of various dilutions of pooled normal adsorbed plasma to correct this deficiency is tested. This provides a reference curve. The ability of the patient's adsorbed plasma to correct the deficient plasma is then tested, and by comparison with the reference curve the level of factor VIII may be estimated. It is simpler, however, to use the partial-thromboplastin time for such assay procedures.
3. The TGT is not a good test of platelet factor 3 activity; however, it will show severe defects. Defective factor 3 activity may be due to absence of factor 3 or to failure to release it from platelets. These possibilities may be separated by comparing the activity of platelets washed and suspended in saline with those washed in saline and artificially ruptured by suspending them in distilled water.

REAGENTS

1. Platelet suspension and platelet-poor plasma

   The citrated blood is lightly centrifuged (approximately 400 *g* for 5 to 10 minutes) to obtain platelet-rich plasma. This plasma is transferred to another test tube, and the platelets are centrifuged down (approximately 1,500 *g* for 10 minutes). The supernatant platelet-poor plasma is removed for use as substrate or for preparation of adsorbed plasma. The platelets are washed 3 times with saline and resuspended in approximately the same volume of saline as the volume of plasma from which they were harvested. A suspension of normal and patient's platelets is prepared and kept under refrigeration until needed. If frozen at −20°C, the platelet remains potent for several weeks.
2. Platelet substitute

   Many commercially available "partial thromboplastins" may be used as platelet substitutes. They may be used at the same concentration recommended for the PTT, or they may be diluted 1:5. A platelet substitute is simpler to prepare and may be used in place of a platelet suspension unless the patient's platelets are to be tested.

3. Serum

   It is essential that serum be obtained from well-clotted blood. Blood drawn into glass should be allowed to stand at 37°C for at least 3 hours, or preferably overnight. The serum is centrifuged to remove all cells, then diluted 1:10 with saline (or buffered saline, pH 7.4). Both normal and patient's serum should be prepared. Keep the diluted serum at 37°C until needed.

4. Adsorbed plasma

   Normal and patient's platelet-poor citrated plasma (obtained during preparation of platelet suspensions) are adsorbed with aluminum hydroxide gel (alumina) by mixing 9 parts plasma with 1 part gel. After standing at room temperature for 10 minutes, the mixture is centrifuged, and the clear supernatant is removed. The one-stage prothrombin time of this supernate should be longer than 1.5 minutes. The supernate is diluted 1:5 with saline (or buffered saline, pH 7.4) and refrigerated until needed. This dilute adsorbed plasma should be used within a few hours.

REFERENCE

Biggs, R., and Douglas, A. S., The Thromboplastin Generation Test. J. Clin. Pathol., *6*, 23, 1953.

Bleeding Time

Ivy Method

PRINCIPLE

A series of small skin punctures is made, and the time it takes for the wounds to stop bleeding is measured.

The object of the test is to measure the efficiency of the vascular and platelet aggregation phases of hemostasis (see p. 187). In order to minimize the effect of the next phase of hemostasis, blood coagulation, the blood is removed as it appears on the skin surface.

NORMAL VALUES

2 to 6 minutes.

PROCEDURE

1. Expose and rest the forearm, flexor surface uppermost.
2. Inflate a sphygmomanometer cuff to 40 mm Hg and maintain it at this pressure throughout the test.
3. Make three punctures in the skin, using a disposable lancet, and start a stop-watch. The area chosen should be devoid of obvious venules, and the punctures should be an inch or more apart.
4. At half-minute intervals gently blot the blood exuding from the punctures with a sheet of filter paper.
5. Measure to the nearest half minute the time taken for each wound to stop bleeding. Report all three results. It is seldom necessary to continue the test beyond 15 minutes.

NOTES

1. Two other methods in common use involve punctures in the earlobe or the fingertip. The fingertip has the disadvantages of being a painful site and varying greatly in skin thickness. The earlobe is an awkward place with which to work, the number of puncture sites is limited to two, and it is not possible to apply standard venous pressure.
2. Although the Ivy method is probably the best available, it still contains many variables. One variable is the end point, which may be defined as that moment when the flow of blood ceases. This must be distinguished from the oozing of serum.
3. Reporting the result of each individual puncture will enable the clinician to form an opinion of the reliability of the result. Thus, a test result such as 2, 4, and 11 minutes is more likely to be normal than 4, 6, and 6 minutes, despite the similarity of the average times. A long bleeding time from one puncture out of three suggests that a small vein may have been punctured.

REFERENCE

Ivy, A. C., Shapiro, P. R., and Melnick, O., The Bleeding Tendency in Jaundice. Surg. Gynecol. Obstet., *60*, 781, 1935.

Assay of Factor VIII (Antihemophilic Globulin)

PRINCIPLE

Almost all assays of single plasma clotting factors are based on a comparison of the ability of the test plasma with that of normal plasma to correct the defect in plasma with a known deficiency. Many different tests may be used, depending on the factor to be assayed. The us of the partial-thromboplastin time (PTT) in the assay of factor VIII will be described. A reference curve is constructed by recording the ability of various dilutions of normal plasma to correct the PTT of known factor VIII-deficient plasma; then, knowing the PTT obtained when the test plasma is used, it is possible to extrapolate the factor VIII content of the test plasma.

NORMAL VALUES

When any single "normal" specimen is compared with a reference curve based on a pool of at least four normals, it may contain from 50 to 200% factor VIII.

SPECIMEN

4.5 ml of whole blood, collected in 0.5 ml of 0.13*M* sodium citrate solution.

PROCEDURE

1. A series of double dilutions of the normal pooled plasma, starting with a 1:10 dilution, is prepared, using buffered saline solution. The 1:10 dilution will arbitrarily represent 100% factor VIII; hence the 1:20 dilution represents 50% factor VIII, and so on to a 1:320 dilution, which represents 3.1% factor VIII.
2. Add 0.1 ml of normal plasma dilution to 0.1 ml of factor VIII-deficient plasma and perform a PTT.
3. Repeat this procedure in duplicate for each dilution of the normal plasma and record the results.
4. Add 0.1 ml of a 1:10 dilution of test plasma to 0.1 ml of factor VIII-deficient plasma and measure its PTT in duplicate.
5. A second dilution of test plasma is similarly tested. The dilution used will depend on the result obtained with a 1:10 dilution. If the latter suggests an approximately normal factor VIII content, then a greater dilution (1:20 or 1:40) should be tested next. If the result obtained with a 1:10 dilution suggests considerable factor VIII deficiency, then a lower dilution, such as 1:5, should be used for the second test.

CALCULATION

The concentration of factor VIII in the various dilutions of normal plasma are plotted against their respective PTT's on semi-logarithmic graph paper. These points should lie on a straight line. The concentration of factor VIII in the unknown can be derived from this reference curve. The results obtained with the two dilutions should fall within 10% factor VIII.

NOTES

1. The PTT of the various dilutions of plasma should be measured as soon as possible after the dilution is made. Both normal and test plasma dilutions should be kept at 5°C until they are needed.
2. This assay procedure is applicable to any factor active in the intrinsic coagulation pathway for which a specifically deficient plasma is available.

REAGENTS

1. Partial thromboplastin and calcium chloride

   As used in the partial-thromboplastin test (see p. 194).
2. Normal plasma

   Fresh citrated plasma pooled from at least four normal donors.
3. Buffered saline

   To 250 ml of a stock solution of tris base (24.30 g tris (hydroxymethyl) aminomethane per liter of aqueous solution) add approximately 42 ml of *N* hydrochloride and make up to 990 ml with distilled water. Add 2.20 g of sodium chloride. Adjust the pH to 7.2 at 37°C, then make up to 1 liter with distilled water.

Deficiency of Factor XIII (Fibrin-Stabilizing Factor)

PRINCIPLE

Clots formed in the absence of factor XIII are soluble in 5*M* urea or in 1% monochloroacetic acid, whereas normal clots are insoluble in these solutions.

SPECIMEN

Blood from a patient and a control subject is collected, using either sodium citrate or oxalate as anticoagulant.

PROCEDURE

1. Centrifuge blood to obtain plasma.
2. Set up three tubes as follows.
   Tube 1: 0.5 ml of patient's plasma.
   Tube 2: 0.5 ml of normal plasma.
   Tube 3: 0.5 ml of a mixture containing 9 parts patient's plasma and 1 part normal plasma.
   Add 0.5 ml of calcium chloride to each tube.
3. Allow the three tubes to stand at 37°C for 30 minutes to ensure complete clotting.
4. Gently loosen the clots from their tubes and tip each into 5 ml of urea solution or monochloroacetic acid.
5. Stand the tubes undisturbed at room temperature and observe at intervals for evidence of dissolution of the clot.

INTERPRETATION

If the patient is deficient in factor XIII, his clot will dissolve in 2 or 3 hours in urea solution, or in 5 to 10 minutes in monochloroacetic acid, whereas the normal clot and the clot from the mixture will remain undissolved for 24 hours or more. If the clot prepared from the plasma mixture and the patient's clot both dissolve, this would suggest that lysis was due to fibrinolysis rather than to factor XIII deficiency.

NOTES

1. The clots must be prepared by adding calcium to the plasma, and not by adding thrombin, since normal clots formed by adding thrombin are soluble in urea.
2. The results appear to be more reliable when monochloroacetic acid is used rather than urea solution.

REAGENTS

1. 5*M* urea solution in water, or 1% monochloroacetic acid
2. Calcium chloride (0.025*M*)

REFERENCE

Barry, A., and Delâge, J. M., Congenital Deficiency of Fibrin-Stabilizing Factor. Observations of a New Case. N. Engl. J. Med., *272*, 943, 1965.

Vitamin B_{12} Absorption (Schilling) Test

PRINCIPLE

The Schilling test is designed to test the patient's ability to absorb vitamin B_{12} (cyanocobalamin). A small dose of radioactive vitamin B_{12} is given by mouth, followed by a large "flushing" dose of unlabeled vitamin B_{12} injected intramuscularly. The flushing dose is so large that most of it is excreted in the urine, regardless of the status of the patient's vitamin B_{12} stores. If any radioactive vitamin B_{12} has been absorbed from the gut, a portion of it will also be excreted in the urine. If less than normal quantities of the radioactive vitamin B_{12} are excreted in the urine, it can be inferred that less than normal quantities were absorbed from the gut.

Failure to absorb vitamin B_{12} from the gut may be due to failure of intrinsic-factor secretion by the stomach, as in pernicious anemia and after total gastric resection, or may be due to malabsorption from the terminal ileum. These two possibilities may be distinguished by repeating the test with intrinsic factor added to the oral dose of radioactive vitamin B_{12}. If this second test shows normal absorption of vitamin B_{12}, this suggests that the patient is unable to produce intrinsic factor and most probably has pernicious anemia. However, if the second test again shows an abnormal result, it indicates that the patient is unable to absorb the vitamin due to disease or excision of the terminal ileum.

NORMAL VALUES

Using the method described here, an excretion of less than 3% of the ingested dose indicates almost complete failure to absorb the vitamin. An excretion of over 8% indicates normal absorption. In the indeterminate range of 3 to 8% the result of a second test with added intrinsic factor may help to clarify the problem.

PROCEDURE

1. The patient fasts for at least 6 hours.
2. The patient swallows a capsule containing 0.5 μc of ^{57}Co-labeled vitamin B_{12}, then must fast for a further 4 hours.
3. Two hours after the patient has swallowed the radioactive vitamin B_{12}, inject 1000 μg of unlabeled vitamin B_{12} intramuscularly.
4. The patient empties his bladder, and the urine specimen is discarded. A 24-hour urine collection is then started.
5. Measure the volume of urine and adjust to 1 liter with water. If the urine volume is greater than 1 liter, use a 1-liter aliquot.
6. Place the urine sample in a 1-liter counting bottle and record its radioactivity in counts/minute.
7. Record the radioactivity of the 1-liter standard in counts/minute.
8. Record the background count in counts/minute.

CALCULATION

1. Subtract the background count from the sample count and from the standard count.
2. Calculate the percentage of the ingested dose that is excreted in the urine in 24 hours as follows:

$$\% \text{ radioactive vitamin } B_{12} \text{ recovered} = \frac{\text{counts recovered} \times 100}{\text{counts administered}}.$$

If the volume of the urine sample was 1 liter or less,

$$\text{counts recovered} = \text{counts in urine};$$

if the volume sample was more than 1 liter,

$$\text{counts recovered} = \text{counts in liter aliquot of urine} \times \frac{\text{urine volume}}{1000};$$

$$\text{counts administered} = \text{counts in standard} \times 5.$$

NOTES

1. A constant geometry of urine and standard bottles must be maintained while counting.
2. The dosage of radioactive vitamin B_{12} must be small, because if more than 1 μg of the vitamin is administered, the proportion absorbed, even by a normal individual, becomes variable.

REAGENTS

1. Radioactive vitamin B_{12}

   ^{57}Co- or ^{60}Co-labeled vitamin B_{12} is commercially available in capsules, which can also be obtained with added intrinsic factor. These capsules contain approximately 0.5 μc. The ^{57}Co label has the advantage of a shorter half-life than ^{60}Co.

2. Standard

   Prepare a 1:5 dilution of the oral dose of radioactive vitamin B_{12} in 1 liter of saline.

REFERENCE

Schilling, R. F., Clatanoff, D. V., and Korst, D. R., Intrinsic Factor Studies. III. Further Observations Utilizing the Urinary Radioactivity Test in the Subject with Achlorhydria, Pernicious Anemia, or a Total Gastrectomy. J. Lab. Clin. Med., *45*, 926, 1955.

HISTOLOGY

Sectional Directory

Introduction

Histology and histologic technics differ from other areas of endeavor in the clinical laboratory in that they deal with bits of solid tissue removed from the human body at surgery or autopsy rather than with secretions and other body fluids, as most clinical laboratory procedures do. The treatment to which such tissues are subjected is essentially a form of applied chemistry. Tissues are largely composed of proteins, carbohydrates and lipids. Utilizing our knowledge of the chemistry of these substances, it is possible to apply suitable reagents to the tissue to make a preparation that can give the experienced observer considerable information. As most of these procedures require the use of appropriate dyes, the considerable lore of the dye chemist must be employed. All of this information, plus experience and care and, we suspect, often a bit of mysticism, will result, when properly used, in the successful demonstration of those features of the tissue that the pathologist wishes to be emphasized. To accomplish this, it is often necessary to remove or alter other elements of the tissue so that the desired appearance is achieved. The different treatments to which serial slides from the same block of tissue may be subjected may cause them to present such diverse appearances that the identity of the different slides is scarcely perceptible.

The importance of good histologic technic cannot be overemphasized. Not only is the pathologist more directly dependent upon his histologic technician's ability than upon the work of almost any other person in the laboratory, but the histologic preparation stands as a permanent record of the patient's illness as well as of the skill and success of the person who prepared it. Often the only reliable evidence given to the clinical staff as to the competency of the technical staff of the laboratory is the excellence of its histology.

The technics presented here lay no claim to originality. However, many have been modified on the basis of experience. It is hoped that the reader will take advantage of this experience and make profitable use of these bench-tried and tested technics.

John W. King, M.D., Ph.D.

Preparation of Solutions and Stains for Use in the Histology Laboratory

FUNDAMENTAL RULES NECESSARY IN PREPARATION OF SOLUTIONS AND STAINS

1. Use standard graduated cylinders and pipettes. Always read the lower meniscus when taking the reading of a liquid.
2. Use chemically clean glassware in order to prevent contamination.
3. Use distilled water for all aqueous solutions.
4. Use accurate weighing equipment and balance the equipment before operation. Weigh caustic material in glass beakers. Use a camel's-hair brush for dusting the weighing equipment before and after use.
5. Use only quality-grade salt and acid reagents.
6. Use certified dyes and stains when possible. Index the dyes according to color index and percentage of dye content or similar standardization for future reference.
7. Use precautions in handling all materials employed in the laboratory. Read the instructions given on the bottles before use.
8. Use care when making solutions from concentrated acids. Remember to add acid to water *slowly*.
9. Label and date all solutions. Some solutions are stable for extended periods, others deteriorate after a limited time.

SOLUTIONS AND THEIR DEFINITIONS

Molar Solution contains 1 gram molecular weight of a compound dissolved in enough solvent to make 1000 ml of solution. Molecular weight (M.W.) is always stated on quality-grade reagent bottles. Example: 1*N* sodium chloride,

NaCl (M.W. 58.45)	58.45 g
solvent (distilled water) to make	1000.00 ml

Molal Solution contains 1 gram molecular weight plus 1000 gram of solvent. Example: 1*N* sodium chloride,

NaCl	58.45 g
distilled water	1000.00 ml

Normal Solution contains 1 gram equivalent weight per liter of solution. Example: 1*N* hydrochloric acid,

HCl, concentrated (Sp. G. 1.19, 39%)	78.4 ml
distilled water (to make 1000.0 ml)	921.6 ml

When using a volumetric flask, add distilled water to the 1000-ml mark.

Saturated Solution consists of dissolved and undissolved salt in a solution. Example: saturated picric acid,

picric acid crystals	1.3 g or until saturated
distilled water	100 ml

Buffer Solution is a substance added to a solution to cause resistance to any change of hydrogen ion concentration when either acid or alkali is added. Example: neutral buffered formalin (pH 7.0),

formaldehyde, 37—40%	100.0 ml
distilled water	900.0 ml
sodium acid phosphate monohydrate	4.0 g
disodium phosphate, dibasic, anhydrous	6.5 g

pH Solution may range from 1 to 14 in pH value, with 7 being neutral; acids are below 7, and bases are above 7.

Acid Solution. Acid in solution will donate hydrogen ions.

Base Solution. Basic solution will accept hydrogen ions.

Distilled Water is water from which minerals and chlorides have been removed by the process of distillation. To test for complete removal of chlorides, add a small crystal of silver nitrate to 40 ml of the distilled water. If any chlorides are present, the water will appear cloudy or milky; in the absence of chlorides the solution remains clear.

Mordant Solution combined with another solution, substance or dyestuff, forms an insoluble compound that fixes the color. Example: 2% phosphotungstic acid is used in the modified Masson trichrome stain to fix the yellow and red dye, so that the fast green does not destroy the other two colors.

Decolorizing Solution is a substance in solution that will remove or bleach out a color. Example: acid alcohol,

hydrochloric acid, concentrated	0.1 ml
alcohol, 70%	99.0 ml

Oxidizing Solution causes an increase of oxygen ions in a solution, or the loss of electrons, with a change toward a more positive valance number (basic in nature). Example: 4% chromic acid.

DILUTIONS FROM STOCK SOLUTIONS

These are prepared by making a lower-percentage solution from a higher-percentage solution. Stock or higher-percentage solutions provide more space in the laboratory, save the technician time, and cut down costs. Examples are given below.

1. Alcohol dilutions made with 95% alcohol instead of absolute alcohol.

Percentage Alcohol Solution	95% Alcohol	Distilled Water
80%	80 ml	15 ml
70%	70 ml	25 ml
50%	50 ml	45 ml
10%	10 ml	85 ml

2. Dilutions made from higher-percentage staining solutions can be determined without the aid of a mathematical formula.

3. Dilutions made from 29% ferric chloride (aqueous).
   (a) Ferric chloride solution (29% aqueous)

ferric chloride	29 g
distilled water	100 ml

   (b) Ferric chloride solution (10% aqueous)

ferric chloride solution, 29%	10 ml
distilled water	19 ml

   If larger quantities are needed, multiply the amounts given.

   (c) Ferric chloride solution (2% aqueous)

ferric chloride solution, 29%	2 ml
distilled water	27 ml

   This dilution can be made from the 10% ferric chloride solution. If larger quantities are needed, multiply the amounts given.

General Preparation of Tissue

10% Formalin Method

General preparation of tissue consists of fixation, dehydration, clearing, infiltration and impregnation, and the embedding process.

Fixation. The process of immediate killing and hardening of tissues in order to preserve and keep the specimen as life-like as possible. Tissue blocks for examination that are to be automatically machine-processed should be approximately 2 to 4 mm thick and are allowed to fix for 3 to 24 hours in a universally used fixative, such as 10% formalin. The remaining specimen may be preserved and stored in the fixative without washing in tap water.

Dehydration. The process of gradually replacing the water in the tissue with a miscible solution to assist in hardening the tissue and at the same time prevent shrinkage; for example, the use of graded alcohols: 80%, 95%, and absolute alcohol. The strength of the dehydrant tends to harden the tissue as well as prepare it to be miscible in a clearing reagent.

Clearing of Tissue. The process of removing a dehydrate, such as alcohol, and replacing it with a reagent that will be miscible in paraffin. A reagent commonly used is xylol. This procedure continues to harden the tissue and to make it more transparent.

Infiltration and Impregnation. The process of replacing the dehydrating reagent with paraffin (M.P. 54—56°C). To remove this reagent thoroughly, it is necessary to use three paraffin changes. The impregnation time can be shortened with the use of a vacuum.

Embedding. The method of placing the prepared tissue in a liquid medium that will solidify into a firm block, such as paraffin (M.P. 56—58°C), to enable the tissue to be cut on a microtome.

FIXATION

100% formalin or 37—40% formaldehyde	100 ml
distilled or deionized water	900 ml
sodium bicarbonate	8 g

Phenol red indicator, pH 6—8, is added to the solution, which should remain pink while being used. Fix the tissue for 3 to 24 hours. Store the remaining tissue in the same solution.

DEHYDRATION, CLEARING, AND EMBEDDING

Dehydration, clearing, and embedding of tissue proceed after proper fixation as follows:

1. 10% formalin: 1 to 3 hours.
2. 80% alcohol: 1 to 2 hours.
3. 95% alcohol: 1 hour.
4. 100% alcohol, I: 1 hour.
5. 100% alcohol, II: 1 hour.

6. 100% alcohol, III: 1 hour.
7. Xylol, I: 1 hour.
8. Xylol, II: 1 hour.
9. Paraffin (54—56°C), I: 1 hour.
10. Paraffin (54—56°C), II: 1 hour.
11. Paraffin (56—58°C), III: embed; if available, vacuum in oven for 15 minutes before embedding.

NOTES

1. When Zenker's fixative is used, it is necessary to remove the mercuric chloride crystals present in the tissue. This is accomplished by deparaffinizing the section (see p. 224) and hydrating to water. Place in Lugol's or Gram's iodine for 15 minutes, transfer to 5% aqueous sodium thiosulfate for 3 minutes, wash well in tap water, then stain as desired.

REFERENCE

Manual of Histologic and Special Staining Technics. Armed Forces Institute of Pathology, Washington, D.C., 1957.

Acid-Fast Stain for Tubercle Bacilli

Verhoeff's Carbol Fuchsin Method (1912), Modified

FIXATION

10% formalin, or Zenker's acetic acid fixative.

TECHNIC

Cut paraffin sections at 4 to 5 microns. Use a known control slide.

PROCEDURE

1. Use known control for acid-fast bacilli.
2. Deparaffinize the slides as for the hematoxylin-and-eosin stain (see p. 224). If Zenker's fixative is used, remove the mercuric chloride crystals (see p. 216).
3. Rinse the slides 3 times in distilled water.
4. Place the slides in Verhoeff's carbol fuchsin staining solution that has previously been heated in a paraffin oven at 56°C.
5. Leave the slides in stain in the paraffin oven at 56°C for at least 1 hour.
6. Remove the slides from the paraffin oven and cool to room temperature.
7. Decolorize the slides in acid-alcohol for exactly 20 seconds.
8. Rinse thoroughly in ammonia water (3 drops of concentrated ammonia to 100 ml of distilled water).
9. Rinse thoroughly in distilled water (at least 5 rinses).
10. Place the slides in 1% potassium permanganate solution for 5 minutes.
11. Rinse well in 3 changes of distilled water.
12. Place the slides in 2% oxalic acid solution for 2 minutes.
13. Rinse well in distilled water.
14. Place the slides in Loeffler's methylene blue solution for approximately 3 seconds.
15. Dehydrate the slides in 95% alcohol and in absolute alcohol.
16. Clear the slides in xylol.
17. Mount in the usual manner.

RESULTS

1. Tubercle bacilli: brilliant red.
2. Background: light blue.

SOLUTIONS

1. Verhoeff's carbol fuchsin stock solution

fuchsin (basic)	2 g
absolute alcohol	50 ml
carbolic acid crystals (melt in paraffin oven at 56°C)	25 ml

Combine the above ingredients, mix, and place overnight in a 56°C incubator. Cool the solution the next day, then filter it. Stock solution does not deteriorate and keeps well at room temperature. The stain is very powerful.

2. Verhoeff's carbol fuchsin staining solution
   Dilute 10 ml of Verhoeff's carbol fuchsin stock solution with 50 ml of distilled water. This stain does not need to be filtered. Prepare fresh each day.
3. Acid-alcohol solution
   Add 1 ml of concentrated hydrochloric acid to 99 ml of 70% alcohol.
4. Potassium permanganate solution (1%)
   Dissolve 1.0 g of potassium permanganate crystals in 100 ml of distilled water.
5. Oxalic acid (2%)
   Dissolve 2.0 g of oxalic acid in 100 ml of distilled water.
6. Loeffler's methylene blue solution

methylene blue solution (saturated in 95% alcohol)	30 ml
sodium hydroxide (0.1% aqueous solution)	100 ml

REFERENCE

Mallory, F. B., Pathological Technic, p. 276. W. B. Saunders, Philadelphia, 1942.

Amyloid Stain

FIXATION

10% formalin, or Zenker's acetic acid fixative.

TECHNIC

Cut paraffin sections at 5 to 6 microns, frozen sections at 15 microns. Use a known control slide.

PROCEDURE

1. Deparaffinize the slides as for the H-and-E (Hematoxylin-and-Eosin) stain (see p. 224). If Zenker's fixative is used, remove the mercuric chloride crystals (see p. 216).
2. Stain in crystal violet solution for 5 to 24 hours or until a bluish-purple color appears. Generally the slides are stained overnight.
3. Rinse the slides in distilled water until excess stain has been removed.
4. Mount in Valnor Mounting Medium, Type ABP*.

RESULTS

1. Amyloid: purple to bluish purple.
2. Mast cells: purple.
3. All other elements: light blue to blue.

NOTES

1. Mast cells will be stained by this method. Staining time varies from 5 to 15 minutes.
2. Frozen sections can be stained by the same method.
3. Avoid excess rinsing in distilled water after staining in crystal violet.

SOLUTIONS

1. Saturated alcohol crystal violet stock
   Dissolve 14.0 g of crystal violet in 100 ml of 95% alcohol.
2. Crystal violet staining solution

hydrochloric acid (concentrated)	1 ml
saturated crystal violet alcoholic stock (filtered)	10 ml
distilled water	300 ml

Combine and mix the above ingredients. Make fresh every day.

REFERENCE

Lieb, Ethel, Permanent Stain for Amyloid. Am. J. Clin. Pathol., *17*, 413, 1947.

*A water plastic mount available from Valnor Corporation, 16 Clinton Street, Brooklyn, New York 11201.

Brown-and-Brenn Stain for Bacteria and Charcot-Leyden Crystals in Tissue

FIXATION

10% formalin, or Zenker's acetic acid fixative.

TECHNIC

Cut paraffin sections at 4 to 5 microns. Use a known control slide.

PROCEDURE

1. Deparaffinize the slides as for the H-and-E stain (see p. 224). If Zenker's fixative is used, remove the mercuric chloride crystals (see p. 216).
2. Place the slides in 1% crystal violet staining solution for 1 minute and agitate.
3. Rinse in 2 changes of distilled water.
4. Rinse with Gram's iodine solution for 1 minute.
5. Rinse in distilled water, then blot with filter paper to complete dryness.
6. Decolorize the slides with a mixture of equal parts of ether and acetone until no more blue color runs off.
7. Stain with 0.1% basic fuchsin solution for 1 minute.
8. Wash in distilled water. Blot gently, but not completely dry.
9. Dip the slides in acetone to start reaction.
10. Differentiate immediately with 0.1% picric acid-acetone solution until the sections are yellowish pink. (Decolorize more for Charcot-Leyden crystals.)
11. Dehydrate in acetone and acetone xylol.
12. Clear in several changes of xylol and mount.

RESULTS

1. Gram-negative bacteria: red.
2. Gram-positive bacteria: blue.
3. Nuclei: red.
4. Charcot-Leyden crystals: pink.
5. Other tissue elements: yellow.

NOTES

1. If the stain is spotty, repeat and blot slide thoroughly.

SOLUTIONS

1. Crystal violet stock solution (1%)
   Dissolve 1 g of crystal violet in 100 ml of distilled water. Filter before use.
2. Sodium bicarbonate stock solution (5%)
   Dissolve 5 g of sodium bicarbonate in 100 ml of distilled water.

3. Crystal violet staining solution
   Combine 40 ml of 1% crystal violet stock solution with 10 ml of 5% sodium carbonate stock solution. Filter and mix just before use.
4. Gram's iodine solution
   Dissolve 1 g of iodine and 2 g of potassium iodide in 300 ml of distilled water.
5. Basic fuchsin solution (0.1%)
   Dissolve 0.5 g of basic fuchsin in 500 ml of distilled water.
6. Picric acid acetone (0.1%)
   Dissolve 0.1 g of picric acid in 100 ml of acetone C.P. Keep covered.

REFERENCE

Brown, J. H., and Brenn, L., Method for Differential Staining of Gram-Positive and Gram-Negative Bacteria in Tissue Sections. Bull. Johns Hopkins Hosp., *48*, 69, 1931. (Modified by Haskell.)

Gridley Fungus Stain (Modified)

FIXATION

10% formalin or any other fixative may be used.

TECHNIC

Cut paraffin sections at 15 microns. Use a known control slide.

PROCEDURE

1. Deparaffinize the slides as for the H-and-E stain (see p. 224).
2. Place the slides in fresh 4% chromic acid for 1 hour.
3. Wash in tap water for 5 minutes.
4. Place in Schiff's reagent for 15 minutes.
5. Rinse in 3 changes of 0.5% sodium bisulfite (1 minute in each).
6. Wash in tap water for 15 minutes.
7. Stain the slides in Gomori's aldehyde fuchsin for 15 minutes.
8. Rinse in 95% alcohol to remove excess stain.
9. Wash well in tap water.
10. Counterstain for 2 to 5 minutes with metanil yellow solution. Control background staining with a microscope.
11. Wash in water, then dehydrate in 95% alcohol and in absolute alcohol.
12. Clear in xylol and mount.

RESULTS

1. Mycelia: deep purple.
2. Conidia: deep rose to purple.
3. Background: yellow.
4. Elastic tissue and mucin: deep purple.

SOLUTIONS

1. Chromic acid (4%)

   Dissolve 4.0 g of chromic acid in 100 ml of distilled water. This solution oxidizes with time. Keep for approximately 2 weeks.

2. Schiff's reagent solution

basic fuchsin	4.0 g
sodium *m*-bisulfite ($Na_2S_2O_5$)	7.6 g
1*N* hydrochloric acid	60 ml
distilled water	340 ml

Shake well for 3 to 6 hours on a mechanical shaker. Add 2 to 3 g of fresh animal charcoal. Shake for 2 minutes more, then filter. The solution should be straw color; if not, make original volume by washing filter paper with distilled water. The solution will be lighter in color the following day. Keep the solution in a refrigerator when not in use.

3. Sodium bisulfite (0.5%)
   Dissolve 5.0 g of sodium bisulfite ($NaHSO_3$) in 1000 ml of distilled water.
4. Gomori's aldehyde fuchsin solution

alcohol, 65%	100.0 ml
basic fuchsin	0.5 g
concentrated hydrochloric acid	1.0 ml
paraldehyde U.S.P. (fresh)	1.0 ml

   The stain is usually ready for use at room temperature in 24 to 48 hours. It changes to a deep purple, similar to the shade of gentian violet. This solution keeps about 2 to 4 weeks or longer in a refrigerator.
5. Metanil yellow stock solution (1%)
   Dissolve 1.0 g of metanil yellow in 100 ml of distilled water.
6. Metanil yellow staining solution
   Dilute 1.5 ml of metanil yellow stock solution in 250 ml of distilled water, adding 0.75 ml of glacial acetic acid. Both stock and staining solution keep well.

NOTES

1. 5% chromic acid can be used in place of 4% chromic acid. It is an oxidizer.
2. Animal charcoal should be purchased once a year to be effective.
3. Gomori's aldehyde fuchsin solution intensifies the fungi (check elastic-staining around vessels for intensity of stain).
4. The metanil yellow is used for background staining only. Its intensity depends on the preference of the pathologist.
5. Use fresh sodium bisulfite solution, so that the red color of the fungi will be distinct under the microscope.

REFERENCE

Gridley, M. F., Stain for Fungi in Tissue Sections. Am. J. Clin. Pathol., *23*, 303, 1953.

Hematoxylin-and-Eosin Stain

TECHNIC

Cut paraffin sections at 5 to 6 microns. Paraffin slides must be oven-dried at 50 to 56°C for at least 20 minutes before deparaffinizing for staining.

PROCEDURE

Deparaffinizing of Slide

1. Xylol I: 4 minutes.
2. Xylol II: 3 minutes. Drain well.
3. Absolute alcohol: 2 minutes.
4. 95% alcohol: 2 minutes.
5. Wash in running water for 1 minute, then rinse in distilled water. Drain well.

Staining

1. Place the slides in Harris' hematoxylin solution for 3 to 5 minutes (the time factor for each batch of stain must be determined by trial). Drain well.
2. Rinse in distilled water.
3. Quickly dip the slides in and out of 0.5% aqueous hydrochloric acid solution.
4. Wash in running water for 1 minute.
5. Place the slides in dilute ammonia water for 1 minute.
6. Wash in running water for 1 minute, then transfer to distilled water.
7. Spot-check the staining microscopically. The nuclei should be dark purple in color and should also be clearly visible. Keep the slides wet during checking. Drain. If the nuclei are not dark enough, rinse the slides in distilled water, replace in Harris' hematoxylin, and repeat steps 2 through 5.
8. Rinse in 95% alcohol.
9. Agitate in eosin staining solution for 10 seconds, then drain for 5 seconds.
10. Rinse in 95% alcohol, using 2 changes of alcohol, 6 times each.
11. Rinse in absolute alcohol, using 2 changes of alcohol, 6 times each.
12. Place the slides in carbol xylol solution for 45 seconds (optional). Use only when absolute alcohol is not available.
13. Rinse in 2 changes of xylol for 2 minutes.
14. Mount with a cover glass. The nuclei should be dark purple, and the cytoplasm should be pink.

NOTES

1. Change xylols twice weekly.
2. Change alcohols when they appear saturated with stain.
3. Slides can be stained longer, if necessary, in Harris' hematoxylin. Decalcified tissue may take 15 minutes to stain with Harris' hematoxylin.
4. Intensity of routine stain should be checked with the pathologist, so that routine staining can be standardized.
5. The AFIP procedure calls for acid alcohol rather than aqueous hydrochloric acid. If this reagent is used, care must be taken not to overtreat.

SOLUTIONS

1. Harris' hematoxylin

hematoxylin	5.0 g
alcohol, 95%	50.0 g
alum (ammonium or potassium)	100.0 g
distilled water	1000.0 ml
mercuric oxide, red, powder	2.5 g

Dissolve the hematoxylin in absolute alcohol. Dissolve the alum in water with the aid of heat, then add the alcoholic solution of the dye. Bring the mixture to a rapid boil, then add the mercuric oxide. The solution assumes at once a dark-purple color, and as soon as this occurs, cool it by plunging the flask into ice-cold water. For use, add glacial acetic acid to make a 4% solution. Filter daily and keep in a refrigerator.

2. Dilute aqueous hydrochloric acid solution (0.5%)

Dilute 5.0 ml of concentrated hydrochloric acid with 100 ml of distilled water.

3. Dilute ammonia water

Dilute 3.0 ml of 28% ammonia with 1000 ml of distilled water.

4. Eosin staining solution for formalin-fixed tissues

eosin Y, water-soluble	2.0 g
distilled water	160.0 ml
alcohol, 95%	640.0 ml
glacial acetic acid	0.8 ml

Keep the staining dish covered to prevent evaporation of the alcohol.

5. Carbol xylol solution (optional)

carbolic acid crystals (phenol)	200 ml
xylol	600 ml

Melt the carbolic acid crystals by placing the bottle in a paraffin oven. Measure the quantity in a graduated cylinder, then add xylol. Exercise care in its use.

REFERENCE

Manual of Histologic and Special Staining Technics. Armed Forces Institute of Pathology, Washington, D.C., 1957.

Iron Stain

FIXATION

10% formalin, or Zenker's acetic acid fixative.

TECHNIC

Cut paraffin sections at 5 to 6 microns. Use a known control slide.

PROCEDURE

1. Deparaffinize the sections as for the H-and-E stain (see p. 224). If Zenker's fixative is used, remove the mercuric chloride crystals (see p. 216).
2. Place the sections in distilled water.
3. Heat the iron-staining solution in a beaker to 60°C. Do not overheat.
4. Pour the solution immediately over the slides. Reaction takes place within 2 minutes; do not leave the slides in the solution any longer, for they may show a false reaction.
5. Wash the slides thoroughly in 4 changes of distilled water.
6. Counterstain quickly in filtered phloxine B solution (in and out).
7. Dehydrate the slides in 95% alcohol.
8. Dehydrate the slides in absolute alcohol.
9. Clear the slides in 2 changes of xylol.
10. Mount the slides in the usual manner.

RESULTS

1. Iron: blue.
2. Cytoplasm: red.

NOTES

1. All glassware must be chemically clean.
2. False reactions result in background staining all blue in color.

SOLUTION

1. Iron-staining solution

   Combine 10 ml of a 2% aqueous solution of potassium ferrocyanide with 30 ml of a 1% aqueous solution of hydrochloric acid. Mix fresh each time.
2. Phloxine B solution (0.5%)

   Dissolve 0.5 g of phloxine B in 100 ml of distilled water.

REFERENCE

Pathological Technic Manual, p. 67 (modified). U.S. Naval Medical School, National Naval Medical Center, Bethesda, Maryland.

Luxol Fast Blue-Periodic Acid Schiff Stain (Myelin-Stain)

FIXATIVE

10% formalin.

TECHNIC

Celloidin, paraffin, or frozen sections. Cut paraffin sections at 15 microns. Use a known control slide.

PROCEDURE

1. Deparaffinize the slides to absolute alcohol as in the H-and-E procedure (see p. 224).
2. Place the slides for 5 minutes in 1% parlodion in a covered Coplin jar. Air-dry quickly, then place them for 10 minutes in 80% alcohol (to harden the parlodion) and then into water.
3. Quickly dip the slides in and out of 95% alcohol.
4. Place the slides in luxol fast blue solution, cover the container, and keep overnight in an oven at 60°C.
5. Next day, rinse off the excess stain in 95% alcohol.
6. Rinse the slides in distilled water.
7. Place the slides for approximately 25 seconds in 0.05% lithium carbonate.
8. Differentiate the slides in 70% alcohol. Do not overdecolorize the myelin, which is blue, while the background is white.
9. Rinse the slides in distilled water.
10. If necessary, place the slides for 25 seconds in a fresh solution of 0.05% lithium carbonate.
11. Differentiate the slides in 70% alcohol. If needed, repeat steps 9, 10 and 11 until contrast is complete.
12. Rinse the slides 3 times in distilled water.
13. Place the slides for 10 minutes in periodic acid solution.
14. Rinse the slides for 5 minutes in running tap water.
15. Place the slides for 10 minutes in Schiff's solution.
16. Place the slides in 3 changes of 0.5% sodium bisulfite, 2 minutes in each change.
17. Wash the slides for 5 minutes in running tap water.
18. Stain the slides with Harris' hematoxylin, using the same timing as for routine staining.
19. Rinse the slides in distilled water.
20. Dip the slides quickly in hydrochloric acid solution for decolorizing excess hematoxylin.
21. Rinse well with tap water.
22. Blue the slides in ammonia water.
23. Rinse the slides several times in tap water.
24. Dehydrate the slides in 2 changes of 95% alcohol and 2 changes of absolute alcohol. (Parlodion will be completely dissolved in the dehydration.)

25. Clear the slides in 2 changes of xylol.
26. Mount in the usual manner.

RESULTS

1. Myelin: blue.
2. Neuroglia: purple.
3. Nuclei: blue.

NOTES

1. Parlodion is used to hold the sections on the slide. Care must be exercised to avoid a parlodion coating that is too thick, because the stain may not penetrate evenly.
2. The luxol fast blue stain is affected by the 60°C temperature and should be discarded after one use.
3. Spot-check the slides microscopically after steps 9, 10, and 11 of the procedure. The slides may all be differentiated and allowed to stand in water before continuing with the procedure.
4. The hematoxylin stain is optional.
5. Allow additional time for dehydration and clearing of slides, since the sections are thicker than usual.

SOLUTIONS

1. Parlodion solution (1%)

luxol fast blue	1 g
alcohol, 95%	1000 ml
acetic acid, 10%	5 ml
ether, U.S.P.	50 ml

Dissolve thoroughly (takes 2 to 3 days). Keep in a well-stoppered bottle. May be used repeatedly; if used more than once, it will need to be thinned with a small amount of the ether-alcohol mixture.

2. Luxol fast blue solution (0.1%)
Dissolve 1.0 g of luxol fast blue in 1000 ml of 95% alcohol, then add 5.0 ml of 10% acetic acid. The solution keeps for 2 months.
3. Lithium carbonate (0.05%)
Dissolve 0.5 g of lithium carbonate in 1000 ml of distilled water. This solution keeps well.
4. Periodic acid in dilute nitric acid

potassium *m*-periodate (KIO_4 crystals)	6.9 g
nitric acid, concentrated	3.0 ml
distilled water	1000.0 ml

Combine the potassium *m*-periodate and nitric acid (all should dissolve). Add water and mix. Keeps well at room temperature.

5. Schiff's reagent solution

basic fuchsin	4.0 g
sodium *m*-bisulfite ($Na_2S_2O_5$)	7.6 g
1*N* hydrochloric acid	60.0 ml
distilled water	340.0 ml

Combine the above ingredients and shake well for 3 to 6 hours in a mechanical shaker. Add 2 to 3 g of fresh animal charcoal. Shake for 2 minutes more, then filter the solution. The solution should be straw color; if not, make up to original volumc by washing the edges of the filter paper with distilled water. The solution will be lighter in color the following day. Keep under refrigeration when not in use. The solution may be reused until a cloudy precipitate forms.

6. Sodium bisulfite (0.5%)

   Dissolve 5.0 g of sodium bisulfite (Na_2HSO_3) in 1000 ml of distilled water. Make up fresh each week.

REFERENCE

Margolis, G., and Pickert, J. P., New Applications of Luxol Fast Blue Myelin Stain. Lab. Invest., *5*, 459, 1956.

Masson Trichrome Stain (Modified)

FIXATION

For best results, use Zenker's acetic acid fixative. 10% formalin may be used.

TECHNIC

Cut paraffin sections at 5 microns. Use liver or testes control.

PROCEDURE

1. Deparaffinize the slides as for the H-and-E stain (see p. 224).
2. Stain for 5 minutes in Weigert's iron hematoxylin.
3. Wash the slides for 5 minutes in running water (check nuclei under a microscope).
4. Transfer the slides for 1 minute to 1% aqueous acetic acid solution.
5. Place the slides for 15 seconds in picric acid stain (5 seconds for testes).
6. Place the slides for 1 minute in 1% aqueous acetic acid solution, using 2 changes.
7. Place the slides for 60 seconds in Ponceau acid fuchsin stain (6 seconds for testes).
8. Place the slides for 2 minutes in 1% aqueous acetic acid solution, using 2 changes.
9. Place the slides for 1½ minutes in 2% aqueous phosphotungstic acid solution.
10. Transfer the slides for 2 minutes to 1% aqueous acetic acid solution.
11. Transfer the slides for 1½ minutes to fast green staining solution.
12. Rinse quickly in 1% aqueous acetic acid solution.
13. Dehydrate quickly in 2 changes of absolute alcohol.
14. Clear in xylol.
15. Mount in the usual manner.

Treatment of Formalin-Fixed Tissue (Optional)

1. Place the mordant slides for 10 minutes in 5% potassium dichromate.
2. Wash for 10 minutes in running water.

RESULTS

1. Collagen: green.
2. Nuclei: brown to black.
3. Cytoplasm and neuroglia fibrils: pink to reddish brown.
4. Blood cells: yellow.

NOTES

1. Nuclei should be stained well; background is usually gray in color.
2. The 1% acetic acid solution is used before each stain to intensify that particular dye.
3. Timing is short in the red and green stain, and the slides should therefore be agitated.
4. Dehydrate the slides in the absolute alcohol quickly to prevent fading of the fast

green stain, then clear in xylol. If the slide is not clear, return it quickly to absolute alcohol for another rinse.

5. The staining solutions other than Weigert's hematoxylin should be changed after approximately 15 slides have been stained.
6. The picric acid staining solution is made up fresh every day.
7. Keep the staining jars covered.

SOLUTIONS

1. Acetic acid solution (1%)
   Dilute 10 ml of glacial acetic acid with 990 ml of distilled water.
2. Weigert's iron hematoxylin

   Solution A:

hematoxylin	4 g
alcohol, 95%	400 ml

   Solution B:

ferric chloride (29% aq. sol.)	16 ml
distilled water	380 ml
hydrochloric acid (concentrated)	4 ml

   Use equal portions of solution A and B and filter. Can be used for 2 days.
3. Saturated picric acid stock solution
   Dissolve 9 g of picric acid in 100 ml of 95% alcohol. Keep covered when not in use.
4. Picric acid staining solution
   Add 15 ml of 95% alcohol to 35 ml of the saturated picric acid stock solution. Keep covered when not in use.
5. Ponceau fuchsin stock solution
   Dissolve 0.75 g of Ponceau xylidin and 0.25 g of acid fuchsin in 100 ml of 1% acetic acid.
6. Azo phloxin stock solution
   Dissolve 0.5 g of azo phloxin in 100 ml of 1% acetic acid.
7. Ponceau acid fuchsin stain
   Add 10 ml of Ponceau fuchsin stock solution and 2 ml of azo phloxin stock solution to 88 ml of 1% acetic acid. Make up fresh every week.
8. Phosphotungstic acid solution (2%)
   Dissolve 2.0 g of phosphotungstic acid in 100 ml of distilled water.
9. Fast green
   Dissolve 0.2 g of fast green FCF in 100 ml of 1% acetic acid.
10. Potassium dichromate solution (5%)
    Dissolve 5.0 g of potassium dichromate in 100 ml of distilled water.

REFERENCES

Masson, P., Some Histological Methods: Trichrome Stainings and Their Preliminary Technique. J. Technol. Methods, *12*, 75, 1939.

McManus, J. F. A., and Mowry, R. W., Staining Methods: Histologic and Histochemical, p. 234. Hoeber Medical Division, Harper and Row, New York, 1960.

Mayer's Mucicarmine Stain for Epithelial Mucin

FIXATION

10% formalin or any other fixative may be used.

TECHNIC

Cut paraffin sections at 5 to 6 microns. Use a known control slide.

PROCEDURE

1. Deparaffinize the sections as for the H-and-E stain (see p. 224). If Zenker's fixative is used, remove the mercuric chloride crystals (see p. 216).
2. Stain for 7 minutes in a working solution of Weigert's hematoxylin.
3. Wash the slides for 5 to 10 minutes in tap water.
4. Place the slides in diluted mucicarmine solution for 30 to 60 minutes or longer. Check the control slide under a microscope after 30 minutes.
5. Rinse quickly in distilled water.
6. Stain for 1 minute in metanil yellow solution.
7. Rinse quickly in 95% alcohol.
8. Dehydrate in 2 changes of absolute alcohol.
9. Quickly clear with 2 to 3 changes of xylol.
10. Mount in the usual manner.

RESULTS

1. Mucin: deep rose to red.
2. Nuclei: black.
3. Other tissue elements: yellow.

NOTES

1. If the control slide stains light in the carmine solution after rinsing quickly in distilled water, try rinsing the slides in 70% alcohol instead.
2. Formalin-fixed tissue usually stains lighter in color.

SOLUTIONS

1. Weigert's iron hematoxylin

Solution A:

hematoxylin	1 g
95% alcohol	100 ml

Solution B:

ferric chloride (29% aq. sol.)	4 ml
distilled water	95 ml
hydrochloric acid (concentrated)	1 ml

Mix equal portions of solutions A and B and filter. Prepare fresh each day.

2. Metanil yellow solution

   Dissolve 0.25 g of metanil yellow in 100 ml of distilled water and add 0.25 ml of glacial acetic acid.

3. Mucicarmine stain

carmine	1.0 g
aluminum chloride, anhydrous	0.5 g
distilled water	2.0 ml
alcohol, 50%	100.0 ml

   Mix the carmine, aluminum chloride and distilled water in a small beaker, then heat carefully for 2 minutes; the liquid becomes syrupy and almost black. Dilute with the alcohol and let the mixture stand for 24 hours. Filter. For use, dilute with tap water 1:3. This solution keeps for 1 week in a refrigerator.

REFERENCE

Mallory, F. B., Pathological Technic, p. 130. W. B. Saunders, Philadelphia, 1942.

Papanicolaou Technic for Smears (Modified)

FIXATION

1. Prepare Carnoy's fixative as follows:

alcohol, 95%	97 ml
glacial acetic acid, C.P.	3 ml

2. Place the fresh wet smears immediately into a bottle of Carnoy's fixative for 15 minutes or longer. Label with a diamond-point pencil.

PROCEDURE

1. Rinse in 95% alcohol.
2. Rinse in 80% alcohol.
3. Rinse in distilled water.
4. Stain in half-strength Harris' hematoxylin solution (dilute 200 ml of the staining solution with 200 ml of distilled water). Check timing with each batch of this stain.
5. Rinse in tap water.
6. Agitate quickly in 0.5% aqueous hydrochloric acid solution.
7. Rinse in tap water.
8. Agitate in dilute ammonia water until blue.
9. Rinse in tap water, then in distilled water.
10. Check the staining microscopically.
11. Rinse in 80% alcohol.
12. Rinse in 95% alcohol.
13. Stain for 1 minute and 45 seconds in orange G-6* solution.
14. Rinse in 2 changes of 95% alcohol.
15. Stain for 1 minute and 45 seconds in eosin A-56*.
16. Rinse in 2 changes of 95% alcohol.
17. Rinse quickly in absolute alcohol.
18. Clear in xylol.
19. Mount from xylol, using Permount® slide mounting medium†.

NOTES

1. Both staining solutions should be changed when the colors fade.
2. The fast green in the eosin A-56 solution fades quickly.

SOLUTIONS

1. Harris' hematoxylin

hematoxylin	5.0 g
absolute alcohol	50.0 ml

*Available in 450-cc quantities from Ortho Pharmaceutical Corporation, Raritan, New Jersey, or in 1-gallon containers from Hartman-Leddon Company, Philadelphia, Pennsylvania. Staining qualities of the products from one source are compatible with those obtained from the other.

†Available from Fisher Scientific Co., Pittsburgh, Pennsylvania.

alum (ammonium or potassium)	100.0 g
distilled water	1000.0 ml
mercuric oxide, red, powder	2.5 g

Dissolve the hematoxylin in the absolute alcohol. Dissolve the alum in water with the aid of heat. Add the alcoholic solution of the dye. Bring the mixture to a rapid boil and add the mercuric oxide. The solution at once assumes a dark-purple color, and as soon as this occurs, cool it by plunging the flask into ice-cold water.

2. Dilute ammonia water

Dilute 12 ml of 28% ammonia with 1000 ml of distilled water.

3. Orange G-6 working solution

orange G	2.5 g
water	25.0 ml
ethyl alcohol	475.0 ml
phosphotungstic acid	0.125 g

Dissolve the orange G in the water with the aid of gentle heat.

4. Light-green stock solution

light green	1.25 g
water	25.0 ml
ethyl alcohol	475.0 ml

5. Eosin stock solution

eosin	2.5 g
water	25.0 ml
ethyl alcohol	475.0 ml

Dissolve the eosin in the water by using heat, then add alcohol.

6. Bismarck brown stock solution

Bismark brown	2.5 g
water	25.0 ml
ethyl alcohol	475.0 ml

Dissolvc the Bismarck brown in the water with the aid of gentle heat, then add alcohol.

7. Eosin A-56 working solution

light-green stock solution	225 ml
Bismarck brown stock solution	50 ml
eosin stock solution	225 ml
phosphotungstic acid	1 g
glacial acetic acid	1 ml

Combine the above ingredients and store at room temperature. Do not filter. Stock solution need not stand; it may be used immediately.

REFERENCE

Papanicolaou, G. M., Atlas of Exfoliative Cytology. Commonwealth Fund, Harvard University Press, Cambridge, Massachusetts, 1954.

Periodic Acid Schiff Stain

FIXATION

Zenker's acetic acid fixative is preferred, but any fixative may be used.

TECHNIC

Cut paraffin sections at 5 to 6 microns. Use a control slide with each fresh mixture of Schiff's reagent.

PROCEDURE

1. Deparaffinize the slides as for the H-and-E stain (see p. 224). If Zenker's fixative is used, remove the mercuric chloride crystals (see p. 216).
2. Stain the slides for 10 minutes in periodic acid solution.
3. Wash the slides for 5 minutes in running water.
4. Rinse well twice with distilled water.
5. Stain the slides for 10 minutes in Schiff's reagent. Agitate 2 or 3 times.
6. Place the slides in 3 changes of 0.5% sodium bisulfite, 2 minutes each change.
7. Wash the slides for 10 minutes in slightly warm running tap water.
8. Stain the slides in Harris' hematoxylin, using the same timing as for routine hematoxylin-eosin staining.
9. Rinse thoroughly in water for approximately 2 minutes.
10. Decolorize in 0.5% aqueous solution of hydrochloric acid.
11. Rinse in tap water, then blue in ammonia.
12. Wash the slides for 2 minutes in running water.
13. Dehydrate in 2 changes of 95% alcohol, then in 2 changes of absolute alcohol.
14. Clear in 2 changes of xylol.
15. Mount in the usual manner.

RESULTS

1. Basement membranes, glycogen, mucin, and mast cells: red.
2. Nuclei: blue.

NOTES

1. The Schiff reaction color will gradually fade from red to pink. When this is the case, change the solution.
2. The color reaction depends on the amount of reactive glycol structure present in the tissue.
3. When staining specifically for glycogen, use the digested PAS stain and a known liver control slide.
4. When staining for mast cells, use a known mast cell control slide.

SOLUTIONS

1. Periodic acid in dilute nitric acid

potassium *m*-periodate (KIO_4) crystals	6.9 g
nitric acid, concentrated	3.0 ml
distilled water	1000.0 ml

Mix the potassium *m*-periodate and nitric acid together until all crystals dissolve, then add water and mix. This solution keeps well at room temperature.

2. Schiff's reagent solution

basic fuchsin	4.0 g
sodium *m*-bisulfite ($Na_2S_2O_5$)	7.6 g
1*N* hydrochloric acid	60.0 ml
distilled water	340.0 ml

Combine and shake the above ingredients well for 3 to 6 hours on a mechanical shaker. Add 2 to 3 g of fresh animal charcoal and shake for 2 minutes more. Filter. The solution should be straw color. If not, make the original volume by washing the filter paper with distilled water. The solution will be lighter in color the following day. Keep under refrigeration when not in use. The solution may be reused until a cloudy precipitate forms.

3. Sodium bisulfite solution (0.5%)
   Dissolve 5 g of sodium bisulfite ($NaHSO_3$) in 1000 ml of distilled water. Make up fresh each week.

REFERENCES

Lillie, R. D., Histopathologic Technic and Practical Histochemistry, 3rd ed. McGraw-Hill, New York, 1965.

McManus, J. F. A., and Mowry, R. W., Staining Methods: Histologic and Histochemical. Hoeber Medical Division, Harper and Row, New York, 1960.

Periodic Acid Schiff Stain, Digested, for Glycogen

FIXATION

10% formalin or any other fixative may be used.

TECHNIC

Paraffin cut at 5 to 6 microns. Use two liver control slides: one for regular staining of glycogen, and one for digestion of glycogen.

PROCEDURE

1. Deparaffinize the slides as for the H-and-E stain (see p. 224). If Zenker's fixative is used, remove the mercuric chloride crystals (see p. 216).
2. Use two sets of slides: one for digestion and one for regular PAS.
3. For staining digested tissue slides,
   (a) take the slides down to distilled water;
   (b) place them for 1 hour in a preheated diastase solution in a 37°C incubator;
   (c) wash in tap water to remove all traces of diastase solution.
4. Proceed to stain both sets of slides, using the periodic acid Schiff staining technic (see p. 236).

RESULTS

1. Digested control and unknown slides: colorless to light pink.
2. Glycogen, regular control and unknown slides: red.
3 Mucin, regular and digested slides: red.
4. Nuclei: blue.

NOTES

1. Care must be taken in handling the digested slides, because the tissue has a tendency to come off after digestion.
2. The liver control should contain an abundant amount of glycogen.

SOLUTIONS

1. Diastase solution

   Dissolve 0.5 g of malt diastase in 100 ml of normal saline. Do not filter. The unused portion may be kept in a refrigerator for 24 hours.

REFERENCE

Lillie, R. D., Histopathologic Technic and Practical Histochemistry, 3rd ed. McGraw-Hill, New York, 1965.

Propylene Glycol-Sudan Method for Lipids

FIXATION

10% formalin.

TECHNIC

Cut frozen sections at 10 to 15 microns.

PROCEDURE

1. Wash the cut frozen sections well to remove the formalin.
2. Mount the sections on albuminized slides and dry them at room temperature.
3. Transfer them for 5 to 7 minutes to the staining solution. Agitate occasionally throughout this period.
4. Transfer the slides for 2 to 3 minutes to 85% propylene glycol and agitate.
5. Transfer the slides for 2 to 3 minutes to 50% propylene glycol.
6. Wash gently for 1 minute in warm running water.
7. Counterstain in Harris' hematoxylin as for routine staining (decolorize in acid and blue in ammonia).
8. Mount in glycerine gelatine mounting medium.

RESULTS

1. Lipids: red if using Sudan IV, black if using Sudan black B.

NOTES

1. Thorough rinsing in propylene glycol after removal from the dye is necessary for even staining and may require up to 10 minutes in steps 4 and 5.

SOLUTIONS

1. Sudan IV or Sudan black B dye solution

Sudan IV	0.7 g, or
Sudan black B	0.7 g, or
oil red O	0.7 g
propylene glycol, pure	100.0 ml

Dissolve the dye in propylene glycol by heating to 100°C and stirring for a few minutes. Filter through Whatman #2 filter paper. Cool to room temperature and filter through a thin film of glass wool by means of a suction filter. The dye solution keeps well at room temperature, but must be filtered before each use.

2. Glycerine gelatin mounting medium

gelatin	15 g
distilled water	70 ml
glycerine	15 ml

Heat the distilled water and add the gelatin. Continue heating to dissolve the gelatin, then add the glycerine and a small crystal of thymol. Keep the medium refrigerated. For use, melt in a hot water bath.

REFERENCE

Pearse, A. G., Histochemistry: Theoretical and Applied, 2nd ed., p. 855. J. and A. Churchill, Ltd., London, England, 1960.

Reticulin Stain

Method of Bielschowsky, Modified by Foot

FIXATION

10% formalin or any other fixative may be used, but Zenker's acetic acid fixative gives especially good results.

TECHNIC

Cut paraffin sections at 5 to 6 microns. Use a known control slide.

PROCEDURE

1. Deparaffinize the slides as for the H-and-E stain (see p. 224). If Zenker's fixative is used, remove the mercuric chloride crystals (see p. 216).
2. Wash for 2 minutes in tap water.
3. Treat the section for 5 minutes with 0.25% aqueous solution of potassium permanganate.
4. Rinse in tap water.
5. Place the sections for 15 to 30 minutes in 5% aqueous solution of oxalic acid to bleach the tissue.
6. Wash for 2 minutes in tap water.
7. Rinse 3 times in distilled water.
8. Leave the sections for 48 hours in 2% aqueous silver nitrate in subdued light, but not in the dark.
9. Wash for a short time in 2 changes of distilled water.
10. Place the slides for 30 minutes in ammoniacal silver solution.
11. Rinse very quickly in distilled water.
12. Reduce for 30 minutes in 5% neutral formalin solution. It is well to change the solution after the first 10 to 15 minutes.
13. Rinse several times in tap water, then twice in distilled water.
14. Tone for 1 hour in 1% aqueous gold chloride.
15. Rinse 3 times in tap water.
16. Remove excess silver by treating the sections for 2 minutes with 5% aqueous solution of sodium thiosulfate.
17. Wash thoroughly for 5 minutes in running tap water.
18. Dehydrate in 95% and in absolute alcohol.
19. Clear in xylol.
20. Mount, using a spray medium.

RESULTS

1. Coarse collagenous fibrils: red to rose.
2. Finer fibrils: black to dark violet.
3. Nuclei: black, blue to brown.

NOTES

1. Use chemically clean glassware for the silver solution. including staining jars.
2. Use fresh potassium permanganate solution.
3. Be accurate in making all solutions.
4. Stain the control slide first for the test run.
5. Since silver stains are unpredictable, it may be necessary to repeat the test. The trouble is due to the way in which the ammoniacal silver solution is made. Silver solutions should be made up each day from fresh stock solutions. 2% silver nitrate solutions can be made from the 10% silver nitrate solution by mixing 2 ml of the 10% solution with 8 ml of distilled water.
6. Be sure that the 30—40% formaldehyde stock is not too old; it becomes acid with age.

SOLUTIONS

1. Potassium permanganate solution

   Dissolve 0.25 g of potassium permanganate in 100 ml of distilled water.
2. Oxalic acid solution (5%)

   Dissolve 5.0 g of oxalic acid in 100 ml of distilled water.
3. Silver nitrate solution (2%)

   Dissolve 2.0 g of silver nitrate crystals, C.P., in 100 ml of distilled water.
4. Silver nitrate solution (10%)

   Dissolve 5.0 g of silver nitrate crystals, C.P., in 50 ml of distilled water.
5. Sodium hydroxide (40%)

   Dissolve 20 g of sodium hydroxide pellets, C.P., in 50 ml of distilled water. Weigh the sodium hydroxide pellets on a watch glass. Gradually add the pellets to the distilled water. The solution is very caustic, and care must be exercised in its preparation.
6. Neutral formalin solution (5%)

   Dilute 5.0 ml of 37—40% neutral formaldehyde with 95 ml of distilled water.
7. Gold chloride solution

   Dissolve 1.0 g of gold chloride in 100 ml of distilled water. Store in a dark bottle. The solution keeps indefinitely. When dirty, it may be filtered and reused.
8. Sodium thiosulfate solution (5%)

   Dissolve 5.0 g of sodium thiosulfate, U.S.P., in 100 ml of distilled water.
9. Ammoniacal silver hydroxide solution

   Using a medicine dropper, add 20 drops of 40% aqueous sodium hydroxide to 20 ml of 10% aqueous silver nitrate. Dissolve the brownish precipitate with about 2 ml of 28% ammonia (leave two particles of precipitate undissolved for best results). Filter into a chemically clean Coplin jar, then add distilled water to 80 ml and filter again.

REFERENCE

Mallory, F. B., Pathological Technique, p. 161. W. B. Saunders, Philadelphia, 1942.

Toluidine Blue Stain, Buffered (pH 4.85), for Connective-Tissue Mucin and Mast Cells

FIXATION

10% formalin, or Zenker's acetic acid fixative.

TECHNIC

Cut paraffin sections at 5 to 6 microns. Use a known control slide.

PROCEDURE

1. Deparaffinize the slides as for the H-and-E stain (see p. 224). If Zenker's fixative is used, remove the mercuric chloride crystals (see p. 216).
2. Stain for 1 minute in toluidine blue buffered solution.
3. Blot the slides quickly with bibulous paper.
4. Dip the slides once into distilled water.
5. Dip the slides twice into 2 changes of 95% alcohol.
6. Dip the slides into 2 changes of absolute alcohol.
7. Rinse the slides in toluene.
8. Rinse the slides in 2 changes of xylol.
9. Mount in the usual manner.

RESULTS

1. Nuclei: blue.
2. Mast cell granules: red.
3. Connective-tissue mucin: purplish red.

NOTES

1. Formalin-fixed tissues stain lighter.

SOLUTIONS

1. Acetic acid stock solution (1/5*M*)

   Dilute 11.58 ml of glacial acetic acid with CO_2-free distilled water to 1 liter.
2. Sodium acetate stock solution (1/5*M*)

   Dissolve 27.21 g of sodium acetate and dilute to 1 liter with CO_2-free distilled water.
3. Buffered toluidine blue (pH 4.85)

toluidine blue (dye content approximately 67%)	2 g
acetic acid (1/5*M*)	70 ml
sodium acetate (1/5*M*)	130 ml

Combine the above ingredients and mix well. This solution does not need to be filtered and keeps well at room temperature for a long period of time. The stain may be used repeatedly until it becomes contaminated.

Van Gieson Stain

FIXATION

Any fixative may be used.

TECHNIC

Cut paraffin sections at 5 to 6 microns.

PROCEDURE

1. Deparaffinize the slides as for the H-and-E stain (see p. 224). If Zenker's fixative is used, remove the mercuric chloride crystals (see p. 216).
2. Stain the section in Harris' hematoxylin somewhat darker than in the routine H and E procedure. This may take 10 minutes.
3. Wash the sections in water.
4. Stain the sections for 5 minutes in Van Gieson (picrofuchsin) solution.
5. Dehydrate the sections quickly in 2 changes of 95% alcohol.
6. Clear the sections in 2 changes of xylol.
7. Mount in the usual manner.

RESULTS

1. Collagen: deep red.
2. Muscle: yellow.
3. Nuclei: brown.

NOTES

1. If the slides are rinsed too long in alcohol after the Van Gieson stain, the picric acid may disappear. In that case repeat the counterstain.

SOLUTIONS

1. Van Gieson (picrofuchsin) solution

acid fuchsin (1% aqueous)	5.0 ml
picric acid solution (sat. aq.)	95.0 ml
hydrochloric acid (concentrated)	0.25 ml

Combine and mix the above ingredients. Filter the solution each time before use. The solution keeps well.

REFERENCE

Lynch, M. J., Raphael, S. S., Meller, L. D., Spore, P. D., and Inwood, M. J. H., Medical Laboratory Technology and Clinical Pathology, 2nd ed. W. B. Saunders, Philadelphia, 1969.

Verhoeff's Elastic-Tissue Stain

FIXATION

10% formalin or any other fixative may be used.

TECHNIC

Cut paraffin sections at 5 to 6 microns. Use a control slide.

PROCEDURE

1. Deparaffinize the slides as for the H-and-E stain (see p. 224).
2. Transfer the slides into Verhoeff's iron hematoxylin and allow to stain for 1 hour.
3. Differentiate the slides directly in 2% aqueous solution of ferric chloride. Differentiation requires only a few minutes. Control differentiation under a microscope. If differentiation has been carried too far, the sections may be restained, provided they have not been treated with alcohol.
4. Wash the slides for 3 minutes in running water.
5. Place the slides for 5 minutes in 95% alcohol.
6. Wash the slides for 5 minutes in running water.
7. Counterstain for 10 seconds in Van Gieson solution.
8. Dehydrate in 2 changes of 95% alcohol.
9. Dehydrate in 2 changes of absolute alcohol.
10. Clear the slides in 2 changes of xylol.
11. Mount in the usual manner.

RESULTS

1. Elastic fibers: intensely blue to black.
2. Nuclei: blue to black.
3. Collagen: red.
4. Other tissue elements: yellow, if Van Gieson is used.

NOTES

1. Prolonged staining in Van Gieson counterstain will fade the iron hemoxatylin.
2. Slow dehydration will remove the picric acid.
3. Slightly overstain the elastic tissue, as the 95% alcohol removes the iodine from the elastic tissue and makes it appear lighter.

SOLUTIONS

1. Verhoeff's iron hematoxylin stock solution

   Dissolve 10 g of hematoxylin in 200 ml of absolute alcohol with the aid of gentle heat.
2. Ferric chloride solution (10%)

   Dissolve 10 g of ferric chloride in 100 ml of distilled water.

3. Iodine solution
   Add 2 g of iodine and 4 g of potassium iodide to 600 ml of distilled water.
4. Verhoeff's staining solution

hematoxylin stock solution	30 ml
10% ferric chloride solution	12 ml
iodine solution	12 ml

   Make up fresh from stock each day. Filter before use.
5. Ferric chloride solution (2%)
   Dissolve 2.0 g of ferric chloride, U.S.P. lump, in 100 ml of distilled water.
6. Acid fuchsin (1%)
   Dissolve 1 g of fuchsin in 100 ml of distilled water.
7. Picric acid solution (sat. aq.)
   Dissolve 1.22 g of picric acid in 100 ml of distilled water.
8. Modified Van Gieson (picrofuchsin) solution
   Dilute 5.0 ml of 1% acid fuchsin in 95 ml of saturated aqueous solution of picric acid. Filter before use. This solution keeps well.

REFERENCE

Mallory, F. B., Pathological Techniques, p. 170. W. B. Saunders, Philadelphia, 1942.

BACTERIOLOGY

Sectional Directory

Introduction

The bacteriological procedures presented here may be incomplete in that many time-honored procedures may have been omitted. However, an attempt has been made to include all of the commonly used test procedures that have clinical usefulness and that the clinical bacteriology laboratory might correctly be expected to be able to do. The procedures lay no claim to originality, but are subject to our own interpretation and modification in the light of our own experiences.

To be clinically useful, a procedure must be accurate, precise, rapid, and reasonable in respect to labor and cost. Any of these criteria may be sacrificed in some instances, but in general the best and most useful procedures attempt to abide by these limitations as closely as possible.

Thomas L. Gavan, M.D.

Initial Preparation of Specimens

Material for Examination	Specimen Required	Isolation Media	Incubation	Remarks
Blood	10 ml of whole blood; transfer immediately to isolation media. If an anticoagulant is required, use sodium polyethylene sulfonate (Liquoid) or heparin.	2 tubes or flasks of brain-heart infusion broth (30—50 ml). 1 tube or flask of thioglycollate medium (30—50 ml). If brucellosis is suspected, a Castaneda bottle.	35°C, aerobically; examine daily for 14 days for evidence of growth. If listeriosis is suspected, incubate 1 tube of brain-heart infusion at 4°C. Subculture weekly for 1 month. Incubate the Castaneda bottle at 35°C in 5—10% CO_2 or in a candle jar.	Subculture on blood agar and on chocolate agar plates; prepare Gram stains at 24 hours and at 14 days incubation. Hold cultures for *Brucella* for 30 days. Examine the agar slant for growth. If no growth is observed, tilt the bottle so that the blood broth flows over the agar surface. Repeat every 3 days.
Body fluids (except CSF)	Aliquot of fluid in a sterile container.	Blood agar plate. MacConkey's agar plate. Thioglycollate medium. Blood agar plate.	35°C, aerobically; incubate the blood agar plate in 5—10% CO_2 or in a candle jar. 35°C, anaerobically.	If fungi of acid-fast bacilli are suspected, inoculate Sabouraud's dextrose agar as well as Lowenstein-Jensen medium. Examine Gram and acid-fast stains. Joint fluid should be inoculated on chocolate agar and incubated at 35°C in 5—10% CO_2 or in a candle jar in addition to the media listed.
Bone marrow	Marrow aspirate.	Inoculate at bedside: blood agar plate, brain-heart infusion broth, thioglycollate medium. If fungi are suspected, 2 Sabouraud's agar slants and 2 brain-heart infusion agar slants. If tuberculosis is suspected, Lowenstein-Jensen medium.	35°C, aerobically, for 24 to 48 hours. 35°C and at room temperature, aerobically. 35°C, aerobically.	

Initial Preparation of Specimens (*cont.*)

Material for Examination	Specimen Required	Isolation Media	Incubation	Remarks
Bronchial aspirate	Bronchoscopic aspirate in a U-tube or in a sterile container.	Blood agar plate. MacConkey's agar plate. Thioglycollate medium. Blood agar plate.	35°C, aerobically; incubate the blood agar plate in 5—10% CO_2 or in a candle jar. 35°C, anaerobically.	If *Haemophilus* is suspected, inoculate in a chocolate agar plate; incubate in 5—10% CO_2 or in a candle jar. If fungi or acid-fast bacilli are suspected, inoculate Sabouraud's dextrose-chloramphenicol agar and Lowenstein-Jensen medium after decontamination (see p. 254).
Ear	Swab of exudate.	Blood agar plate. MacConkey's agar plate. Thioglycollate medium.	35°C, aerobically.	If fungi are suspected, inoculate Sabouraud's dextrose-chloramphenicol agar.
Eye	Swab of exudate.	Blood agar plate. Chocolate agar plate. MacConkey's agar plate. Thioglycollate medium.	35°C, aerobically: incubate the chocolate agar plate in 5—10% CO_2 or in a candle jar.	
Nasopharynx	Swab on a wire applicator.	Blood agar plate. Chocolate agar plate. Thioglycollate medium.	35°C, aerobically; incubate the chocolate agar and blood agar plates in 5—10% CO_2 or in a candle jar.	If pertussis is suspected, inoculate a freshly prepared Bordet-Gengou blood agar plate. If diphtheria is suspected, make a smear and stain with Loeffler's methylene blue (see p. 273); inoculate a Loeffler serum agar slant and a potassium-tellurite blood or chocolate agar plate.
Nose	Swab in a sterile container.	Blood agar plate. Thioglycollate medium.	35°C, aerobically; incubate the blood agar plate in 5—10% CO_2 or in a candle jar.	If only staphylococci are of importance for survey studies, inoculate a mannitol salt agar (MSA) plate.
Pus	Swab of exudate in a sterile container.	Blood agar plate. Thioglycollate medium. MacConkey's agar plate. Blood agar plate.	35°C, aerobically. 35°C, anaerobically.	

Initial Preparation of Specimens (*cont.*)

Material for Examination	Specimen Required	Isolation Media	Incubation	Remarks
Spinal fluid	Spinal fluid in a sterile container.	Blood agar plate. Chocolate agar plate. Thioglycollate medium.	35°C, aerobically; incubate the blood and chocolate agar plates in 5—10% CO_2 or in a candle jar.	If cryptococcosis is suspected, make an India ink preparation (see p. 274); inoculate 2 Sabouraud's, dextrose agar slants; incubate at 35°C and at room temperature. If tuberculosis is suspected, inoculate Lowenstein-Jensen medium.
Sputum	Deep-cough specimen in a sterile container.	Blood agar plate. MacConkey's agar. Thioglycollate medium. Blood agar plate.	35°C, aerobically: incubate the blood agar plate in 5—10% CO_2 or in a candle jar. 35°C anaerobically.	If tuberculosis is suspected, inoculate Lowenstein-Jensen medium after decontamination (see p. 293) If fungi are suspected, inoculate Sabouraud's dextrose-chloramphenicol agar. If *Haemophilus* is suspected, inoculate a chocolate agar plate; incubate in 5—10% CO_2 or in a candle jar.
Stool	Feces in a clean container.	MacConkey's agar plate. SS* agar plate (XLD† agar plate). Selenite broth (GN‡ broth).	35°C, aerobically.	Subculture growth in an enrichment broth (selenite or GN broth) on MacConkey's agar plate and on SS agar (or XLD agar) after 24 hours.
Throat	Swab in a sterile container.	Blood agar plate (sheep blood).	35°C, in 5—10% CO_2 or in a candle jar.	Place a low-concentration (0.02 unit) bacitracin disc in the inoculated portion of the plate. If *Haemophilus* is suspected, inoculate a chocolate agar plate; incubate in 5—10% CO_2 or in a candle jar.

* SS = *Salmonella-Shigella*.
† Available from BBL.
‡ Available from BBL and Difco Laboratories.

Initial Preparation of Specimens (*cont.*)

Material for Examination	Specimen Required	Isolation Media	Incubation	Remarks
Tissue	Tissue from surgery or autopsy in a sterile container.	Blood agar plate. MacConkey's agar plate.	35°C, aerobically.	Homogenize the tissue in a tissue grinder prior to inoculating the isolation media.
		Thioglycollate medium. Blood agar plate.	35°C, anaerobically.	If fungi or acid-fast bacilli are suspected, inoculate 2 Sabouraud's dextrose agar slants; incubate at 35°C and at room temperature, aerobically; inoculate Lowenstein-Jensen medium.
Urine	Clean, midstream-voided urine in in a sterile container.	Blood agar plate. MacConkey's agar plate.	35°C, aerobically.	Inoculate the blood agar plate with a loop calibrated to deliver 0.001 ml of urine; streak the plate evenly with a sterile bent-glass rod; each colony represents 1,000 organisms per ml of the original specimen.
Vaginal-cervical	Swab.	Blood agar plate. MacConkey's agar plate. Chocolate agar plate Thioglycollate medium.	35°C, aerobically; incubate the blood and chocolate agar plates in 5—10% CO_2 or in a candle jar.	If gonococcus is suspected, Thayer-Martin medium is preferred to chocolate agar. If anaerobic infection is suspected, inoculate a blood agar plate; incubate at 35°C, anaerobically.

Decontamination of Sputum and Bronchial Secretions in Preparation for Culture of Mycobacteria

PRINCIPLE

Since most media suitable for the growth of mycobacteria also support other rapid-growing microorganisms, it is necessary to treat contaminated specimens with agents that reduce the non-mycobacterial population to negligible numbers, yet at the same time do not significantly reduce the chances for successful culture of mycobacterial species. The sodium hydroxide decontamination procedure adequately fills this requirement.

PROCEDURE

1. Transfer a portion of the sputum or bronchial-secretion specimen to a sterile disposable petri dish placed over a black background.
2. Break a sterile wood applicator in half and use the two pieces to tease and divide the specimen. Select small bits of purulent, bloody, or caseous material. Twirl this between the two pieces of the stick and rapidly transfer it to a screw-capped sterile disposable 50-ml centrifuge tube until 2 to 5 ml of sputum are accumulated. If the specimen is watery, transfer it with a Pasteur pipette and rubber bulb.
3. Transfer a selected particle to a new, clean slide, press another slide on top of this, then squeeze together and slide apart. Label both slides and flame them as soon as they are dry. Stain, using an acid-fast technic (see pp. 271–272).
4. Add to the centrifuge tube from step 2 a volume of 4% sodium hydroxide containing phenol red indicator equal to the volume of specimen in the tube. Do not allow the final concentration of sodium hydroxide to exceed 2%.
5. Homogenize the specimen by shaking vigorously for 15 minutes in a mechanical shaker.
6. Centrifuge the tube for 15 minutes at 3,000 rpm.
7. Remove the cap and discard all but 0.1 to 1 ml of the supernatant fluid into a container of dilute Cresyline®* or similar disinfectant. Wipe the lip of the tube with an alcohol sponge.
8. Immediately neutralize the sediment. Under no circumstances should the specimen be in contact with sodium hydroxide for more than 40 minutes. Add sterile 2*N* hydrochloric acid drop by drop until a yellow end point is reached.
9. Mix well, then transfer approximately 0.1 ml of the resulting sediment to a Lowenstein-Jensen slant or to Middlebrook's 7H10 agar.
10. A smear of the sediment may be prepared and examined microscopically for acid-fast bacilli.
11. Incubate at 35—37°C. Examine the slants at weekly intervals for 8 weeks. If no growth appears by that time, they may be discarded as negative. It is essential that the screw caps of the media bottles or tubes be loosened weekly to permit an exchange of air. If 7H10 agar is used, incubation in an atmosphere containing 5% CO_2 is necessary.

*Hunt Manufacturing Company, Cleveland, Ohio.

REAGENTS

1. Phenol red indicator stock solution (0.4%)
   Dissolve 0.1 g of phenol red in 25 ml of 4% sodium hydroxide. Store this solution in the dark.
2. Sodium hydroxide digestant (4%)
   Dissolve 40 g of sodium hydroxide in 1 liter of distilled water. Add 1 ml of phenol red indicator to every 99 ml of sodium hydroxide solution (0.004% indicator concentration). Sterilize the solution by autoclaving. Prepare fresh at least once each month.
3. Hydrochloric acid (2*N*)
   Dilute 167.2 ml of concentrated hydrochloric acid with distilled water to a total volume of 1 liter. Distribute the solution into small screw-capped tubes and sterilize by autoclaving. Use one tube for each day's work and discard the unused portion.

Outlines for the Identification of Medically Important Bacteria

PRINCIPLE

The following outlines indicate the principal biological and biochemical criteria for the identification of medically important bacteria. Only passing mention is made of cellular and colonial morphology. While it is recognized that these characteristics are extremely helpful in characterizing colonies seen on isolation media, they can vary considerably with the media selected and with other conditions of growth. It is felt that these outlines would serve more universally if only well-defined and reliably expected biologic and biochemical characteristics were used. The starting point for each group is the Gram-stained appearance of the organism when first isolated. From this point, characteristics expected to be present or absent in 90% or more of the strains are used in defining the genera or species.

Where necessary, supplementary tables of confirmatory tests are included. These outlines are meant to be used as keys to the identification of bacteria to a level consistent with the clinical relevance of the organism. For research purposes a more definitive scheme may be desirable or necessary.

FAMILY *ENTEROBACTERIACEAE*

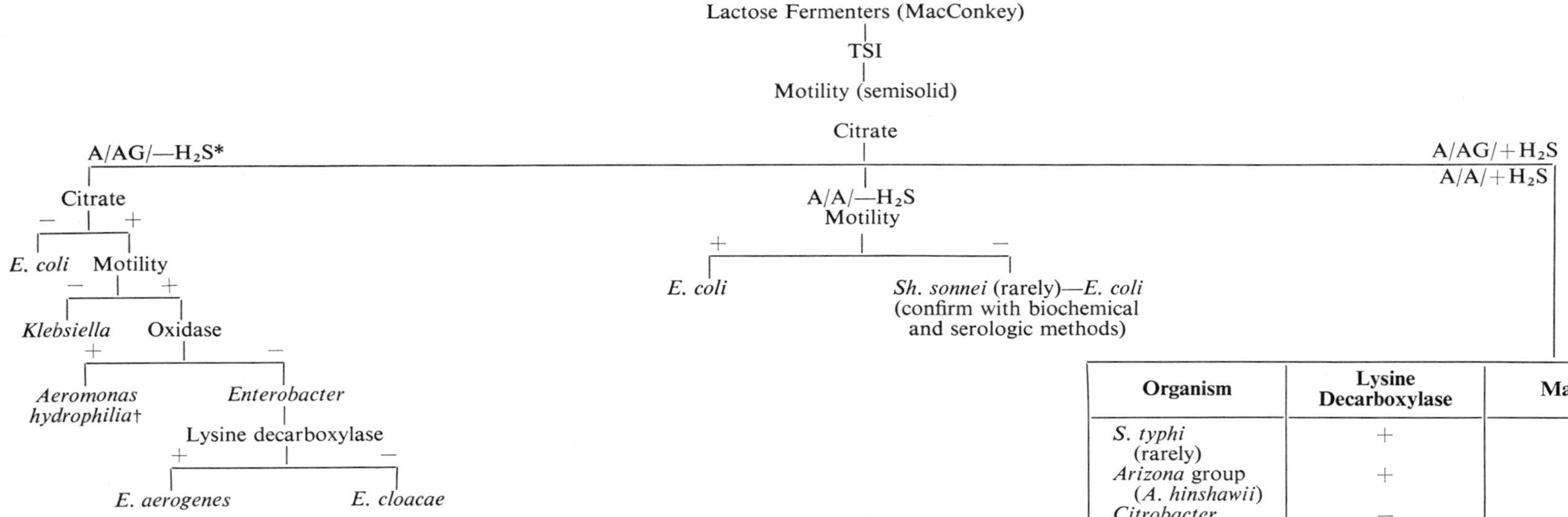

Organism	Lysine Decarboxylase	Malonate
S. typhi (rarely)	+	—
Arizona group (*A. hinshawii*)	+	+
Citrobacter freundii	—	—

*TSI reactions: slant/butt/H_2S; k = alkaline, A = acid, AG = acid and gas.
†Not a member of *Enterobacteriaceae*, but included because of similar reactions.

FAMILY *ENTEROBACTERIACEAE*

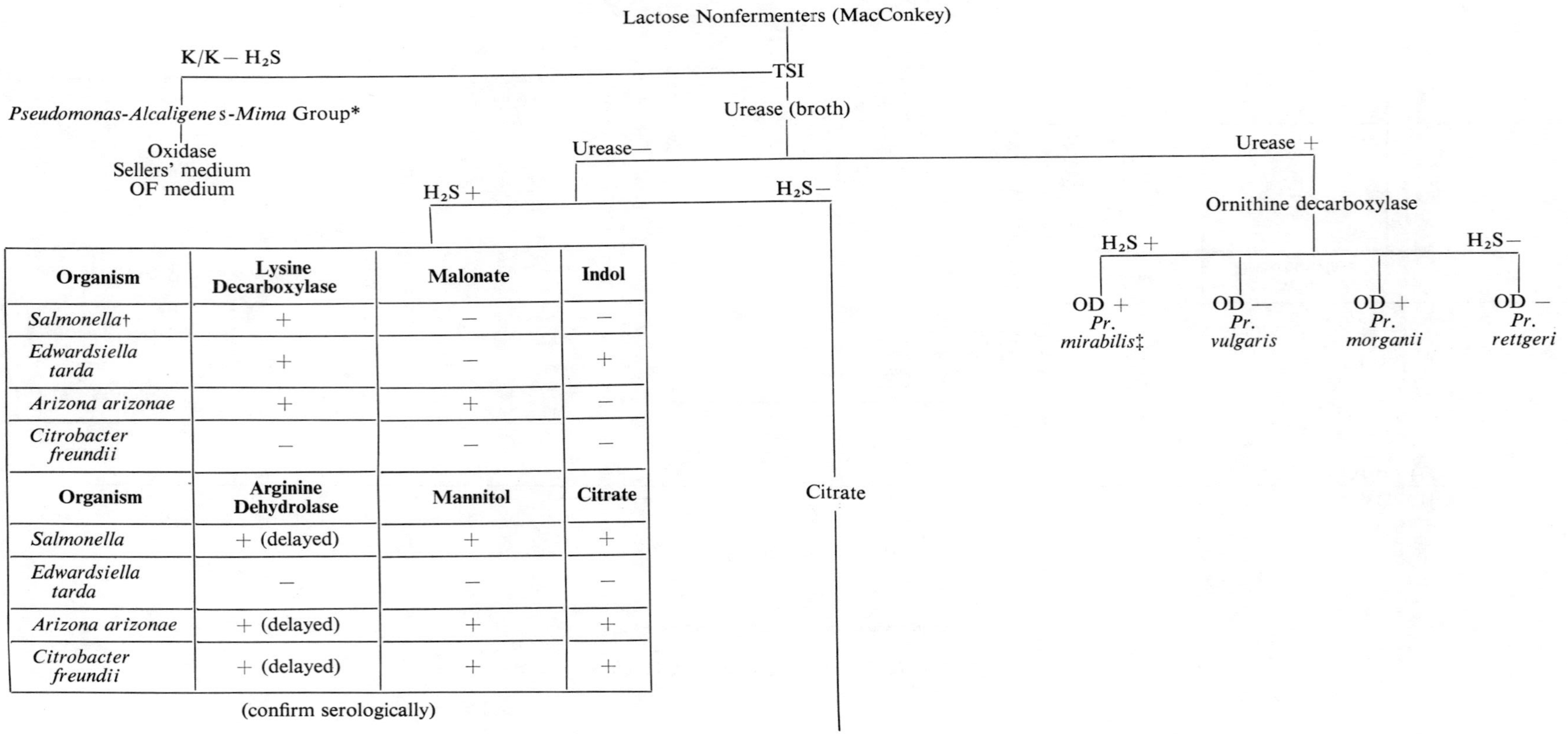

Organism	Lysine Decarboxylase	Malonate	Indol
Salmonella†	+	–	–
Edwardsiella tarda	+	–	+
Arizona arizonae	+	+	–
Citrobacter freundii	–	–	–
Organism	**Arginine Dehydrolase**	**Mannitol**	**Citrate**
Salmonella	+ (delayed)	+	+
Edwardsiella tarda	–	–	–
Arizona arizonae	+ (delayed)	+	+
Citrobacter freundii	+ (delayed)	+	+

(confirm serologically)

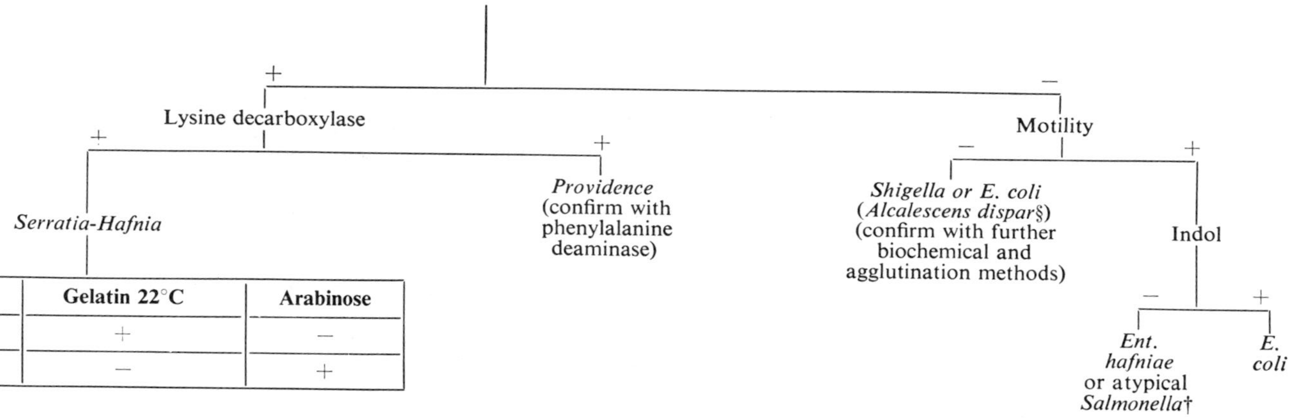

Organism	MR	V-P 37°C	Gelatin 22°C	Arabinose
Serratia	−	+	+	−
Hafnia	+	−	−	+

BIOCHEMICAL REACTIONS OF *SALMONELLA* SPECIES

Organism	Hydrogen Sulfide	Gas from Glucose	Citrate	Motility	LD	OD
S. typhi	±	−	−	+	+	−
S. gallinarum	+	−	−	−	+	−
S. pullorum	+	+	−	−	+	+
S. paratyphi A	−	+	−	+	− (+)	+
S. cholerae-suis	−	+	−	+	+	+

*Not members of the family *Enterobacteriaceae*.
†*Salmonella* species not giving typical biochemical reactions.
‡*Proteus mirabilis* is usually indol-positive, whereas other *Proteus* species are indol-negative.
§With few exceptions, the biochemical reactions given by the *Alcalescens dispar* biotypes are similar to those given by typical *E. coli* cultures; i.e., + lysine decarboxylase, etc.

GRAM-POSITIVE COCCI

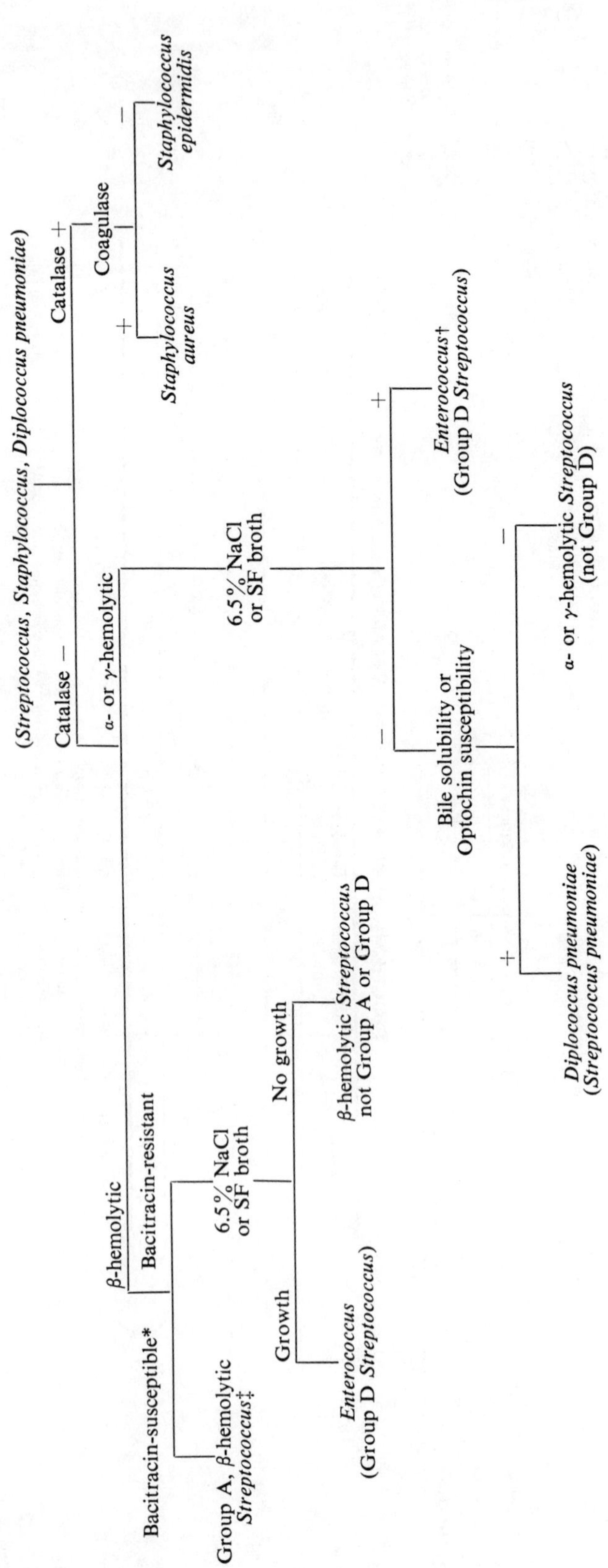

*0.02-unit disc.
†This category may contain some non-catalase-producing strains of *Aerococcus*. These can be distinguished from *Enterococcus* by their inability to grow at 45°C.
‡May be confirmed by the Lancefield precipitin test or the direct fluorescent-antibody technic, using group-specific serum.

GRAM-NEGATIVE COCCI

(*Neisseria* and *Viellonella*)

- Aerobic
  - Growth on unenriched media without CO_2
    - −
    - +
- Anaerobic
  - *Viellonella*

Growth on unenriched media without CO_2: −

Organism	Glucose (acid)	Maltose (acid)	Sucrose (acid)
N. meningitidis	+	+	−
N. gonorrhoeae	+	−	−

Growth on unenriched media without CO_2: +

Organism	Glucose (acid)	Maltose (acid)	Sucrose (acid)	Yellow Pigment
N. flavescens	−	−	−	+
N. flava	+	+	−	+
N. perflava	+	+	+	+
N. sicca	+	+	+	−
N. catarrhalis	−	−	−	−

FAMILY *BRUCELLACEAE*

Because of the complex nature of this family of bacteria, no simple flow diagram is practical. The following tables list the principal characteristics of the clinically important *Brucellaceae*.

PASTEURELLA

Organism	Growth on Blood Agar	Optimal Growth at 25—30°C
P. pestis	+	+
P. tularensis	−	−
P. multocida	++	−

BORDETELLA

Organism	Bordet-Gengou Medium Required	Urease	Citrate	Motility	Glucose (acid)
B. pertussis	+	−	−	−	+
B. parapertussis	−	+	+	−	−
B. bronchiseptica	−	++	+	+	−

BRUCELLA

Organism	5% CO_2 Required	Hydrogen Sulfide (Lead Acetate)	Urease	Growth	
				Thionine	Basic Fuchsin
Br. melitensis	−	−/+	— or slow	+	+
Br. abortus	+	+	— or slow	−	+
Br. suis	−	+	+ rapid	+	−

HAEMOPHILUS

Organism	Usual Infection Site	Requires X Factor	Requires V Factor	Hemolysis
H. influenzae	Respiratory tract, CSF, blood	+	+	−
H. aegypticus	Conjunctiva	+	+	−
H. haemolyticus	Respiratory tract	+	+	+
H. parainfluenzae	Respiratory tract	−	+	−
H. parahaemolyticus	Respiratory tract	−	+	+
H. ducreyi	Genitalia	+	−	+

MISCELLANEOUS GRAM-NEGATIVE BACILLI

(*Pseudomonas, Mima, Herellea, Alcaligenes, Vibrio*)

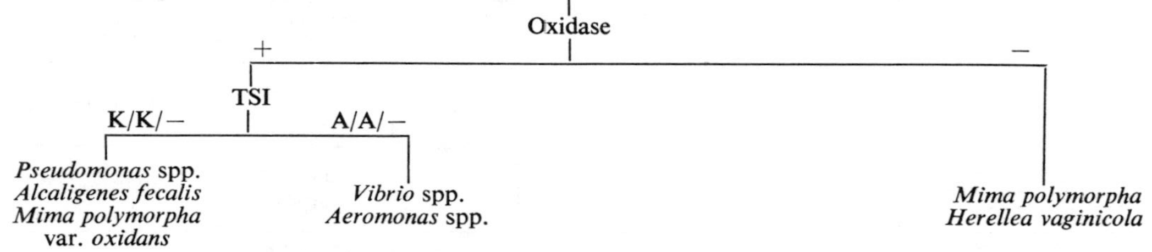

Organism	Sellers' Medium					OF Medium		
	Slant	Butt	Band	Fluorescent Slant	N_2 Gas	Glucose	Lactose	Sucrose
Ps. aeruginosa	blue	blue or green	−	yellow-green	+	O	−	−
Ps. pseudomallei	blue	blue or green	variable	−	+	O	O	O
Mima polymorpha	blue	green	−	−	−	−	−	−
Herellea vaginicola	blue	green	yellow	−	−	O	− or O + late	−
Alcaligenes fecalis	blue	blue or green	−	−	+	−	−	−
Vibrio comma	blue or yellow	yellow	not applicable	−	+ (slight)	F	−	F
*Vibrio fetus**	green	green	−	−	−	−	−	−
Aeromonas hydrophilia	yellow	yellow	not applicable	−	−	F	F	F

*Microaerophilic.

O = oxidation; F = fermentation.

GRAM-POSITIVE SPORE-FORMING RODS

(Bacillus, Clostridium)

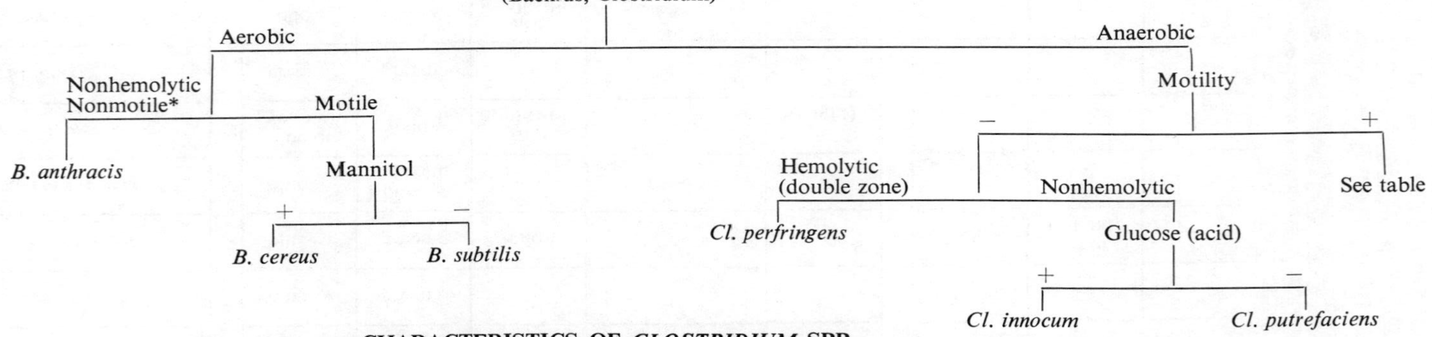

CHARACTERISTICS OF *CLOSTRIDIUM* SPP.

Organism	Spores	Glucose (acid)	Lactose (acid)	Indol	Nitrate Reduction	Cooked-Meat Medium
Cl. septicum	Oval, eccentric	+	+	−	+	Gas, no digestion
Cl. novyi	Oval, eccentric	+	−	−	−	Gas, no digestion
Cl. sordelli	Oval, eccentric	+	−	+	−	Gas, blackening
Cl. sporogenes	Oval, eccentric	+	−	−	+	Gas, blackening, digestion
Cl. botulinum	Oval, eccentric	+	−	−	−	Gas, blackening, digestion
Cl. histolyticum	Oval, subterminal	−	−	−	−	Gas, blackening
Cl. tetani	Round, terminal	−	−	−	−	Slight gas, slow blackening

**B. cereus* var. *mycoides* and nonrhizoid variants may be nonmotile.

NON-ACID-FAST, NON-SPORE-FORMING GRAM-POSITIVE RODS

Catalase

− (negative)

- Nonmotile
  - *Corynebacterium pyogenes*
  - *Lactobacillus* spp.
  - *Erysipelothrix* spp.
- Motile
  - *Lactobacillus* spp. (rare)

+ (positive)

- Nonmotile
  - *Corynebacterium* spp. (see table for differentiating criteria)
- Motile
  - *Listeria monocytogenes* (see table for characteristics)
  - *Corynebacterium* spp. (plant pathogens)

CRITERIA FOR DIFFERENTIATING SPECIES OF *CORYNEBACTERIUM*

Organism	Arginine Hydrolysis	Glucose (acid)	Maltose (acid)	Sucrose (acid)	Trehalose (acid)	Lactose (acid)	Nitrate Reduction	Urease	Pink Pigment	Hemolysis	Anaerobic	Starch (acid)
C. diphtheriae var. *gravis*	−	+	+	−	−	−	+	−	−	−	−	+
C. diphtheriae var. *mitis*	−	+	+	−	−	−	+	−	−	+	−	−
C. diphtheriae var. *intermedius*	−	+	+	−	−	−	+	−	−	−	−	−
C. ulcerans	−	+	d	−	+	−	−	+	−	+	−	+
C. xerosis	−	+	+	+	−	−	+	−	−	−	−	−
C. murium	−	+	+	+	+	−	+	d	−	−	−	+
C. renale	+	+	d	−	−	d	+	+	−	d	−	d
C. ovis	+	+	+	d	−	d	d	+	−	d	−	+
C. bovis	−	−	−	−	−	−	−	−	−	−	−	−
C. epui	−	−	−	−	−	−	+	+	+	−	−	−
C. hofmannii	−	−	−	−	−	−	+	+	−	−	−	−
C. haemolyticum	−	+	+	+	−	+	−	−	−	+	−	d
C. pyogenes	−	+	+	d	−	+	−	−	−	+	−	+
C. acnes	x	+	−	d	x	−	+	−	+*	−	+	x

Key: + = positive in 80 to 100% of strains
— = negative in 80 to 100% of strains
d = 21 to 79% positive
x = not determined

*In thioglycollate broth.

CHARACTERISTICS OF *L. MONOCYTOGENES*

Catalase	+	**Dulcitol**	−
Motility 4°C 20°C 37°C	 + ++++ ++	**B-D Galactosidase**	+
		Nitrate Reduction	−
		Urease	−
Glucose (OF Medium)	F	**Hemolysis**	β
Glucose (acid)	+	**6.5% NaCl**	+
Lactose	+*	**40% Bile**	+
Maltose	+	**KCN**	−
Sucrose	+*	**Gelatin Liquefaction**	−
Trehalose	+	**Malonate**	−
Mannitol	−	**Citrate**	−
Arabinose	−	**Oxidase**	−
Raffinose	−	**Decarboxylases**	
Salicin	+	Lysine Arginine Ornithine	− − −
Adonitol	−		

*Delayed.

CHARACTERISTICS OF GRAM-NEGATIVE ANAEROBIC OR MICROAEROPHILIC BACILLI

Organism	Micro-aerophilic	Pleo-morphic	Gas Production	Foul Odor	Indol	Black Pigment	10—30% Ascitic Fluid Required in Thioglycollate Broth for Growth
Bacteroides fundiliformis	−	+++	+	+	+	−	−
Bacteroides fragilis	−	−	+	+	−	−	−
Bacteroides melaninogenicum	−	−	+	+	+	+	−
Fusibacterium fusiforme	−	−	−	−	x	−	−
Streptobacillus moniliformis	+	++++	−	−	x	−	+

Key: x = not determined

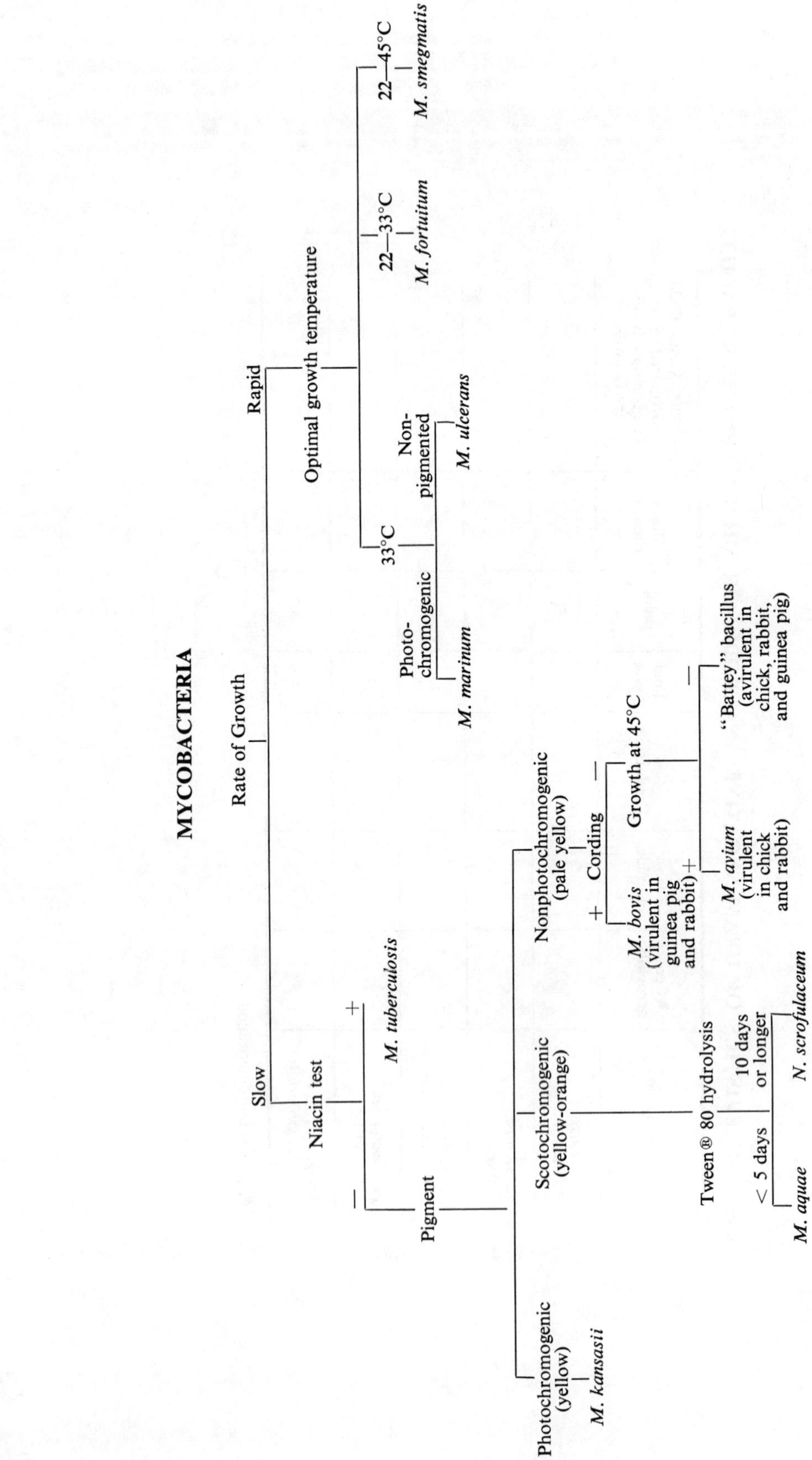
MYCOBACTERIA
Rate of Growth
Slow
Rapid
Niacin test
+
−
M. tuberculosis
Pigment
Photochromogenic (yellow)
M. kansasii
Scotochromogenic (yellow-orange)
Tween® 80 hydrolysis
< 5 days
10 days or longer
M. aquae
N. scrofulaceum
Nonphotochromogenic (pale yellow)
Cording
+
−
M. bovis (virulent in guinea pig and rabbit)
Growth at 45°C
M. avium (virulent in chick and rabbit)
"Battey" bacillus (avirulent in chick, rabbit, and guinea pig)
Optimal growth temperature
33°C
Photo-chromogenic
Non-pigmented
M. marinum
M. ulcerans
22—33°C
M. fortuitum
22—45°C
M. smegmatis

Gram Stain

Hucker's Modification

PRINCIPLE

Both Gram-positive and Gram-negative organisms form a complex of crystal violet and iodine within the bacterial cell during the Gram-staining procedure. Gram-positive organisms resist decolorization by alcohol or acetone because cell wall permeability is markedly decreased as a result of dehydration by these solvents and the dye complex is entrapped within the cell. Cell wall permeability of Gram-negative organisms is increased, resulting in the removal of the crystal violet-iodine complex from the cell. The decolorized Gram-negative cell can then be rendered visible with a suitable counterstain.

PROCEDURE

1. Stain thinly spread smears for 1 minute with ammonium oxalate crystal violet. (If overstaining results in improper decolorization of known Gram-negative organisms, use less crystal violet.)
2. Wash in tap water no longer than 2 seconds.
3. Flood the smears with Gram's iodine. Allow them to remain for 1 minute.
4. Decolorize with 95% ethyl alcohol until the blue dye no longer flows from the smear. (Acetone may be used as a decolorizing agent with caution, since this solvent very rapidly decolorizes the smear.)
5. Wash for 2 seconds in tap water.
6. Flood the smears with safranin O counterstain. Allow them to remain for 1 minute.
7. Wash with tap water.
8. Blot dry between sheets of clean bibulous paper, then examine.

RESULTS

1. Gram-positive organisms: blue.
2. Gram-negative organisms: red.

REAGENTS

1. Crystal violet (Hucker's)

Solution A

crystal violet, certified	2.0 g
ethyl alcohol, 95%	20.0 ml

Solution B

ammonium oxalate	0.8 g
distilled water	80.0 ml

Mix solutions A and B. Store for 24 hours before use. The resulting stain is stable.

2. Gram's iodine
   Dissolve 1.0 g of iodine and 2.0 g of potassium iodide in 300 ml of distilled water.
3. Ethyl alcohol (95%)
4. Counterstain stock solution
   Dissolve 2.5 g of certified safranin O in 100 ml of 95% ethyl alcohol.
5. Counterstain working solution
   Dilute 10 ml of the stock solution with distilled water to 100 ml.

Acid-Fast Stain

Kinyoun Method

PRINCIPLE

This differential staining technic, useful for identification of the tubercle bacillus, other mycobacteria, and *Nocardia*, depends on the chemical composition of the bacterial cell wall. Because of the difficulty in staining these organisms with ordinary dyes, basic dyes in the presence of controlled amounts of acid are used. Generally, heat must be applied during the staining procedure, or wetting agents must be used, to aid dye penetration. Organisms exhibiting the property of acid-fastness, once stained, are not easily decolorized by acid alcohol.

PROCEDURE

1. Stain the fixed smear for 3 to 5 minutes in carbolfuchsin (no heat is necessary).
2. Wash in running tap water.
3. Decolorize to a faint pink with acid alcohol until no more stain comes off in the washings. (If washing is not thorough, false positive results may be obtained.)
4. Wash with tap water.
5. Counterstain for 30 seconds with methylene blue.
6. Wash with tap water, dry in air, then examine under an oil immersion lens.

RESULTS

1. Acid-fast organisms retain a brilliant red color.
2. All other organisms and cellular material stain blue.

NOTES

1. If *Mycobacterium leprae* or *Nocardia* sp. are suspected, use 1% sulfuric acid as a decolorizing agent, since these organisms are overdecolorized by the usual acid alcohol.

REAGENTS

1. Carbolfuchsin

basic fuchsin	4 g
phenol (melted crystal)	8 ml
ethyl alcohol, 95%	20 ml
distilled water	100 ml
Tergitol® 7*	3 drops

2. Acid alcohol
   Dilute 3 ml of concentrated hydrochloric acid with 97 ml of ethyl alcohol.
3. Counterstain
   Dissolve 0.3 g of methylene blue in 100 ml of distilled water.

*Union Carbide Corporation, New York, New York.

Acid-Fast Stain

Ziehl-Neelsen Method

PRINCIPLE

This differential staining technic, useful for identification of the tubercle bacillus, other mycobacteria, and *Nocardia*, depends on the chemical composition of the bacterial cell wall. Because of the difficulty in staining these organisms with ordinary dyes, basic dyes in the presence of controlled amounts of acid are used. Generally, heat must be applied during the staining procedure, or wetting agents must be used, to aid dye penetration. Organisms exhibiting the property of acid-fastness, once stained, are not easily decolorized by alcohol.

PROCEDURE

1. Flood the slides with carbolfuchsin stain. Heat to steaming with a low flame; do not boil and do not permit drying.
2. Allow to stand for 5 minutes without further heating.
3. Wash in running tap water.
4. Decolorize to a faint pink with acid alcohol until no more stain comes off in the washings. (If washing is not thorough, false positive results may be obtained.)
5. Wash with tap water.
6. Counterstain for 30 seconds with methylene blue.
7. Wash with tap water, dry in air, then examine under an oil immersion lens.

RESULTS

1. Acid-fast organisms retain a brilliant red color.
2. All other organisms and cellular material stain blue.

NOTES

1. If *Mycobacterium leprae* or *Nocardia* sp. are suspected, use 1% sulfuric acid as a decolorizing agent, since these organisms are overdecolorized by the usual acid alcohol.

REAGENTS

1. Carbolfuchsin

basic fuchsin	0.3 g
ethyl alcohol, 95%	10.0 ml
phenol (melted crystals)	5.0 ml
distilled water	95.0 ml

2. Acid alcohol

   Dilute 3.0 ml of concentrated hydrochloric acid with 97 ml of 95% ethyl alcohol.

3. Counterstain

   Dissolve 0.3 g of methylene blue in 100 ml of distilled water.

Methylene Blue Stain

PRINCIPLE

While the Gram stain is extremely useful in differentiating various bacteria, the morphologic features of the individual cells are not as clearly defined as with the methylene blue stain. This simple stain permits a rapid evaluation of the morphology of bacteria in exudates. It is particularly useful in determining the presence of *Corynebacterium diphtheriae* on morphologic grounds. Classically, Loeffler's methylene blue required the addition of alkali to counteract acid impurities in dye; today's dyes are sufficiently pure, however, and do not require the addition of alkali.

PROCEDURE

1. Flood the smear with methylene blue stain and allow to remain for 1 minute.
2. Wash with tap water, blot dry with clean bibulous paper, then examine under an oil immersion lens.

RESULTS

1. The metachromatic granules take up the dye and appear deep blue.

NOTES

1. Contrast may be lost if the preparation is overstained.

REAGENTS

1. Methylene blue stain

    Dissolve 0.3 g of methylene blue in 100 ml of distilled water.

India Ink Preparation

PRINCIPLE

While not a staining procedure, this technic permits visualization of the usually transparent and unstainable capsule of many organisms, most importantly *Cryptococcus neoformans*. India ink consists of a suspension of fine particles of carbon. These form a dark background, against which capsules are clearly seen as a result of displacement of the carbon particles.

PROCEDURE

1. To a loopful of cerebrospinal fluid, or to a light aqueous or saline suspension of growth from an agar culture, add a loopful of India ink. Mix well and cover with a thin cover glass. If only a few organisms are present, centrifugation of the cerebrospinal fluid may be necessary.
2. Examine promptly with a high dry lens. The light may have to be reduced by lowering the condenser. Oil immersion may be used if higher magnification is required.

RESULTS

1. Capsules, when present, will stand out against a dark background of carbon particles as clear halos surrounding the microorganism.

NOTES

1. When India ink preparations are made from young cultures *C. neoformans*, capsules may be absent or atypical.

REAGENTS

1. India ink

   India ink precipitates on standing and usually must be replaced every 6 months. Pelikan India ink (Günther-Wagner, Hanover, Germany) is recommended.

Antibiotic-Susceptibility Testing

Standardized Disc Method of Bauer and Kirby

PRINCIPLE

The single-paper disc method of antibiotic-susceptibility testing used in most clinical microbiology laboratories has been found to correlate well with the results of dilution technics and is, therefore, recommended. It is important to standardize the technic and, if possible, to correlate it with dilution studies in each laboratory. The method described is suitable for most rapidly growing pathogens.

MEDIA

1. Brain-heart infusion (BHI) broth or equivalent
2. Mueller-Hinton agar
   5 to 6 mm deep in petri dishes with a diameter of 15 cm.

PROCEDURE

1. Transfer a few colonies (3 to 10) of the organism to be tested to 4 ml of a nutrient broth (e.g., BHI). Incubate for 2 to 5 hours to produce a distinct turbidity.
2. Dilute the broth, if necessary, with sterile water or saline to the density of a standard consisting of 0.5 ml of 1% anhydrous barium chloride in 99.5 ml of 1% sulfuric acid. This standard can be prepared, and an aliquot sealed in a tube of similar size as that used for the broth medium.
3. Using a sterile cotton swab, evenly streak Mueller-Hinton agar in 15-cm plates with inoculum from the broth culture.
4. Firmly place antibiotic-containing discs in contact with the inoculated agar surface.
5. Incubate the plates overnight at 35°C. (If a preliminary report is desired, zones of inhibition can frequently be detected at 6 hours.)
6. After overnight incubation, determine the size of the zone of inhibition to the nearest millimeter. A reading of 6 mm indicates the diameter of the standard antibiotic disc when no zone of inhibition is observed.

SIGNIFICANCE

The table on the next page suggests standards for evaluating the zones of inhibition in terms of susceptibility of the organism to clinically obtainable levels of drugs.

NOTES

1. Other media may be substituted for those listed, but the observed inhibition-zone diameters may differ from those given in the table.
2. Swarming of *Proteus* strains may not be inhibited by all antibiotics, and a veil of growth into the zone can be ignored.
3. If several colonies are present in the zone of inhibition, they should be checked for purity and retested. If they are still present on retest, they are regarded as significant.

4. Standard control organisms of known susceptibility should be tested daily as a check on the activity of the discs and the reproducibility of the test.

ZONE SIZES AND THEIR INTERPRETATION FOR FREQUENTLY USED CHEMOTHERAPEUTICS

Antibiotic or Chemotherapeutic Agent	Disc Potency	Inhibition Zone Diameter to Nearest Millimeter		
		Resistant	Intermediate	Sensitive
Ampicillin				
S. aureus	10 μg	20 or less	21—28	29 or more
all other organisms	10 μg	11 or less	12—13	14 or more
Bacitracin	10 units	8 or less	9—12	13 or more
Cephalothin	30 μg	14 or less	15—17	18 or more
Chloramphenicol	30 μg	12 or less	13—17	18 or more
Colistin	10 μg	8 or less	9—10	11 or more
Erythromycin	15 μg	13 or less	14—17	18 or more
Kanamycin	30 μg	13 or less	14—17	18 or more
Lincomycin*	2 μg			17 or more
Methicillin	5 μg	9 or less	10—13	14 or more
Nalidixic acid†	30 μg	13 or less	14—18	19 or more
Neomycin	30 μg	12 or less	13—16	17 or more
Nitrofurantoin†	300 μg	8 or less	9—12	13 or more
Novobiocin‡	30 μg	17 or less	18—21	22 or more
Oleandomycin	15 μg	13 or less	14—17	18 or more
Penicillin-G	10 units	20 or less	21—28	29 or more
Polymyxin-B	300 units	8 or less	9—11	12 or more
Streptomycin	10 μg	11 or less	12—14	15 or more
Sulfonamides§	300 μg	12 or less	13—16	17 or more
Tetracycline	30 μg	14 or less	15—18	19 or more
Vancomycin	30 μg	9 or less	10—11	12 or more

*Tentative standard.
†Standards apply to urinary-tract infections only.
‡Zone sizes not applicable when blood is added to medium.
§Any of the commercially available 300- or 250-μg sulfonamide discs may be used with the same standards of zone interpretation.

REFERENCE

Bauer, A. W., Kirby, W. M. M., Sherris, J. C., and Turck, M., Antibiotic Susceptibility Testing. by a Standardized Single Disc Method. Am. J. Clin. Pathol., *45*, 493, 1966.

Antibiotic-Susceptibility Testing

Tube Dilution Method

PRINCIPLE

The standardized disc method of antibiotic-susceptibility testing gives acceptable estimates of *in-vitro* susceptibility of organisms to various antibiotics in most situations. In cases of serious infection, a close estimate of the minimum inhibitory concentration (MIC) and of the minimum bactericidal concentration (MBC) of a drug must be determined. Serial dilutions of standard antibiotic solutions and observation of the effects of various concentrations on the growth and viability of organisms provide a means for such evaluation.

MEDIA

1. Brain-heart infusion (BHI) broth or equivalent

REAGENTS

1. Standard antibiotic stock solutions

   For each antibiotic to be tested, make a stock solution in brain-heart infusion (BHI) broth, with a concentration of active drug of 1000 μg/ml. Secondary reference standards of antibiotics can be obtained from various drug manufacturers.

   (a) Weigh out enough standard to provide 25.000 mg of active antibiotic. (Note the ratio of active antibiotic in the sample to the total weight of the sample. This information is usually supplied with each batch of standard; e.g., methicillin 900 μg/mg = 27.777 mg total for 25.000 mg of active drug.) For drugs measured in units (i.e., polymixin-B and penicillin), calculate the weight required to provide 25.000 units.

   (b) Dissolve the antibiotic in a 25-ml volumetric flask with sufficient brain-heart infusion broth to make 25 ml. This solution will contain 1000 μg or units per ml.

   (c) Sterilize the solution by filtration, then dispense it aseptically in aliquots of 0.5 or 1 ml into sterile cork-stoppered tubes. Store in a freezer at —20°C.

2. Working antibiotic solutions

   Thaw the needed amount of stock solution. Dilute it 1:5 with brain-heart infusion broth. This results in an antibiotic concentration of 200 μg/ml.

3. Culture for inoculum

   Make an overnight culture of the organism to be tested in brain-heart infusion broth.

4. Inoculum

   Use a 1:1000 dilution of the overnight culture as the inoculum.

PROCEDURE

1. Set up twelve 13 × 75 mm sterile test tubes in a rack.
2. Add 1 ml of the working antibiotic solution to tube 1.

3. Add 0.5 ml of BHI broth to each remaining tube (tubes 2 through 12).
4. Using a sterile pipette, transfer 0.5 ml from tube 1 to tube 2. Mix well by drawing fluid into the pipette and expelling it several times.
5. Remove 0.5 ml from tube 2 and transfer it to tube 3 (for greater accuracy, a separate pipette may be used for this and each succeeding transfer). Mix as before.
6. Repeat step 5 through tube 11. Remove and discard 0.5 ml from this tube. Use tube 12 as a control.
7. Add 0.5 ml of the inosulum to each of the twelve tubes.
8. Incubate the tubes overnight at 35°C, then read. In some cases readings may be required at 12, 48, or 72 hours, depending on the drug and/or organism.
9. The following table summarizes the technical procedure.

Tube No.	Working Solution (ml)	BHI (ml)	From Previous Tube (ml)	Inoculum (ml)	Final Antibiotic Concentration (μg/ml)
1	1	0	0	0.5	100
2	0	0.5	0.5	0.5	50
3	0	0.5	0.5	0.5	25
4	0	0.5	0.5	0.5	12.5
5	0	0.5	0.5	0.5	6.25
6	0	0.5	0.5	0.5	3.12
7	0	0.5	0.5	0.5	1.56
8	0	0.5	0.5	0.5	0.78
9	0	0.5	0.5	0.5	0.39
10	0	0.5	0.5	0.5	0.19
11	0	0.5	0.5	0.5	0.095
12	0	0.5	0	0.5	0.0

INTERPRETATION

1. After overnight incubation, examine the tubes for growth.
2. Read the minimum inhibitory concentration (MIC) as the lowest concentration of the antibiotic that produces complete inhibition of growth.
3. To determine the minimum bactericidal concentration (MBC), subculture the contents of the clear tubes. The MBC is the lowest concentration of antibiotic that results in a sterile subculture.

Bacitracin Disc Test for Group A Beta-Hemolytic Streptococci

PRINCIPLE

Bacitracin in low concentration appears to be specifically active against a high percentage of Lancefield group A streptococcus strains. Other groups of beta-hemolytic streptococci are not usually inhibited.

REAGENTS

1. Bacitracin-impregnated discs (0.02 units)

PROCEDURE

1. Using straight wire or a loop, pick several colonies of the organism to be tested.
2. Transfer the colonies to a blood agar plate. Spread evenly over a section of the plate.
3. Place a low-concentration (0.02 units) bacitracin disc in the center of the inoculated section. Two to four tests can be placed on one plate.

SIGNIFICANCE

If the streptococcus is group A, zones of inhibition ranging from 15 to 20 mm will be seen around the disc.

NOTES

1. The area of inoculation around the disc must be larger than the zone of inhibition, or there may be no growth at all.
2. Some alpha streptococci may be inhibited by the bacitracin disc.
3. Inhibition indicates group A only if the organism being tested is beta-hemolytic and is not an enterococcus.
4. Up to 5% of group A streptococci strains are not inhibited by this low concentration.
5. A heavy inoculum must be used; otherwise some non-Group A streptococci may show larger zones of inhibition.

Bile Solubility

PRINCIPLE

Pneumococci are quickly lysed by bile salts, due to activation of autolytic enzymes of the cell. Streptococci are not lysed by bile salts, and inhibition of their growth requires much higher concentrations than pneumococci.

MEDIA

1. Dextrose broth

REAGENTS

1. Phosphate buffer (0.5*M*, pH 7.6)
   This solution contains 2% sodium chloride and 0.05% sodium desoxycholate.

PROCEDURE

1. Centrifuge the growth from a 5-ml culture of the organism in dextrose broth.
2. Resuspend the growth in sodium desoxycholate phosphate buffer solution, using enough reagent to make a moderately turbid suspension of cells.
3. Incubate for 60 minutes at 37°C, then examine the specimen. Pneumococci are lysed under these conditions.

SIGNIFICANCE

1. Clearing of the solution indicates the presence of pneumococcus.
2. If the solution does not clear, pneumococcus is not present.

NOTES

1. This new method overcomes several of the problems encountered in older methods, which employed higher concentration of sodium desoxycholate and no buffer. When sodium desoxycholate is added to broth that contains dextrose, the increased acidity causes precipitation and gelling of the broth.
2. If the solution is too dense, it tends to obscure the clearing, because the presence of cell fragments gives the appearance of continued turbidity.

Catalase Activity

PRINCIPLE

Catalase is an enzyme produced by a wide variety of Gram-positive and Gram-negative organisms. It decomposes hydrogen peroxide to form free oxygen and water. The test for catalase activity is most widely applied in the differentiation of staphylococci and streptococci as well as in the preliminary genus identification of Gram-positive non-spore-forming, non-acid-fast rods.

REAGENTS

1. Hydrogen peroxide (3%)
   The activity of the hydrogen peroxide, which is commercially available in this strength, can be checked by testing against a culture known to be catalase-positive.

PROCEDURE

Method A

1. On a nutrient agar culture, cover the colony to be tested with a drop of 3% hydrogen peroxide.
2. An immediate production of bubbles indicates a positive reaction.

Method B

1. Remove a small amount of growth from an agar surface and smear it over an area 2 mm in diameter on a clean glass slide.
2. Place a drop of 3% hydrogen peroxide over the smeared area and observe for gas bubbles.
3. The sensitivity of this method can be increased by carefully placing a clean cover glass over the preparation, so that small, slowly forming bubbles can be seen more easily.

SIGNIFICANCE

Catalase activity can usually be demonstrated in all aerobic and facultatively anaerobic organisms except streptococci, lactobacilli, erysipelothrix, and some strains of *Shigella dysenteriae*.

NOTES

1. The presence of blood in an agar medium renders the interpretation of the catalase test difficult, since erythrocytes also contain the enzyme. If a test must be done on blood agar, only the immediate vigorous production of gas bubbles is significant; delayed bubbling can be due to erythrocytes in the agar as well as to bacterial growth. Method B is more appropriate if only blood agar is available. However, one must be certain that small fragments of medium containing erythrocytes are not transferred to the slide with the colony to be tested.

Catalase Test in the Identification of Mycobacteria

PRINCIPLE

Demonstration of catalase activity has been utilized as an aid in classifying certain groups of mycobacteria. Organisms normally possessing this enzyme tend to lose activity when they acquire resistance to the drug isoniazid.

MEDIA

1. Middlebrook 7H10 agar
   In 16 × 150 mm tubes, ½-inch butt (no slant).

REAGENTS

1. Tween® 80*-hydrogen peroxide mixture
   Mix equal parts of 10% Tween® 80 and 30% hydrogen peroxide.

PROCEDURE

1. Inoculate the surface of the 7H10 medium and incubate at 37°C until a 3—4+ growth is obtained.
2. Add 1.0 ml of Tween® 80-hydrogen peroxide mixture.
3. Measure the height of the column of bubbles resulting. Be ready to discard the tube quickly into a disinfectant if the bubbles should overflow. Record the maximum height obtained at or before 5 minutes.

SIGNIFICANCE

More than 45 mm of bubbles indicate a strong catalase reaction, and less than 45 mm a weak reaction. *M. tuberculosis, M. bovis, M. gastri*, and some strains of *M. kansasii* possess only a weak-reacting, heat-labile catalase. These organisms lose catalase activity upon development of resistance to isoniazid. Clinically significant strains of *M. kansasii* produce a strong reaction.

NOTES

1. As 30% hydrogen peroxide is a powerful oxidizing agent, it should be handled with care and stored under refrigeration.

REFERENCE

Wayne, L. G., Diaz, G. A., and Doubek, J. R., Acquired Isoniazid Resistance and Catalase Activity of Mycobacteria. Amer. Rev. Resp. Dis., 97, 909, 1968.

*Tween Emulsifiers, Atlas Chemical Industries, Inc., Wilmington, Delaware.

Coagulase, Bound

Slide Test

PRINCIPLE

Coagulase is an enzyme capable of clotting plasma. The coagulase test is generally accepted as the best single criterion of the pathogenicity of *Staphylococcus aureus.*

MEDIA

1. Fresh human plasma
2. Reconstituted rabbit plasma (alternatively)

PROCEDURE

1. Place two small drops of water on a slide and emulsify in each a colony of the organism to be tested. Thorough emulsification is essential. A preparation that exhibits autoagglutination before plasma is added is unsatisfactory for the test.
2. Add 1 loopful of physiological saline to the first suspension and mix for 5 to 15 seconds. This serves as a negative control and should be a uniformly turbid suspension with no clumping.
3. Add 1 loopful of fresh human plasma or of reconstituted rabbit plasma to the second suspension and mix for 5 to 15 seconds. Compare this with the negative control. Easily visible clumps represent a positive reaction. Delayed clumping is not an indication of a positive test.

SIGNIFICANCE

The demonstration of coagulase activity is the best single test for identifying pathogenic strains of *Staphylococcus aureus. Staphylococcus epidermidis* and other members of the family *Micrococcaceae* fail to produce a positive reaction.

NOTES

1. The slide method requires some skill in performing and reading the test; it should be performed only after familiarity has been gained by an extensive series of tests in parallel with coagulase tube tests (see p. 284).
2. Colonies that do not emulsify well may give false positive results. Occasionally false negative results occur, as the slide test measures bound rather than free coagulase. All questionable results should be checked by the tube test.
3. The slide test is particularly useful as a screening test.
4. Since there are other organisms besides staphylococci that produce coagulase, pure cultures must be used.
5. Not all samples of human plasma give clear-cut results; it is, therefore, important that adequate controls be employed when plasma from this source is used.

Coagulase, Free

Tube Test

PRINCIPLE

Coagulase is an enzyme capable of clotting plasma. The coagulase test is generally accepted as the best single criterion of the pathogenicity of *Staphylococcus aureus.*

MEDIA

1. Fresh human plasma
2. Reconstituted rabbit plasma (alternatively)

PROCEDURE

1. Place 0.5 ml of fresh human plasma or of reconstituted rabbit plasma in a clean sterile test tube.
2. Suspend 1 loopful of growth from an 18- to 24-hour agar culture in the plasma, or add 0.1 ml of an overnight culture in nutrient broth.
3. Set up controls with known coagulase-positive and coagulase-negative cultures in the same manner.
4. Incubate at 35°C and examine at intervals. Many cultures form a clot within 1 hour. If satisfactory plasma is used, cultures may be considered negative if there is no clotting after 4 hours; occasional strains, however, do not produce clots in less than 24 hours. When growth is taken directly from agar cultures, overnight incubation may be required before negative results are considered reliable.

SIGNIFICANCE

The demonstration of coagulase activity is the best single test for identifying pathogenic strains of *Staphylococcus aureus. Staphylococcus epidermidis* and other members of the family *Micrococcaceae* fail to produce a positive reaction.

NOTES

1. Since there are other organisms besides staphylococci that produce coagulase, pure cultures must be used.
2. Some potentially pathogenic staphylococci that produce coagulase may also produce staphylokinase. Unless the tube is checked at frequent intervals, a clot may form and then lyse, giving a false negative result.
3. Not all samples of human plasma give clear-cut results; it is, therefore, important that adequate controls be employed when plasma from this source is used.

Decarboxylase Reactions

PRINCIPLE

Many organisms of the family *Enterobacteriaceae* can be differentiated on the basis of their ability or inability to decarboxylate or otherwise attack various amino acids. Such reactions produce end products sufficiently alkaline to overcome any acid produced by fermentation of a small quantity of glucose incorporated in the basal medium. Accordingly, a positive reaction is indicated by an alkaline reaction (purple, no change from the uninoculated medium), and a negative reaction is indicated by an acid reaction (yellow, due to the unneutralized acid produced from glucose fermentation). It is to be noted that, because of the slower rate of the decarboxylase reaction, a positive reaction may first form acid and then revert to an alkaline pH.

MEDIA

1. Moeller's decarboxylase basal medium

peptone	5.0 g
beef extract	5.0 g
pyridoxal	5.0 mg
glucose	0.5 g
bromthymol blue (0.2%)	5.0 ml
cresol red (0.2%)	2.5 ml
distilled water	1000.0 ml

   Dissolve the solids in water by heating. Adjust the pH to 6.0, then add the indicator solution. Add amino acids as indicated below. Autoclave for 20 minutes at 115°C. If necessary, readjust the pH to 6.0.

2. Falkow's decarboxylase basal medium (alternatively)

peptone	5 g
yeast extract	3 g
glucose	1 g
bromcresol purple (0.2%)	10 ml
distilled water	1000 ml

   Dissolve the solids in water by heating. Adjust the pH to 6.7 and add the indicator solution. Add amino acids as indicated below. Autoclave for 20 minutes at 115°C. If necessary, readjust the pH to 6.0.

3. Amino acids
   Add 10 g of L-lysine, L-arginine, or L-ornithine per liter of basal medium. If DL-amino acids are used, use 20 g rather than 10. The pH may have to be readjusted after the addition of ornithine.

PROCEDURE

1. Inoculate the test medium or media as well as a control medium containing no amino acid with well-isolated colonies from an overnight growth on an agar plate or slant.
2. Overlay each culture with sterile mineral oil to exclude air.
3. Incubate at 37°C for at least 18 hours. Delayed reactions may require 4—5 days incubation.

SIGNIFICANCE

The following table presents the decarboxylase reactions for various members of the family *Enterobacteriaceae*.

DECARBOXYLASE REACTIONS OF *ENTEROBACTERIACEAE*

Organism	Lysine	Arginine	Ornithine
Salmonella			
S. typhi	+	−	−
S. paratyphi A	−	− or (+)	+
S. gallinarium	+	−	+
other types	+	(+)	+
Shigella			
subgroups A, B, C	−	− or (+)	−
subgroup D	−	±	+
Arizona	−	(+)	+
Citrobacter	−	(+)	+
Edwardsiella tarda	+	−	+
Serratia	+	−	+
Enterobacter			
subgroup A	−	+	+
subgroup B	+ or (+)	−	+
Klebsiella	+	−	−
Proteus			
P. mirabilis	−	−	+
P. vulgaris	−	−	−
P. morganii	−	−	+
P. rettgeri	−	−	−
Escherichia coli	±	±	±

− or (+) = 90% or more strains positive or negative.
(+) = delayed positive reaction (2—5 days).
± = variable results; 11—89% of strains positive or negative.

NOTES

1. A control must be run with each test to verify the ability of the test organism to produce acid from glucose. Glucose nonfermenters may produce a final reaction that is alkaline regardless of the presence or absence of a decarboxylase, leading to false positive reactions. It is best to use a sterile mineral-oil seal to prevent any oxidation of acid by oxygen in the air, which can also lead to false positive reactions.
2. If Falkow's basal medium is used, reactions encountered in the *Enterobacter–Klebsiella* group may not be typical.

IMViC Tests

IMViC reactions are helpful in identifying members of the family *Enterobacteriaceae*. These reactions are used primarily to distinguish between coliform bacteria, but may also be applied advantageously to other organisms in the family. The word "IMViC" is derived from the initial letters of Indol, Methyl red, Voges-Proskauer, and Citrate reactions.

Indol Reaction

PRINCIPLE

This is a test to determine the ability of bacteria to produce indol from tryptophan. Both Kovac's and Ehrlich's test for indol are commonly used.

MEDIA

A. Kovac's Test

1. Tryptophan broth
   1% solution of tryptone (Difco Laboratories), or 1% solution of trypticase (BBL).

B. Ehrlich's Test

1. Tryptophan broth
   1% solution of tryptone (Difco Laboratories), or 1% solution of trypticase (BBL).
2. SIM medium (alternatively)
3. Semisolid medium (alternatively)
   Add 3 parts infusion broth to 1 part infusion agar.

REAGENTS

A. Kovac's Test

1. Kovac's reagent

pure amyl or isoamyl alcohol	150 ml
para-dimethylaminobenzaldehyde	10 g
hydrochloric acid, concentrated	50 ml

Dissolve the aldehyde in the alcohol and slowly add the acid. Prepare in small quantities and store in a refrigerator.

B. Ehrlich's Test

1. Ether
2. Ehrlich's reagent

ethyl alcohol, 95%	190 ml
para-dimethylaminobenzaldehyde	2 g
hydrochloric acid, concentrated	40 ml

Dissolve the aldehyde in the alcohol and slowly add the acid. Prepare in small quantities and store in a refrigerator.

PROCEDURE

A. Kovac's Test

1. Add 0.2 to 0.3 ml of Kovac's reagent to 5 ml of a 24- to 48-hour culture of the organism under investigation (see Note 1).
2. A dark-red color in the surface layer constitutes a positive test; the original yellow color of the solution indicates a negative test when this reagent is used.

B. Ehrlich's Test

1. Add 1 ml of ether to a 24- to 48- hour broth culture (see Note 1). Shake well and allow to stand until the ether rises to the surface.
2. Gently add 0.5 ml of Ehrlich's reagent down the sides of the tube so that it forms a ring between the medium and the ether.
3. If a brilliant-red ring appears just below the ether layer within 5 minutes, the test is positive. If indol is not produced, no color will develop.
4. When SIM or emisolid smedium is used, the ether can be eliminated and the 0.5 ml of Ehrlich's reagent can be added directly to the culture. Interpretation is the same as with broth cultures.

NOTES

1. Unless the culture medium can be relied upon to support indol production uniformly, the results of the test are misleading. The test for indol can be made as soon as good growth appears. If this is done, 1 or 2 ml of culture should be removed aseptically from the tube and the test performed on this sample; if the result is negative, the remaining portion can be reincubated. An occasional organism may need 48-hour incubation if a 24-hour test is equivocal.
2. To test anaerobic organisms for indol, thioglycollate medium without added glucose may be used. Incubate for 3 days and test with the usual indol reagents.

Methyl Red Reaction

PRINCIPLE

Methyl red is used solely as a pH indicator in this test. Some organisms produce sufficient acidity from glucose to stop growth and to give a red color with methyl red. Others do not produce sufficient acidity to stop growth, and subsequent attack on peptone in the medium results in a rise in pH, giving a yellow color with methyl red. Methyl red is red at pH 4.2 and yellow at pH 6.3.

MEDIA

1. Buffered glucose-peptone broth (MR-VP or Clark and Lubs medium)

REAGENTS

1. Methyl red

ethyl alcohol	300.0 ml
methyl red	0.1 g
distilled water	200.0 ml

Dissolve the methyl red in the alcohol, then add the distilled water.

PROCEDURE

1. Inoculate 5 ml of culture medium.
2. Incubate at 35°C for 48 hours; for the majority of cultures this is sufficient to determine MR reaction.
3. Use 5 or 6 drops of reagent per 5 ml of culture.
4. Read the reactions immediately. Positive tests are bright red; negative tests are yellow; intermediate colors are equivocal.

Voges-Proskauer Reaction

PRINCIPLE

The Voges-Proskauer reaction detects the formation of acetylmethylcarbinol from dextrose. If acetylmethylcarbinol is present in the culture, it is oxidized to diacetyl when alkali is added; the diacetyl combines with the proteose peptone medium to give a reddish color.

MEDIA

1. Buffered glucose-peptone broth (MR-VP or Clark and Lubs medium)

REAGENTS

1. Alpha-naphthol (5%) in absolute ethyl alcohol
2. Potassium hydroxide (40%) containing 0.3% creatine

PROCEDURE

1. Inoculate the culture medium with a pure culture of the organism to be tested.
2. Incubate for 48 hours at the optimum temperature for the organism.
3. Pipette 1 ml of the culture medium into a clean test tube and add 0.6 ml of 5% alpha-naphthol.
4. Add 0.2 ml of 40% potassium hydroxide-creatine mixture, shake well, and allow to stand for 10 to 30 minutes.
5. In a positive test a bright orange-red color will develop at the surface of the medium. A negative test will show no change, or it may develop a copper or faint-brown color.

Citrate Reaction

PRINCIPLE

This test is used to determine the utilization of citrate as the sole carbon source.

MEDIA

1. Simmons' citrate agar

PROCEDURE

1. Prepare the medium as agar slants inoculated by stab and/or streak and incubate at 37°C. (Some workers prefer to use the medium in petri dishes.)
2. Growth is clearly indicated by colony formation accompanied by a color change of the bromthymol blue indicator due to alkali production. In a positive test the color changes to a deep blue in 24 to 48 hours; in a negative test there is no growth and no color change.

NOTES

1. It is important that the containers in which this agar is tubed be scrupulously clean, as traces of alkali or acid will disturb the pH of the medium in that tube.
2. If equivocal results are obtained, the test should be repeated and incubated at room temperature for 7 days.

SIGNIFICANCE OF THE IMViC REACTIONS

Organism	Indol	Methyl Red	Voges-Proskauer	Citrate
Escherichia coli	+	+	−	−
Shigella sp.	variable	+	−	−
Salmonella sp.	−	+	−	variable
Edwardsiella tarda	+	+	−	−
Arizona hinshawii	−	+	−	+
Citrobacter	−	+	−	+
Klebsiella sp.	−	−	+	+
Enterobacter sp.	−	−	+	+
Hafnia group	−	− (22°C)	+ (22°C)	variable
Serratia group	−	−	+	+
Proteus mirabilis	−	+	−	variable
Proteus vulgaris	+	+	−	variable
Proteus morganii	+	+	−	−
Proteus rettgeri	+	+	−	+
Providence group	+	+	−	+

Kligler Iron Agar and Triple-Sugar Iron Agar

PRINCIPLE

Kligler iron agar contains two sugars: dextrose (glucose) and lactose. It also contains phenol red indicator to indicate fermentation, and ferrous sulfate or other iron salts to demonstrate hydrogen sulfide production (by blackening of the medium). The dextrose concentration is one-tenth that of lactose, so that fermentation of this latter carbohydrate alone may be detected. The small amount of acid produced by dextrose fermentation aerobically on the slant is rapidly oxidized, and if lactose is not fermented, the slant will quickly revert to alkaline (red). In contrast, under lower oxygen tension in the butt, the acid reaction is maintained and cannot revert to alkaline. An acid (yellow) butt with an alkaline (red) slant, therefore, indicates fermentation of dextrose alone. If lactose is fermented, both the butt and the slant will be yellow. *Pseudomonas* and related organisms ferment neither dextrose nor lactose; they show no change, or only slightly alkaline reactions. The production of gas in the fermentation of dextrose is shown by bubbles in the butt, or sometimes by splitting the medium.

Triple-sugar iron agar differs from Kligler iron agar only in the addition of sucrose (saccharose). Sucrose is present in the same concentration as lactose; its fermentation, as that of lactose, is shown by an acid (yellow) slant and butt. Most of the enteric bacilli have the same fermentation pattern for lactose and sucrose. The incorporation of sucrose permits the exclusion of certain coliform and *Proteus* strains that have the ability to attack sucrose in a 24- to 48-hour incubation period, but give delayed or negative (*Proteus*) lactose reactions in screening for pathogenic *Salmonella* and *Shigella*. These latter organisms always are both lactose- and sucrose-negative.

MEDIA

1. Kligler iron agar
2. Triple-sugar iron agar

PROCEDURE

1. Inoculate with a pure culture of the organism to be identified by streaking the slant and stabbing the butt.
2. Incubate overnight at 35°C and determine the fermentation group into which the organism falls.

SIGNIFICANCE

This is probably the most important test in differentiating the enteric bacilli. It combines several biochemical reactions in one (see Outlines for the Identification of Medically Important Bacteria, pp. 256–268).

NOTES

1. In order to get a correct reaction in the slant, there must be an exchange of air in the tube. If screw-cap tubes are used, loosen the cap one turn before incubation.
2. It is important to read the reaction after 18 to 24 hours of incubation. Extended incubation may give erroneous results.

Malonate

PRINCIPLE

Malonate liquid medium has as its only source of carbon sodium malonate and as its only source of nitrogen ammonium sulfate. Certain bacteria capable of metabolizing sodium malonate will change the color of bromthymol blue indicator.

This test is best used to separate the *Enterobacter-Klebsiella* group (utilizers of malonate) from *E. coli* (nonutilizer), and *Arizona* (utilizer) from *Salmonella* species (nonutilizers). *Hafnia* and, more rarely, *Citrobacter* and *Serratia* can give positive reactions.

MEDIA

1. Malonate broth

ammonium sulfate	2.0 g
dipotassium phosphate	0.6 g
monopotassium phosphate	0.4 g
sodium chloride	2.0 g
sodium malonate	2.0 g
bromthymol blue	0.025 g

Add the ingredients to 1000 ml of distilled water, distribute to tubes, and autoclave. The final pH should be 6.7.

PROCEDURE

1. Inoculate the liquid medium with a loopful of the culture to be tested.
2. Incubate at 35°C for 18 to 24 hours.
3. A positive reaction is indicated by a color change from green to blue.

SIGNIFICANCE

The majority of strains of *Enterobacter-Klebsiella-Hafnia* utilize sodium malonate, whereas *E. coli* does not. Simmons' citrate gives a better percentage of positive results for *Enterobacter*, but not for *Klebsiella* or *Hafnia*. Malonate is, therefore, an alternative to Simmons' citrate in this differentiation.

Malonate is especially significant in differentiating all members of *Salmonella*, including *S. typhi*, from *Arizona*, which is similar in most biochemical characteristics.

NOTES

1. Ewing has modified this medium by the addition of yeast extract.

Niacin Test for *Mycobacterium tuberculosis*

Runyon Modification

PRINCIPLE

The niacin test depends on the formation of a complex colored compound when a nicotinic acid (niacin) produced by *M. tuberculosis* reacts with cyanogen bromide (CNBr) and a primary or secondary amine.

CULTURES

1. *Mycobacterium* culture

   A mature and fairly heavy growth on a solid medium, such as Lowenstein-Jensen, is needed. If the original culture has these characteristics, it may be used. If not, a subculture must be made.

REAGENTS

1. Cyanogen bromide (10% aqueous)

   Store in a brown bottle in a refrigerator. Make up fresh each month.
2. Aniline (4%) in 95% ethyl alcohol

   Store in a brown bottle in a refrigerator. Make up fresh each month.

PROCEDURE

1. Add 1 ml of sterile distilled water to the slant and allow to stand for 10 minutes in a horizontal position.
2. Transfer the water into a small tube and add 1 ml of each of the test reagents (cyanogen bromide and aniline).
3. The production of a yellow color indicates a positive test.

SIGNIFICANCE

Human tubercle bacilli give a positive test, whereas bovine, avian, and unclassified mycobacteria give negative tests. A positive test does not indicate virulence; it distinguishes human strains from other acid-fast bacilli.

NOTES

1. The tests are carried out under a chemical fume hood, since both reagents are toxic and tear gas forms from cyanogen bromide.
2. Negative and positive controls should be run with each set of determinations.

Nitrate

PRINCIPLE

Bacteria vary in their capacity to reduce nitrates. The reduction proceeds to nitrites, or further to elemental nitrogen or ammonia. Some aerobic bacteria can utilize nitrates under anaerobic conditions in order to derive their oxygen.

Free nitrogen is detected as gas-bubble formation; nitrites are detected by a color reaction.

MEDIA

1. Nitrate agar

beef extract	3 g
peptone	5 g
potassium nitrate	1 g
agar	12 g

Add the above mixture to 1000 ml of cold distilled water. Heat to boiling to dissolve, distribute in tubes, and autoclave. Allow the medium to harden as slants. The pH of the medium is 6.8.

REAGENTS

1. Sulfanilic acid
   Dissolve 8 g of sulfanilic acid in 1000 ml of 5*N* acetic acid.
2. alpha-Naphthylamine
   Dissolve 5 g of alpha-naphthylamine in 1000 ml of 5*N* acetic acid.

PROCEDURE

1. Inoculate the medium by streaking the slant and stabbing deeply into the butt.
2. Incubate at 35°C together with an uninoculated tube of nitrate medium as a control.
3. Nitrogen gas may be produced over several days and will split the medium.
4. Nitrites can be identified by adding a few drops each of the sulfanilic acid and alpha-naphthylamine reagent to both the tube containing the test medium and to that containing the control medium. A distinct pink or red color indicates the presence of nitrites; the control should be colorless.

SIGNIFICANCE

All members of the family *Enterobacteriaceae* reduce nitrates, as do many other medically important bacteria. Important exceptions are all streptococci, *Listeria monocytogenes, Bordetella pertussis*, and *Clostridium botulinum*. Certain *Corynebacteria* species that do not reduce nitrates may be differentiated from *Corynebacteria diphtheria*, which does reduce nitrates. Members of the tribe *Mimeae* do not reduce nitrates.

Optochin Disc Test

PRINCIPLE

Growth of pneumococcus is inhibited by optochin (ethylhydrocupreine hydrochloride), whereas the growth of streptococci is not affected unless very large concentrations of the compound are used.

REAGENTS

1. Paper discs containing optochin

PROCEDURE

1. Using a straight wire, transfer several colonies to be tested to blood agar; spread evenly over a section of the plate with a sterile swab or loop.
2. Place an optochin disc in the center of the area and incubate overnight. Two or three tests can be run on one plate.
3. If the organism is pneumococcus, zones of inhibition ranging from 15 to 30 mm in diameter will be observed.

NOTES

1. If a very light inoculum is used, small zones of inhibition may be seen around streptococci; the proper amount of growth needed to obtain good results will be learned quickly with experience.
2. The area of growth must be large enough to prevent inhibition of the entire area; otherwise no zone will be seen and the organism will appear to be nonviable.
3. Some strains of alpha-streptococci are capable of producing zones of inhibition less than 15 mm in diameter, even when a heavy inoculum is used.

Oxidative-Fermentative (OF) Medium

PRINCIPLE

The oxidative and fermentative metabolism of carbohydrates by bacteria may be distinguished by the use of this medium. In the presence of smaller than usual amounts of peptone, certain organisms that fail to produce acid from carbohydrates by fermentation will do so by oxidative metabolism. Two tubes of a suitable medium for each carbohydrate used are inoculated with the test organism. The medium in one tube of each pair is covered with sterile mineral oil to exclude oxygen; the medium in the other tube is left exposed to the air within the tube. If the carbohydrate is metabolized by oxidation, acid will form only in the open tube. If fermentative metabolism takes place, both tubes will show an acid reaction.

MEDIA

1. Hugh and Leifson's oxidative-fermentative (OF) basal medium

trypticase or tryptone	2.0 g
sodium chloride	5.0 g
dipotassium phosphate	0.3 g
agar	2.5 g
bromthymol blue, 1% aqueous solution	3.0 ml

Suspend the above ingredients in 1000 ml of distilled water, using heat and frequent agitation to effect dissolution. Adjust the pH to approximately 7.1, then autoclave at 121°C for 15 minutes. To this sterile basal medium aseptically add sterile solutions of any carbohydrate to be tested (usually glucose, lactose, and sucrose) in a final concentration of 1%. Dispense the medium in 5-ml quantities into sterile tubes. The resulting medium is semi-solid.

PROCEDURE

1. Inoculate two tubes of each carbohydrate to be used by stabbing with the organism to be tested. Add 2 ml of sterile mineral oil to one of each pair of tubes.

SIGNIFICANCE

The following table lists representative results with various organisms.

Organism	Glucose		Lactose		Sucrose	
	Open	Closed	Open	Closed	Open	Closed
Alcaligenes faecalis	—	—	—	—	—	—
Pseudomonas aeruginosa	A	—	—	—	—	—
Bacterium anitratum	A	—	A	—	—	—
Pseudomonas pseudomallei	A	—	A	—	A	—

NOTES

1. If organisms fail to grow in the OF medium, repeat the test, using a basal medium enriched with 2% serum or 0.1% yeast extract.

REFERENCE

Hugh, R., and Leifson, E., The Taxonomic Significance of Fermentative versus Oxidative Metabolism of Carbohydrates by Various Gram-Negative Bacteria. J. Bacteriol., *66*, 24, 1953.

Oxidase Test for *Neisseria*

PRINCIPLE

Cytochromes are iron-porphyrin pigments important in the transfer of electrons to oxygen. Ferric iron of cytochrome may be reduced to the ferrous state by certain flavoproteins. The reoxidation of this reduced cytochrome by molecular oxygen is then catalyzed by the enzyme cytochrome oxidase. The presence of this enzyme can be detected in bacteria by a color change when certain reagents are applied.

REAGENTS

1. *para*-Aminodimethylaniline monohydrochloride (1% solution)
   This reagent is unstable, losing its activity after a few hours. It should be prepared fresh daily. If a black precipitate forms, it is not suitable for use. Alternatively, the oxalate salt may be used. It is less toxic for gonococcus and more stable in solution than the monohydrochloride. The oxalate salt, however, is harder to get into solution and usually must be heated gently to do so.

PROCEDURE

1. Apply the reagent directly to the plate with a dropper, or use a nasal atomizer to spray the plate.
2. Reactions should take place within approximately 2 minutes, if the reagents are fresh. Oxidase-positive colonies first turn pink, then maroon, and finally black. Picking of the subcultures from the treated colonies must be done quickly when the colony is just pink, as the organisms are no longer viable after the colony turns black. Oxidase-negative colonies show no change.
3. Because other organisms are also oxidase-positive, make a Gram stain to ascertain whether these are Gram-negative diplococci. The colonies are suitable for Gram staining even after they turn black.

NOTES

1. A reagent variation suggested by Edwards and Ewing calls for a 1% solution of alpha-naphthol in 95% ethyl alcohol to be added in equal amounts with the monohydrochloride solution. In this case oxidase-positive colonies turn blue in 30 to 120 seconds; oxidase-negative colonies show no change.

SIGNIFICANCE

This test has its greatest values in detecting colonies of pathogenic neisseria when only a few colonies are present in a heavy growth of other flora, as is often the case with gonococcus infections. However, as all neisseria are oxidase-positive, the test will not differentiate meningococcus from normal throat neisseria.

Oxidase Test for *Pseudomonas*

PRINCIPLE

Cytochromes are iron-porphyrin pigments important in the transfer of electrons to oxygen. Ferric iron of cytochrome may be reduced to the ferrous state by certain flavoproteins. The oxidation of this reduced cytochrome by molecular oxygen is then catalyzed by the enzyme cytochrome oxidase. The presence of this enzyme can be detected in bacteria by a color change when certain reagents are applied.

REAGENTS

1. Tetramethyl *para*-phenylenediamine dihydrochloride (1% solution)

   This reagent is unstable, losing its activity after a few hours. It should be prepared fresh daily. If a black precipitate forms, the reagent is not suitable for use. Alternatively, 1% solution of *para*-aminodimethylaniline monohydrochloride may be used.

PROCEDURE

1. Place 2 or 3 drops of reagent in a 6-cm square piece of Whatman #1 filter paper.
2. Remove a suspected colony from the plate and smear with a loop on the reagent-saturated paper.
3. A positive reaction, recognized by a dark-purple color, develops in 5 to 10 seconds.
4. Alternatively, the plate may be flooded with the reagent, as in the oxidase test for neisseria (see p. 298).

SIGNIFICANCE

This test is used to differentiate cultures of pseudomonas that fail to produce pigment or the typical fruity odor from other morphologically similar Gram-negative rods. Some strains of *Mima polymorpha* are also oxidase-positive.

Phenylalanine Deaminase Test

PRINCIPLE

Certain members of the family *Enterobacteriaceae* are able to form phenylpyruvic acid from phenylalanine by deamination. The addition of an acidified ammonium sulfate, ferric ammonium sulfate mixture, or 10% ferric chloride solution produces a characteristic green color.

MEDIA

1. Phenylalanine agar

yeast extract	3 g
DL-phenylalanine	2 g
disodium phosphate	1 g
sodium chloride	5 g
agar	12 g

Add the above to 1 liter of cold distilled water and heat to boiling to effect dissolution. Distribute in tubes, autoclave for 15 minutes at 15 pounds (121°C), and allow the agar to harden as slants.

REAGENTS

1. Reagent for phenylalanine agar

   Dissolve 2 g of ammonium sulfate and 1 ml of 10% sulfuric acid in 5 ml of saturated ferric ammonium sulfate.

PROCEDURE

1. Inoculate the slant with organism and incubate at 35—37°C for 18 to 24 hours.
2. Add 5 drops of the test reagent to cover the slant and loosen the colonies.
3. A positive test is indicated by the production of a green color within 1 to 5 minutes.

SIGNIFICANCE

Members of *Proteus* and *Providence* are phenylalanine deaminase-positive, whereas all other members of *Enterobacteriaceae* are not. The reaction is useful when used with the urease reaction for identification of *Proteus* or *Providence*.

Potassium Cyanide (KCN) Medium

PRINCIPLE

Some organisms are capable of growth in the presence of potassium cyanide.

MEDIA

1. Potassium cyanide (KCN) medium

KCN broth base (Difco or BBL)	1 liter
potassium cyanide solution, 0.5%	15 ml

Prepare 0.5% potassium cyanide solution by adding 0.5 g of potassium cyanide to 100 ml of cold sterile distilled water. Add 15 ml of this reagent to 1 liter of chilled sterile KCN broth base. CAUTION: DO NOT PIPETTE WITH YOUR MOUTH. Dispense the medium in 1-ml quantities into sterile tubes and stopper quickly with corks sterilized by heating in paraffin. The tubed medium can be stored safely for 2 weeks at 4°C.

PROCEDURE

1. Inoculate tubes with a loopful (3-mm loop) of a 24-hour broth culture grown at 37°C.
2. Observe daily for 2 days.
3. Positive results are indicated by growth in the presence of KCN.

SIGNIFICANCE

This test has become of increasing importance with the new taxonomic scheme of Edwards and Ewing. *Shigella, Escherichia, Salmonella,* and *Arizona* give negative results. *Proteus, Providence, Citrobacter, Klebsiella, Enterobacter, Hafnia,* and *Serratia* are positive. This test is especially important in differentiating *Citrobacter* from *Arizona* and *Salmonella.*

NOTES

1. Care should be taken not to inoculate the medium too heavily, as it may make it difficult to determine whether or not growth is present.
2. Handling of potassium cyanide should be done carefully, as it is poisonous. It should never be added to hot solutions.
3. The medium should be discarded after 2 weeks, as it is relatively unstable. It should be stored under refrigeration.

REFERENCE

Edwards, P. R., and Ewing, W. H., Identification of *Enterobacteriaceae*. Burgess Publishing Co., Minneapolis, 1962.

Sellers' Medium

PRINCIPLE

This medium provides a variety of reactions that are helpful in differentiating and identifying nonfermentative Gram-negative bacteria, which produce a completely alkaline reaction on triple-sugar iron agar. In addition to enabling oxidative organisms to produce acid from glucose, the medium is useful in detecting the reduction of nitrate to gaseous nitrogen by the formation of bubbles within the agar butt. The medium enhances the production of fluorescein by *Pseudomonas aeruginosa*; under ultraviolet light, a typical apple-green fluorescence can be observed.

MEDIA

1. Sellers' differential agar (Difco or BBL)

yeast extract	1.000 g
peptone	20.000 g
L-arginine	1.000 g
D-mannitol	2.000 g
sodium chloride	2.000 g
sodium nitrate	1.000 g
sodium nitrite	0.350 g
magnesium sulfate	1.500 g
dipotassium phosphate	1.000 g
bromthymol blue	0.040 g
phenol red	0.008 g

   Suspend the above ingredients in 1000 ml of distilled water and heat to boiling to effect complete dissolution. Autoclave for 15 minutes at 121°C, then dispense into test tubes with cotton plugs or loose-fitting caps. Allow the tubes to solidify in a slanted position with a 1½-butt and a 3-inch slant.

2. Sterile glucose (50% in water)
   Prepare enough solution so that you have 0.15 ml for each tube of Sellers' medium prepared. The solution may be sterilized by autoclaving for 15 minutes at 121°C. Do not overheat.

PROCEDURE

1. Just prior to inoculation, add 0.15 ml of sterile 50% glucose solution to the tube, allowing it to run down the side opposite the slant so that it accumulates between the tube wall and the base of the slant without wetting the upper portion of the slant.
2. Inoculate the medium with a deep stab and streak the surface of the slant.
3. Incubate at 35°C for 18 to 24 hours.

SIGNIFICANCE

The reactions produced by nonfermenting Gram-negative organisms are listed in the following table.

Organism	Slant Color	Butt Color	Band Color	Fluorescent Slant	Nitrogen Gas
Pseudomonas aeruginosa	green or blue	blue or no change	sometimes blue	greenish yellow	+
Bacterium anitratum	blue	no change	yellow	—	—
Herellea vaginicola	blue	no change	yellow	—	—
Mima polymorpha	blue	no change	—	—	—
Alcaligines faecalis	blue	blue or no change	—	—	+

REFERENCE

Sellers, W., Medium for Differentiating the Gram-Negative Bacilli of Medical Interest. J. Bacteriol., *87*, 46, 1964.

Serological Identification of Group A Beta-Hemolytic Streptococci

PRINCIPLE

Strains of beta-hemolytic streptococci may be definitely identified by the determination of their specific serologic groups and types. In most clinical laboratories, the most important question that arises when such a streptococcus is isolated from the upper respiratory tract is whether or not the strain belongs to the serologic group A. Infections with streptococci in this group may be associated with the subsequent development of rheumatic fever and acute glomerulonephritis.

MEDIA

1. Todd-Hewitt broth (Difco or BBL)

REAGENTS

1. Hydrochloric acid (*N*/5) in 0.85% sodium chloride
2. Sodium hydroxide (*N*/5)
3. Thymol blue (0.01%)
4. Phenol red (0.01%)
5. Group-specific antiserum (Difco or BBL)

PROCEDURE

Preparation of Antigen Extract

1. Inoculate the organism into 40 ml of Todd-Hewitt broth and incubate overnight at 35°C.
2. Centrifuge the culture, then discard the supernatant fluid.
3. Add 0.4 ml of *N*/5 hydrochloric acid in 0.85% sodium chloride to the sediment.
4. Transfer 1 loopful of the acidified suspension to a spot plate and add 1 drop of 0.01% thymol blue. This should result in an orange-red color (pH 2.0—2.4). If necessary, add additional *N*/5 hydrochloric acid to obtain the desired color.
5. Place the suspension in a boiling water bath for 10 minutes. Shake at 3-minute intervals.
6. Cool, centrifuge, then decant the supernatant into a clean tube.
7. Add a small drop of 0.01% phenol red to the supernatant. This should result in a distinct yellow color.
8. Add *N*/5 sodium hydroxide drop by drop to obtain a pH of 7.0—7.2 (orange). The optimum pH is 7.0—7.6; a pH above 7.6 may result in a false positive reaction. If the mixture is too alkaline, the pH can be adjusted by adding *N*/2 hydrochloric acid.
9. Centrifuge, then pipette the supernatant fluid into a clean tube for the precipitin test.

Precipitin Test (Capillary-Tube Method)

1. Dip a capillary tube of 0.1—1.0 mm ID and 75—90 mm length into the rehydrated group-specific antiserum. Allow the antiserum to rise 2 to 3 cm into the tube.

2. Close the end of the capillary tube with the forefinger and remove it from the antiserum. Wipe the excess antiserum from the tip of the tube.
3. Insert the tube into the prepared antigen extract and allow it to rise 2 to 3 cm into the tube.
4. Remove the tube from the antigen extract and allow the contents to rise further, until there is an equal air space at each end.
5. Wipe any excess fluid from the outside of the tube, then insert the tube in vertical position into a plasticine or clay block.
6. The antigen extract derived from an organism belonging to the streptococcal group corresponding to the specific antiserum used will produce a precipitate at the junction of the antiserum and antigen extract in 10 to 15 minutes.

SIGNIFICANCE

The serologic group of beta-hemolytic streptococci can be defined with the greatest accuracy by this method. While a complete battery of antisera is required for epidemiologic studies, clinically significant group A organisms can be identified with assurance by using antiserum specific for this group.

The procedure is time-consuming, requiring the preparation of an overnight broth culture. This further delays a report to the physician. Because the bacitracin disc test (see p. 279) has been shown to be accurate in identifying at least 95% of group A strains, this method is recommended for routine use. The precipitin test can be used to evaluate negative results obtained by the bacitracin disc test, thus identifying those strains in the 5% not susceptible to small quantities of bacitracin.

NOTES

1. Upon standing, the precipitate formed in 10 to 15 minutes may redissolve or clump and fall to the bottom of the serum.
2. Always include known positive and negative control extracts.
3. Because the antigen extracts contain large amounts of group-specific carbohydrates, difficulties from antigen excess may arise, especially if weak antisera are used. In this case dilution of the extract 1:4 or 1:16 with 0.85% sodium chloride may be required to produce a precipitate.

REFERENCE

Lancefield, R. C., The Antigenic Complex of *Streptococcus haemolyticus*. I. Demonstration of a Type-Specific Substance in Extracts of *Streptococcus haemolyticus*. J. Exp. Med., *47*, 91, 1928.

Tween® 80 Hydrolysis

PRINCIPLE

The rate of hydrolysis of phosphate-buffered Tween® 80*, using neutral red as an indicator, has been shown to be useful in the classification of mycobacteria other than *M. tuberculosis*. Neutral red in 0.5% Tween® 80 at pH 7.0 presents a yellow color. As the Tween® 80 is hydrolyzed and oleic acid is produced, a change from yellow to red occurs.

REAGENTS

1. Substrate solution

phosphate buffer (*M*/15, pH 7.0)	100.0 ml
Tween® 80	0.5 ml
neutral red solution (1 mg/ml)	2.0 ml

Prepare the neutral red solution with distilled water; be sure to take into account the actual dye content of the dye in use. Dispense the substrate solution in 4-ml quantities into screw-capped tubes. Autoclave at 121°C for 15 minutes. Store in a refrigerator, protected from light.

PROCEDURE

1. Emulsify a 3-mm loopful of mycobacteria, actively growing on a solid medium, in the substrate.
2. Incubate at 37°C.
3. Compare the color of the substrate with that of an uninoculated control tube after 4 hours, then once daily for 10 days. A change in color from amber to red is a positive reaction.

SIGNIFICANCE

Pathogenic members of the Group II scotochromogenic mycobacteria are unable to hydrolyze Tween® 80 rapidly, or indeed at all. The species designation *M. scorfulaceum* has been suggested for this group. Those members of Group II that produce rapid hydrolysis (*M. aquae*) are usually nonpathogenic and are encountered as contaminants in gastric washings and in urine.

The following table lists the expected reactions for various mycobacteria.

*Tween Emulsifiers, Atlas Chemical Industries, Inc., Wilmington, Delaware.

REACTION PATTERNS OF TWEEN® 80 HYDROLYSIS OF VARIOUS SPECIES OF MYCOBACTERIA

Runyon Group	Species or Subgroup	Tween® 80 Hydrolysis at	
		1 to 5 Days	10 Days
—	*M. tuberculosis*	−	+
—	*M. bovis*	−	+
I	*M. kansasii*	+	+
II	*M. scrofulaceum* *M. aquae*	− +	− +
III	Battey-*M. avium* Radish "J"	− + +	− + +
IV (Rapid Growers)	*M. fortuitum* *M. smegmatis* *M. phlei* *M. rhodochrous* Other rapid growers	+ + + + +	+ + + + +

NOTES

1. During 37°C incubation the tubes should be protected from light to minimize spontaneous decolorization of the neutral red.

REFERENCE

Wayne, L. G., Doubek, J. R., and Russell, Ruth L., Classification and Identification of Mycobacteria. I. Tests Employing Tween® 80 as Substrate. Am. Rev. Resp. Dis., *90*, 588, 1964.

Urease

PRINCIPLE

Urease, an enzyme produced by various microorganisms, catalyzes the decomposition of urea, forming ammonia as an end product. Urea is incorporated in a buffered medium containing phenol red as an indicator. A positive reaction is indicated by a color change from yellow (pH 6.8) to red or cerise (pH 8.1 or more alkaline).

MEDIA

1. Rustigian and Stuart urea broth medium
2. Christensen urea agar medium

PROCEDURE

A. Rustigian and Stuart Medium

1. Inoculate Rustigian and Stuart urea broth with a straight needle from the organism to be tested.
2. Incubate at 35°C.
3. *Proteus* organisms produce a red color in 2 to 4 hours. Generally, urease-positive organisms other than *Proteus* species do not produce a sufficient amount of ammonia to render the strongly buffered Rustigian and Stuart broth alkaline.

B. Christensen Medium

1. Tube Christensen urea agar as agar slants and inoculate heavily over the entire surface. The butt should not be inoculated.
2. Incubate at 35°C.
3. *Proteus* gives a red slant in 2 to 4 hours. The color penetrates into the medium, and at 24 hours the entire tube shows an alkaline reaction. Other urease-positive organisms, in contrast, hydrolyze urea much more slowly, showing only slight penetration of the alkaline reaction into the butt in 6 hours and requiring 3 to 5 days to change the reaction of the entire butt. Some Gram-positive bacilli, diphtheroids and others, can give a positive reaction on this medium; these cultures should be held for 4 days before discarding them as negative. *Salmonella* and *Shigella* species fail to produce any trace of alkalinity on this medium.

SIGNIFICANCE

Proteus species are probably the most troublesome and common lactose-nonfermenting organisms encountered in searching for enteric pathogens. The urease test is valuable in ruling out confusing colonies that mimic *Salmonella* on many types of media.

OTHER ORGANISMS EXHIBITING UREASE ACTIVITY

Gram-Positive Organisms	Gram-Negative Organisms
Bacillus species	*Actinobacillus* species (variable)
Clostridium botulinum (variable)	*Bordetella bronchiseptica*
Clostridium histolyticum	*Enterobacter* (variable)
Clostridium sordellii	*Klebsiella*
Clostridium tetani (variable)	*Pasteurella pseudotuberculosis*
Corynebacterium species	*Proteus*
Rapid-growing mycobacteria	*Pseudomonas aeruginosa*

NOTES

1. The main concern in this test is to prevent contamination of the medium, which may give false positive reactions.
2. Urea cannot be autoclaved; it must be filter-sterilized.
3. Christensen urea agar medium contains nutrients and is weakly buffered. Not only *Proteus* can be detected in this medium, but also some members of the *Klebsiella, Enterobacter* and *Serratia* groups that give weak delayed reactions.

REFERENCES

Christensen, W. B., Urea Decomposition as a Means of Differentiating *Proteus* and Paracolon Cultures from Each Other and from *Salmonella* and *Shigella* Types. J. Bacteriol., *52*, 461, 1946.

Rustigian, R., and Stuart, C. A., Decomposition of Urea by *Proteus*. Proc. Soc. Exp. Biol. Med., *47*, 108, 1941.

Urine Colony Count

Pour-Plate Method

PRINCIPLE

An estimate of the number of viable bacteria in urine or other fluid media can be made by appropriate dilution procedures. The original fluid is serially diluted, and the resultant dilution is incorporated in a pour plate of a suitable growth medium. The number of colonies present after appropriate incubation is counted, and the appropriate dilution factor is applied to determine the number of organisms in an aliquot of the original urine.

MEDIA

1. Nutrient agar

PROCEDURE

1. Dilute 0.1 ml of a well-mixed fresh urine specimen in 99.9 ml of sterile water. This results in a 1:1000 (10^{-3}) dilution.
2. Transfer 1.0 ml of the 1:1000 dilution to a sterile petri dish. Pour 15 ml of melted and cooled (50°C) nutrient agar into the dish, mix well with the specimen, and allow to solidify.
3. Incubate the plate at 35°C for 18 to 24 hours.
4. Count the number of colonies produced. The number of organisms present in 1 ml of the original specimen equals the number of colonies counted times 1000.

SIGNIFICANCE

Most authorities agree that bacteriuria exceeding 100,000 organisms per ml indicates true urinary-tract infection. Counts of less than 10,000 organisms per ml are usually associated with contamination. Counts between these limits are of indeterminate significance.

NOTES

1. The urine specimen must be fresh, no more than 2 hours old. Prompt refrigeration extends this time considerably. Bacterial counts on old specimens that were not refrigerated are of no clinical value in estimating the level of significance of bacteriuria.
2. Care must be taken to use cooled agar, since even short exposure to temperatures above 50°C may be fatal to many organisms.

Urine Colony Count

Calibrated-Loop Method

PRINCIPLE

An alternative method for estimating the number of viable bacteria in urine is to take an extremely small amount of the specimen and plate it on the surface of a suitable medium. The number of colonies present after appropriate incubation is counted and multiplied by the appropriate factor to determine the number of organisms in an aliquot of the original specimen.

An advantage of the calibrated-loop method, aside from speed and convenience, is the ability to estimate the relative numbers of organisms when mixed organisms of differing colonial morphology are present.

MEDIA

1. Blood agar

PROCEDURE

1. Dip a calibrated platinum loop designed to deliver 0.001 ml into a well-mixed fresh specimen of urine.
2. Streak the droplet across the surface of a blood agar plate.
3. Using a flamed, bent glass rod, spread the inoculum evenly over the entire surface of the blood agar.
4. Incubate the plate at 35°C for 18 to 24 hours.
5. Count the resulting colonies. The number of organisms per ml of the original specimen is calculated by multiplying the number of colonies counted by 1000.

SIGNIFICANCE

Most authorities agree that bacteriuria exceeding 100,000 organisms per ml indicates true urinary-tract infection. Counts of less than 10,000 organisms per ml are usually associated with contamination. Counts between these limits are of indeterminate significance.

NOTES

1. The urine specimen must be fresh, no more than 2 hours old. Prompt refrigeration extends this time considerably. Bacterial counts on old specimens that were not refrigerated are of no clinical value in estimating the level of significance of bacteriuria.

SEROLOGY

Sectional Directory

Introduction

Any compilation of serologic procedures must accept the fact that serologic methods, in particular syphilis serology, are the most rigorously standardized and most carefully controlled of all laboratory procedures. Not only do the various states regulate the conduct of these test procedures, but the Public Health Service has published a manual of syphilis serology that serves as the rule and guide of conduct for the conscientious serologist. The present compilation serves to contribute by presenting these procedures in the light of our own experience and by describing how these tests have been performed in our own laboratories.

The inclusion of the Kline test was decided upon prior to the publication of the current edition of the PHS Manual*, which omitted the Kline test from its pages, thus stripping it of any official blessing. After considerable discussion it was decided to continue presentation of this procedure in the CRC Manual as a salute to a time-honored procedure that—in our minds, at least—still has usefulness and as yet has not achieved complete emeritus status.

Thomas L. Gavan, M.D.

*Manual of Tests for Syphilis, 1969. U.S. Department of Health, Education and Welfare, Public Health Service, National Communicable Disease Center, Venereal Disease Program, Atlanta, Georgia 30333.

Serologic Tests for Syphilis

VDRL

PRINCIPLE

Reagin, an antibody-like substance in the serum, combines with particles of cardiolipin and lecithin, which make up the antigen. Cholesterol is added to increase the effective reacting surface of the antigen. The clumping of these substances is seen microscopically.

SPECIMEN

Serum.

SPECIAL EQUIPMENT

1. Glass-stoppered bottle, 30 ml capacity
2. Slides with ceramic rings
3. Syringe, 1 ml or 2 ml capacity
4. Needles, bevels removed
   (a) 23-gauge
   (b) 18-gauge
   (c) 19-gauge

PROCEDURE

Preparation of Antigen Suspension

1. Mix 0.4 ml of buffered saline* and 0.5 ml of antigen* in a 30-ml glass-stoppered bottle. The antigen is added rapidly to the saline, so that about 6 seconds are allowed for the mixing. Rotate the bottle on the tabletop during the mixing process.
2. Continue rotating and add 4.1 ml of buffered saline to give a total volume of antigen emulsion of 5 ml. This is stable for use during the day.

Preparation of Serum

1. Obtain clear serum from centrifuged clotted blood.
2. Inactivate the clear serum in a 56°C water bath for 30 minutes before starting the test.

Qualitative Determination

1. Pipette 0.05 ml of heated serum into one ring of the slide.
2. Add 1 drop of antigen suspension onto each serum, using a syringe with a 18-gauge needle with the point cut or ground off ($\frac{1}{60}$ ml of antigen).
3. Rotate the slides for 4 minutes at 180 rpm.
4. Immediately read microscopically with 100× magnification.

*Buffered saline diluent and antigen are available commercially from a number of sources.

Quantitative Slide Test

1. Pipette inactivated serum undiluted into the first three rings as indicated below:

   Ring 1: 0.04 ml
   Ring 2: 0.02 ml
   Ring 3: 0.01 ml

2. Dilute serum 1:8 (1 part serum, 7 parts physiological saline), mix well in the tube, then pipette from this dilution into the next three rings as follows:

   Ring 4: 0.04 ml
   Ring 5: 0.02 ml
   Ring 6: 0.01 ml

3. Using a 23-gauge needle, add 2 drops of physiological saline to the second and fifth rings, holding the syringe in vertical position.
4. Add 3 drops of physiological saline to the third and sixth rings in the same manner.
5. Rotate the slide by hand for 15 seconds to mix serum and saline. Using a 19-gauge needle, add 1 drop of antigen into each ring.
6. Rotate the slide at 180 rpm for 4 minutes and read at once. Report only the greatest dilution producing reactive results.

INTERPRETATION

Qualitative Determination

1. Medium and large clumps: reactive (R).
2. Small clumps: weakly reactive (WR).
3. No clumping or very slight roughness: nonreactive (N).

Quantitative Slide Test

Report as reactive in the highest dilution showing flocculation.

Example

1:1	1:2	1:4	1:8	1:16	1:32
R	R	R	***R***	WR	WR

is reported as "reactive, 8 dils", or

1:1	1:2	1:4	1:8	1:16	1:32
WR	R	***R***	WR	N	N

is reported as "reactive, 4 dils".

NOTES

1. All sera are examined when removed from the water bath, and those found to contain particulate debris are centrifuged.
2. Serum to be tested more than 4 hours after the original heating period should be reheated at 56°C for 10 minutes.
3. The antigen emulsion should be tested against known positive and negative sera. Care must be taken to work in a cool or air-conditioned room; there is a tendency for the antigen to evaporate if the laboratory is too warm.

Serologic Tests for Syphilis

Method of Kline

PRINCIPLE

Reagin, an antibody-like substance in the serum, combines with particles of cardiolipin and lecithin, which make up the antigen. Cholesterol is added to increase the effective reacting surface of the antigen. The clumping of these substances is seen microscopically when the antibody is present.

SPECIMEN

Serum.

SPECIAL EQUIPMENT

1. Glass-stoppered bottle, 30 ml capacity
2. Slides with ceramic rings
3. Hypodermic needles, bevels removed
   22- or 25-gauge, whichever delivers 140 drops ± per ml of antigen.

REAGENTS

1. Antigen emulsion

distilled water	0.85 ml
cholesterol, 1%, in absolute alcohol	1.00 ml
cardiolipin-natural lecithin Kline antigen	0.10 ml
saline, physiological	2.45 ml

(a) Pipette the distilled water to the bottom of a glass-stoppered bottle.
(b) Pipette the cholesterol solution slowly, drop by drop, into the water, holding the bottle at a 20-degree angle. Rotate the bottle vigorously, but cautiously, on a flat surface.
(c) Continue to rotate for 20 seconds.
(d) Using a 0.2-ml pipette, add the cardiolipin antigen against the side of the bottle above the solution, avoiding the ground-glass area.
(e) Stopper immediately and shake vigorously for 1 minute; throw the fluid from top to bottom.
(f) Quickly add the saline and immediately, but less vigorously, shake for 30 seconds.
(g) Store under refrigeration. Make fresh every other day.

This antigen is ready and usable for 1 day. Mix the antigen gently each time it is used; do not force it through the needle. Double quantities may be prepared.

PROCEDURE

Preparation of Serum

1. Serum must be unhemolyzed and free of visible particles. Recentrifuge, if necessary.
2. Inactivate at 56°C for 30 minutes. If retested after 24 hours or later, heat at 56°C for 5 minutes just before testing.

Qualitative Determination

1. Pipette 0.05 ml of serum into the well on a glass slide.
2. Add 1 drop (0.007 ml) of antigen emulsion with a Kline antigen pipette (1-ml or 2-ml syringe held vertically).
3. Rotate on a machine at 180 rpm for 4 minutes.
4. Examine microscopically at 100× magnification.

Quantitative Test

1. Place 0.3 ml of saline in five test tubes.
2. Add 0.3 ml of serum to tube 1 and mix.
3. Remove 0.35 ml of diluted serum and measure 0.05 ml into the well of the slide.
4. Add the remaining 0.3 ml to tube 2 and mix.
5. Proceed in this manner through the entire series, making twofold serial dilutions and pipetting 0.05 ml of the dilution onto the slide.
6. Add 1 drop (0.007 ml) of antigen.
7. Rotate at 180 rpm for 4 minutes.
8. Examine microscopically at 100× magnification.

INTERPRETATION

Qualitative Determination

1. Medium and large clumps: reactive.
2. Definite clumps, but small: weakly reactive.
3. No clumping: nonreactive.

Quantitative Test

Report the highest serum dilution that gives reactive results as "reactive in serum dilution ———".

NOTES

1. Failure to use distilled water of the proper pH (6.0—6.8) and free of salts may be responsible for unsatisfactory results. If the distilled water is too acid, the antigen will be coarse; if the distilled water is too alkaline, the antigen will be undersensitive and give nonspecific reactions.
2. If the qualitative determination presents irregular, feathery clumping (atypical reaction), retest the serum quantitatively, using dilutions 1:2 to 1:64.
3. In any serologic test for syphilis it is essential to have adequate controls of serum known to be positive and negative for the test being carried out. In most instances it is useful to have serum of varying degrees of positive reactions. This may be achieved by selecting positive controls of varying degrees of reactivity or by diluting strongly positive controls.

REFERENCE

Serologic Test for Syphilis. U.S. Department of Health, Education and Welfare, Public Health Service, Communicable Disease Center, Venereal Disease Branch, 1964.

Serologic Tests for Syphilis

Fluorescent Treponemal Antibody Test (FTA-ABS)

PRINCIPLE

Demonstration of specific antibodies to *Treponema pallidum* is considered the most reliable means of establishing laboratory evidence of present or past infection with syphilis. At the present time, the most specific and sensitive procedure for the detection of treponemal antibodies is the fluorescent treponemal antibody test by the absorption technic.

SPECIMEN

Serum.

SPECIAL EQUIPMENT

1. Incubator (adjustable to 35—37°C)
2. Dark-field fluorescence microscope assembly.
3. Bibulous paper
4. Diamond-point pencil (optional)
5. Template (optional)
   Used as a guide for cutting circles 1.0 cm in diameter on glass slides.
6. Slide board or holder
7. Moist chamber
   Any convenient cover for slides may be made into a moist chamber by placing wet paper inside.
8. Bacteriological loop (standard 2 mm, 26 gauge platinum wire)
9. Immersion oil (low fluorescence, nondrying)

Glassware

1. Microscope slides (1″ × 3″, approximately 1 mm thick, frosted end)
   Glass slides with two etched circles 1 cm in diameter are available from Clay-Adams, Inc., 141 East 25th Street, New York, New York 10010 (Catalog No. A-1447/10).
2. Cover slips (No. 1, 22 mm square)
3. Staining dish (glass or plastic, with removable slide carriers)
4. Glass rods (approximately 100 × 4 mm, both ends fire-polished)

REAGENTS

1. *Treponema pallidum* antigen* (either A or B)
   A. Nichols strain, extracted from rabbit testicular tissue
      This is the antigen for the FTA test. The suspension should contain a minimum of 30 organisms per high dry field. Store at 6—10°C. If the antigen becomes bacterially contaminated or does not demonstrate the proper reactivity with control sera, it should be discarded.

*Baltimore Biological Laboratory, Baltimore, Maryland 21204. Difco Laboratories, Detroit, Michigan 48201. The Sylvana Company, Millburn, New Jersey, 07041

B. Nichols strain, extracted from rabbit testicular tissue, freeze-dried
Reconstitute according to manufacturer's directions, then store at 6—10°C. A satisfactory antigen should contain a minimum of 30 organisms per high dry field in the liquid state.

2. FTA-ABS test absorbent*
A standardized product prepared from cultures of Reiter treponemas that may be purchased in lyophilized or liquid state. Store and use according to manufacturer's directions.

3. Fluorescein-labeled anti-human globulin (conjugate)*†
Use a product of proven quality. Rehydrated conjugate should be stored in not less than 0.3-ml quantities at −20°C or lower. For practical purposes, a conjugate with a titer of 1:400 or higher may be diluted 1:10 with sterile phosphate-buffered saline (containing Merthiolate‡ in a concentration of 1:5000) before storage. When thawed for use, it should not be refrozen, but can be stored at 6—10°C as long as satisfactory reactivity is obtained with test controls.

4. Phosphate-buffered saline (PBS)

sodium chloride	7.650 g
disodium phosphate	0.724 g
potassium hydrogen phosphate	0.210 g

Dissolve the above ingredients in 1 liter water. This solution yields pH-meter readings of pH 7.2 ± 0.10. Several liters may be prepared and stored in a large polethylene or Pyrex bottle.

5. Tween® 80§ solution (2% in PBS)
To prepare PBS containing 2% Tween® 80, add 2 ml of Tween® 80 to 98 ml of PBS, measuring from the bottom of the pipette, and rinse the pipette. Heat the two reagents in a 56°C water bath. The 2% Tween® 80 solution should be pH 7.0—7.2. The pH should be checked periodically, since the solution may become acid. This solution keeps well at refrigerator temperature, but should be discarded if a precipitate develops or if the pH changes.

6. Mounting medium
Add 1 part PBS, pH 7.2, to 9 parts glycerine (reagent grade).

7. Acetone (ACS)

Check Testing of New Lots of Reagents

1. *Treponema pallidum* antigen
   (a) A new lot of antigen should be compared with an antigen of known reactivity before being placed in routine use. Testing should be performed on more than one testing day, using control sera, individual sera of graded reactivity, and nonreactive sera.
   (b) Results obtained on testing of controls and individual sera with both antigens should be comparable.
   (c) A sufficient number of organisms should remain on the slide after staining to permit reading of the test without difficulty.
   (d) The antigen should not stain nonspecifically with a conjugate of known quality at its working titer.

*Baltimore Biological Laboratory, Maryland 21204. Difco Laboratories, Detroit, Michigan 48201. The Sylvana Company, Millburn, New Jersey 07041.
†Hyland Division Travenol Laboratories, Los Angeles, California 90039.
‡Eli Lilly and Company, P.O. Box 618, Indianapolis, Indiana 46206.
§Hill Top Laboratories, Inc., 250 William H. Taft Road, Cincinnati, Ohio 45219.

(e) The antigen should not contain background material that stains to the extent of interference with the reading of the test.

2. FTA-ABS test sorbent
   (a) A new lot of sorbent should be compared with a sorbent of known activity before being placed in routine use. Testing should be performed on more than one testing day, using control sera, individual sera of graded reactivity, and nonsyphilitic sera demonstrating nonspecific reactivity.
   (b) The new sorbent should remove nonspecific reactivity of the nonspecific serum control. It should not materially reduce the reactivity from a known syphilis serum (reactive control).
   (c) Results obtained on testing of controls and individual sera with both sorbents should be comparable.
   (d) Nonspecific staining controls should be nonreactive.
   (e) The sorbent should be usable rehydrated to the indicated volume or according to the manufacturer's directions.

3. Fluorescein-labeled anti-human globulin (conjugate)

   Before being placed into routine use, each new lot of conjugate, whether prepared in the laboratory or obtained from a commercial source, should first be titered and then check-tested in parallel with a known standard conjugate.

Titration

(a) The titer of each new lot of conjugate should be determined, using the particular dark-field fluorescence microscope assembly available.

(b) Prepare dilutions of the unknown conjugate in PBS containing 2% Tween® 80 to include the titer indicated by the manufacturer. For example:

1 : 10, 1 : 20, 1 : 40, 1 : 80, 1 : 160,

or

1 : 10, 1 : 25, 1 : 50, 1 : 100, 1 : 1200.

Higher dilutions may be prepared, if necessary.

(c) Each conjugate dilution is tested with the reactive (4+) control serum diluted 1 : 5 in PBS.

(d) A nonspecific staining control is run with undiluted as well as with each dilution of unknown conjugate.

(e) A known conjugate, at its titer, is set up at the same time with the reactive (4+) control serum, a minimally reactive (1+) control serum, and a nonspecific staining control, for the purpose of controlling reagents and test conditions. An example is given in the table on p. 323.

(f) The titer of the conjugate selected for use is the dilution that is one doubling dilution lower than the highest dilution giving maximum fluorescence (4+). In the example given, the dilution selected for use is 1 : 160.

(g) A satisfactory conjugate should show no staining on an acceptable antigen at three doubling dilutions below the established titer of the conjugate. In the example of titration given, this conjugate would meet the criterion and be considered satisfactory, since there is no nonspecific staining with the 1 : 20 dilution.

Check-Testing

(a) Each new lot of conjugate should be tested in parallel with a known

TITRATION OF UNKNOWN CONJUGATE

Conjugates	Controls		
	Nonspecific Staining Control	Reactive (4+) Control Serum 1:5 in PBS	Reactive (1+) Control Serum
Known Conjugate			
Titer 1:80	–	4+	1+
Unknown Conjugate			
Undiluted	1+	4+	
Diluted:			
1:10	±	4+	
1:20	–	4+	
1:40	–	4+	
1:80	–	4+	
1:160	–	4+	
1:320	–	4+	
1:640	–	3+	

conjugate before being placed in routine use. Testing should be performed on more than one testing day, using control sera, individual sera of graded reactivity, and nonreactive sera.

(b) Individual sera tested in parallel with a known and a new conjugate are read against the minimally reactive (1+) controls set up with the respective conjugates.

(c) A new conjugate is considered to be satisfactory when comparable test results are obtained with both conjugates.

PROCEDURE

Preparation of Serum

1. Both test and control serum should be heated at 56°C for 30 minutes before testing.
2. Previously heated serum should be reheated at 56°C for 10 minutes on the day of testing.

Preparation of Controls

Control sera are used and stored according to directions. The following controls must be included in each test run.

1. Reactive (4+) control*
   Reactive serum or a dilution of reactive serum demonstrating strong (4+) fluorescence when diluted 1:5 in PBS and only slightly reduced fluorescence when diluted 1:5 in sorbent.
   (a) Using a 0.2-ml pipette, measuring from the tip, add 0.05 ml of reactive control serum into a tube containing 0.2 ml of PBS. Mix well, at least 8 times.
   (b) Using a 0.2-ml pipette, measuring from the tip, add 0.05 ml of reactive control serum into a tube containing 0.2 ml of sorbent. Mix well, at least 8 times.

*Baltimore Biological Laboratory, Baltimore, Maryland 21204. Difco Laboratories Detroit, Michigan 48201. The Sylvana Company, Millburn, New Jersey 07041.

2. Minimally reactive (1+) control
Dilution of reactive serum demonstrating the minimal degree of fluorescence reported as "reactive", for use as a reading standard.
Dilute reactive (4+) control serum in PBS according to the manufacturer's directions to obtain minimally reactive (1+) control.
3. Nonspecific serum control.
A nonsyphilitic serum known to demonstrate at least 2+ nonspecific reactivity in the FTA test at a dilution of 1 : 5 or higher in PBS.
   (a) Using a 0.2-ml pipette, measuring from the tip, add 0.05 ml of nonspecific control serum into a tube containing 0.2 ml of PBS. Mix well, at least 8 times.
   (b) Using a 0.2-ml pipette, measuring from the tip, add 0.05 ml of nonspecific control serum into a tube containing 0.2 ml of sorbent. Mix well, at least 8 times.
4. Nonspecific staining control
   (a) Antigen smear treated with 0.03 ml of PBS.
   (b) Antigen smear treated with 0.03 ml of sorbent.

CONTROL PATTERN ILLUSTRATION

Control	Reaction
Reactive control	
(a) 1:5 PBS dilution	R 4+
(b) 1:5 sorbent dilution	R
Minimally reactive (1+) control	R 1+
Nonspecific serum control	
(a) 1:5 PBS dilution	R (2+—4+)
(b) 1:5 sorbent dilution	N
Nonspecific staining controls	
(a) antigen, PBS, and conjugate	N
(b) antigen, sorbent, and conjugate	N

Note: test runs in which the above control results are not obtained are considered unsatisfactory and should not be reported.

Preparation of *Treponema pallidum* Antigen Smears

1. Mix antigen suspension well by drawing it into and expelling it from a disposable pipette with rubber bulb at least 10 times in order to break the treponemal clumps and insure an even distribution of treponemas. Determine by dark-field examination that the treponemas are adequately dispersed before making slides for the FTA test. Additional mixing may be required.
2. On clean slides, cut two circles 1 cm in diameter with a diamond-pointed pencil. The slides should be wiped with clean gauze to remove loose glass particles.
3. Smear 1 loopful of *Treponema pallidum* antigen evenly within each circle, using a standard 2-mm, 26-gauge platinum wire loop. Allow to air-dry for at least 15 minutes.
4. Fix the smears in acetone for 10 minutes and allow to air-dry thoroughly. Not more than 60 slides should be fixed with 200 ml of acetone. Acetone-treated slides may be stored at −20° or below. Fixed frozen smears are usable indefinitely, provided that satisfactory results are obtained with the controls. Frozen smears should not be thawed and refrozen.

Test

1. Identify previously prepared slides by numbering the frosted end with a lead pencil.
2. Number the tubes to correspond to the sera and control sera being tested and place in racks.
3. Prepare reactive (4+), minimally reactive (1+), and nonspecific control serum dilutions in sorbent and/or PBS according to directions.
4. For each test serum pipette 0.2 ml of sorbent into a test tube.
5. Using a 0.2-ml pipette, measuring from the bottom, add 0.05 ml of the heated test serum into the appropriate tube and mix at least 8 times.
6. The interval between preparing serum dilutions and placing them on the antigen smears should not exceed 30 minutes.
7. Cover the appropriate antigen smears with 0.03 ml of the reactive (4+), minimally reactive (1+), and nonspecific control serum dilutions.
8. Cover the appropriate antigen smears with 0.03 ml of the PBS and 0.03 ml of the sorbent for the respective nonspecific staining controls.
9. Cover the appropriate antigen smears with 0.03 ml of the test serum dilutions.
10. Place the slides into a moist chamber to prevent evaporation.
11. Incubate at 35—37°C for 30 minutes.
12. Rinse as follows:
    (a) place the slides in slide carriers and rinse for approximately 5 seconds with running PBS;
    (b) place the slides for 5 minutes in a staining dish containing PBS;
    (c) agitate the slides by dipping them in and out of the PBS at least 10 times;
    (d) using fresh PBS, repeat steps (b) and (c);
    (e) rinse the slides for approximately 5 seconds in running distilled water.
13. Gently blot the slides with bibulous paper to remove all water drops.
14. Dilute conjugate to its working titer in PBS containing 2% Tween® 80.
15. Place approximately 0.03 ml of diluted conjugate on each smear and spread uniformly with a glass rod to cover the entire smear.
16. Repeat steps 10, 11, 12, and 13.
17. Immediately mount the slides by placing a small drop of mounting medium on each smear and applying a cover slip.
18. Examine the slides as soon as possible. If a delay in reading is necessary, place the slides in a darkened room and read within 4 hours.
19. Study the smears microscopically, using an ultraviolet light source and a high-power dry objective. A combination of a BG-12 exciting filter not more than 3 mm thick and OG-1 barrier filter (or their equivalents*) has been found to be satisfactory for routine use.
20. Check nonreactive smears, using illumination from a tungsten light source, to verify the presence of treponemas.
21. Record the intensity of fluorescence of the treponemas according to the interpretation chart given on p. 326, using the minimally reactive (1+) control slide as the reading standard.

*Filter equivalents: exciting filter BG-12—AO 702; barrier filter OG-1—AO 724 or 1124, B&L Y-8, Zeiss 50/-(II/0).

INTERPRETATION

Reading	Intensity of Fluorescence	Report
2+ to 4+	Moderate to strong	Reactive (R)
1+	Equivalent to minimally reactive (1+) control	Reactive (R)*
<1+	Weak, but definite; less than minimally reactive (1+) control	Borderline (B)*
—	None or vaguely visible	Nonreactive (N)

*Note: retest all specimens with an intensity of fluorescence of 1+ or less; when a specimen initially read as 1+ is retested and subsequently read as 1+ or greater, the test is reported as "reactive"; all other results on retest are reported as "borderline"; it is not necessary to retest nonfluorescent (nonreactive) specimens.

Reporting Scheme

Test Reading	Repeat	Report
4+		R
3+		R
2+		R
1+	1+ or greater	R
	<1+ or N	B
1+	1+, <1+, or —	B
—		N

Suggested Attachment to Reports of Borderline Test Results

The borderline report of the FTA-ABS test performed in our laboratory on the specimen obtained from ____________ (patient's name) means that the result cannot be interpreted as either reactive or nonreactive.

If this is the first specimen you have submitted for FTA-ABS testing on this patient, another specimen should be submitted for retesting.

If this is the second specimen from this patient that gives a borderline result on FTA-ABS testing, it is impossible to state whether the patient does or does not have serologic evidence of syphilitic infection. A careful review of the patient's history and physical findings is suggested; in view of the borderline serologic findings, diagnosis will necessarily rest upon the clinical findings.

NOTES

1. Bacterial contamination or excessive hemolysis may render specimens unsatisfactory for testing.
2. Reactive (4+) control, nonspecific serum control, and nonspecific staining control are included for the purpose of controlling reagents and test conditions; minimally reactive (1+) control serum is included as the reading standard.

REFERENCES

Deacon, W. E., Lucas, J. B., and Price, Eleanor V., Fluorescent Treponemal Antibody-Absorption (FTA-ABS) Test for Syphilis. J. Am. Med. Assoc., *198*, 624, 1966.

Hunter, Elizabeth F., Deacon, W. E., and Meyer, Patricia E., An Improved FTA Test for Syphilis, the Absorption Procedure (FTA-ABS). Public Health Rep., *79*, 410, 1964.

Stout, Genevieve W., Kellog, D. S., Jr., Falcone, Virginia H., McGrew, Betty E., and Lewis, J. S., Preparation and Standardization of the Sorbent Used in the Fluorescent Treponemal Antibody-Absorption (FTA-ABS) Test. Health Lab. Sci., *4*, 5, 1967.

Febrile Agglutinations

Rapid Slide Test

PRINCIPLE

When certain disease-producing agents are present in the body, specific antibodies are produced in response to them. These antibodies can be demonstrated by exposure to antigens *in vitro*, and thus the type and severity of infection can be determined.

SPECIMEN

Serum.

REAGENTS

1. Stock febrile antigens

PROCEDURE

1. Use stock febrile antigens in the form in which they are supplied by the manufacturer.
2. Perform the test on a glass plate with ceramic circles (11 × 6 rows). A sheet of plain glass ruled in 1½-inch squares with a wax pencil can be substituted.
3. Use clear unheated serum and proceed as indicated in the table below.

Febrile Antigens (1 drop per circle)	Serum (ml)*					
	0.08 ↓	0.04 ↓	0.02 ↓	0.01 ↓	0.005 ↓	0.002 ↓
Salmonella Group A →						
Salmonella Group B →						
Salmonella Group C →						
Salmonella Group D →						
Salmonella Group E →						
Paratyphoid A →						
Paratyphoid B →						
Paratyphoid C →						
Typhoid H →						
Proteus 0X19 →						
Brucella abortus →						

*Dispense with a 0.2 ml pipette.

4. Mix the contents of each circle with a clean wooden applicator stick. Use a new stick for each circle.
5. Hold the plate near a light source. Rock slowly and tilt. Observe for a period not to exceed 3 minutes.
6. Record all agglutination as follows:

Percent Agglutination	Reported as
100	4+
75	3+
50	2+
25	1+
25	± (trace)
None	Negative

INTERPRETATION

The smallest quantity of serum that exhibits a 2+ reaction is the end point or titer.

EQUIVALENT DILUTIONS

Serum (ml)	Final Dilution
0.08	1:20
0.04	1:40
0.02	1:80
0.01	1:160
0.005	1:320
0.002	1:640

NOTES

1. Disregard reactions after 3 minutes.
2. Do not allow heat from the light source to evaporate the serum-antigen mixture.
3. Equivalent dilutions are determined by the manufacturer of the antigen and are somewhat arbitrary. The 0.08-ml dose of serum gives a reaction that appears similar to that expected with a 1:20 dilution of serum, and the 0.002-ml dose of serum will give the same results as expected in a 1:640 dilution of the original serum.

Febrile Agglutinations

Tube Method

PRINCIPLE

When certain disease-producing agents are present in the body, specific antibodies are produced in response to them. These antibodies can be demonstrated by exposure to antigen *in vitro*, and thus the type and severity of infection can be determined.

SPECIMEN

Serum.

REAGENTS

1. Normal saline
2. Phosphate-buffered saline
3. Antigen solutions (commercially available)

PROCEDURE

1. Put 0.9 ml of saline in the first tube of a series of ten 13 × 100 mm tubes and 0.5 ml in each of the remaining nine tubes.
2. Using a 1-ml pipette, place 0.1 ml of clear unheated serum in tube 1. Mix well.
3. Remove 0.5 ml from tube 1 and transfer to tube 2. Mix well.
4. Continue this procedure until the contents of tube 10 have been mixed. Discard 0.5 ml from tube 10.
5. Use a tube containing 0.5 ml of saline only as an antigen control.
6. Dilute each febrile antigen with saline as indicated by the manufacturer. Shake well and add 0.5 ml to each tube in the series (a complete series of tubes will be required for each febrile antigen used), including the control.
7. Final dilutions will be 1 : 20, 1 : 40, 1 : 80, etc., through 1 : 10,240.
8. Shake the tubes to mix antigen and serum mixture, then incubate at 48—50°C (37°C for *Brucella abortus*) for 18 to 24 hours (2 hours for paratyphoid A, B, and C, and for typhoid H).
9. Remove the racks of tubes and allow them to stand at room temperature while the results are read. Hold two or three tubes at a time in front of a suitable light source and estimate the degree of agglutination as follows:

complete agglutination and clear supernatant	4+
75% clear supernatant	3+
50% clear supernatant	2+
25% clear supernatant	1+
slight sedimentation	±
no evidence of agglutination	negative

The end point is the highest serum dilution exhibiting 50% agglutination (2+).

INTERPRETATION

A single test result is not diagnostically significant unless unusually high. It is best to demonstrate a changing (rising) titer in successive specimens. A negative test does not exclude infection.

Disease	Febrile Antigen	Serum Agglutinins		
		Appear	Maximum	Titer
Typhoid	*Salmonella* Group D (typhoid O)	7—10 days	3—5 weeks	1:80 (early) suspicious 1:160 indicative
	Typhoid H	Late	Late	1:40 suspicious 1:80 indicative
Paratyphoid fever and other *Salmonella* infections	*Salmonella* Groups A, B, C, and E	Variable	Variable	1:80—1:160 suspicious
	Paratyphoid A, B, and C	Variable	Variable	Try to demonstrate a rising titer
Typhus	*Proteus* 0X19	7—10 days	14th day	1:40—1:80 suspicious 1:160 indicative
Rocky Mountain spotted fever	*Proteus* 0X19	7—10 days	14th day	Peak titer not above 1:160—1:320
Brucellosis	*Brucella abortus*	2—3 weeks	3—5 weeks	1:80—1:160 indicative 1:320 or more conclusive

C-Reactive Protein

PRINCIPLE

C-reactive protein is a specific protein that appears in the blood at times of infection or with tissue necrosis. It is detected by use of a specific antiserum. The amount present is an indication of the severity of the infection.

SPECIMEN

Serum.

REAGENTS

1. C-reactive protein antiserum (commercially available)
2. Plastic sealant (commercially available)

PROCEDURE

1. Mark a capillary tube at about 30 and 60 mm from one end.
2. Dip into C-reactive protein antiserum and allow to fill to the first (30 mm) mark.
3. Close the capillary tube with the finger and remove from the antiserum.
4. Wipe off excess serum.
5. Dip the tube into the patient's serum and allow to fill to the second (60 mm) mark. The two sera must be in contact; avoid air bubbles.
6. Remove the tube from the serum, then tip the capillary tube and run the fluid back and forth several times to mix.
7. Wipe the outside of the tube clean. With the fluid at about the middle of the tube, close one end with the finger and stick the tube upright in plastic sealant. The bottom meniscus of the fluid must be above the level of the plastic.
8. Allow to stand overnight at room temperature.
9. Examine for presence of white precipitate.

INTERPRETATION

Report according to the following scale:

no precipitate	negative
approximately 1 mm of sedimented precipitate	+
approximately 2 mm of sedimented precipitate	++
approximately 3 mm of sedimented precipitate	+++
approximately 4 mm or more	++++

Cold Agglutination

PRINCIPLE

Cold agglutinins are antibodies that manifest their effect at low temperatures, usually below 5°C. They occur during and following many viral diseases and most often are used as a diagnostic criterion for primary atypical pneumonia. The reaction is reversible, and cells agglutinated at 5°C may be resuspended if the preparation is warmed to room temperature.

NORMAL VALUES

Titers up to 1 : 32 may occur in normal subjects.

SPECIMEN

Serum. This should not be left on the clot, but should be separated as soon as practical. Until this is done, the specimen should be kept at room temperature and not refrigerated.

REAGENTS

1. Antigen—Group O human erythrocytes
   Collect in sterile citrate and store in a refrigerator. Do not keep more than 1 week. Do not use if hemolysis is present. Prepare for use by washing 3 times. Make a 1% suspension in normal saline.
2. Normal saline

PROCEDURE

1. Number eight test tubes.
2. To each tube add 0.5 ml of saline solution.
3. Add 0.5 ml of serum to the first tube and mix.
4. Transfer 0.5 ml of the serum dilution to tube 2 and mix. Continue the dilution through tube 7.
5. Discard 0.5 ml of the serum dilution from tube 7 to keep the volumes uniform.
6. Add 0.5 ml of cell suspension to each tube. The final dilutions are as follows:

Tube No.	Dilution
1	1:4
2	1:8
3	1:16
4	1:32
5	1:64
6	1:128
7	1:256

7. Incubate overnight at 5°C or lower.
8. Remove from the refrigerator and read immediately for agglutination.
9. Incubate at 37°C for 30 minutes, or allow to stand at room temperature for 1 hour, then read again.

INTERPRETATION

Read agglutination as negative to 4+. If the incubated dilutions that show agglutination do not reverse their reaction, then it is not true cold agglutination and should not be reported as such.

REFERENCE

Case Western Reserve University, Unpublished Method.

Heterophile Agglutination Test

Presumptive Test

PRINCIPLE

In infectious mononucleosis, heterophile antibodies are found in the patient's serum. The presence of antibodies can be determined by their ability to agglutinate sheep red blood cells. This test is nonspecific, since the antibodies also may be Forssman or serum-sickness types.

SPECIMEN

Serum inactivated at 56°C for 30 minutes.

REAGENTS

1. Normal saline
2. Sheep red blood cells

   Wash 3 times with normal saline and make a 2% suspension. No hemc should result. Prepare daily.

PROCEDURE

1. Set up eleven test tubes, numbering them 1 to 11.
2. Add 0.1 ml of serum to tube 1.
3. Add 0.4 ml of normal saline to tube 1 and mix well.
4. Pipette 0.25 ml of saline into each of the remaining tubes.
5. Pipette 0.25 ml of solution from tube 1 to tube 2 and mix well.
6. Repeat step 5 from tube 2 to tube 3 and continue through tube 10.
7. Pipette 0.25 ml of the solution from tube 10 and discard.
8. Add 0.1 ml of the 2% suspension of sheep cells to tubes 1 through 11.
9. Incubate at room temperature. A positive result may show agglutination after 15 minutes, but negative results should be reported only after 2-hour incubation.
10. To read the results, shake the tubes to resuspend the sediments. Record as follows:

++++	one large clump
+++	large and small clumps
++	small clumps seen distinctly with the naked eye
+	microscopic (scanning lens) clumps
−	no microscopic clumps

The titer is the greatest dilution showing 1+ agglutination.

Tube No.	Dilution
1	1:7
2	1:14
3	1:28
4	1:56
5	1:112
6	1:224
7	1:448
8	1:896
9	1:1792
10	1:3584
11	control

INTERPRETATION

Individuals with infectious mononucleosis have heterophile-antibody titers that range from 1 : 28 to 1 :14,336, with a mean of 1 : 646. In general, sheep agglutinin titers in healthy persons are rarely above 1 :56. Other conditions may produce titers of 1 : 112 or higher. These are listed in the table below.

Titer	Condition
1:56	Upper normal
1:112	Aplastic anemia, agranulocytosis, splenic thrombocytopenia, polycythemia, chronic nephritis, migraine
1:224	Hodgkin's disease, myelogenous leukemia, allergy, staphylococcal infection
1:448	Sarcoma, infectious hepatitis, tuberculosis
1:896	Acute leukemia, injection of liver extract or blood group substance A
1:3584	Monocytic leukemia, serum sickness

A presumptive test with a titer of 1 : 112 or higher in a patient with typical clinical and hematologic findings may be considered positive for infectious mononucleosis. Otherwise a differential test is essential.

REFERENCE

Davidsohn, I., and Henry, J. B., Todd-Sanford Clinical Diagnosis by Laboratory Methods, 14th ed. W. B. Saunders, Philadelphia, 1969.

Heterophile Agglutination Test

Davidsohn Differential Test

PRINCIPLE

When serum is mixed with guinea pig kidney antigen, the antigen absorbs all heterophile antibodies except the infectious-mononucleosis type. Heterophile antibodies of the infectious-mononucleosis type are absorbed by beef cells, whereas those due to other causes are not. The absorbed serum is then tested for the heterophile antibody remaining by agglutination titrations as in the screening procedure.

SPECIMEN

Serum inactivated at 56°C for 30 minutes.

REAGENTS

1. Boiled-beef erythrocytes (20% suspension)
2. Guinea pig kidney antigen (20% suspension)
3. Normal saline
4. Sheep red blood cells
   Wash 3 times with normal saline, then make a 2% suspension.

PROCEDURE

Absorption of Serum

1. Place 0.2 ml of the patient's serum and 1.0 ml of guinea pig kidney antigen in a test tube.
2. Shake and allow to stand for 3 minutes at room temperature.
3. Centrifuge at 1,500 rpm for 10 minutes or longer (full speed), until the supernatant is clear.
4. Remove the supernatant carefully with a capillary pipette and bulb and place in a properly marked test tube. This is now a 1 : 5 dilution of serum.

Serum Dilutions

1. Set up as many tubes (75 × 10 mm) as needed according to the titer of the presumptive test. Add 0.25 ml of physiological saline to all tubes except tube 1.
2. Add 0.25 ml of the absorbed serum to tubes 1 and 2.
3. Mix the contents of tube 2, then transfer 0.25 ml to tube 3. Continue in this manner, discarding 0.25 ml from the last tube.

Test

1. Add 0.1 ml of 2% sheep cell suspension to each tube of serum dilutions. The final dilutions are 1 : 7, 1 : 14, etc.
2. Repeat the absorption of serum, using 1.0 ml of the mixed 20% suspension of boiled-beef erythrocytes in place of guinea pig kidney antigen.
3. Incubate at room temperature. A positive result may show agglutination in 15 minutes, but negative results should be reported only after 2-hour incubation.

Tube No.	Dilution
1	1:7
2	1:14
3	1:28
4	1:56
5	1:112
6	1:224
7	1:448
8	1:896
9	1:1792
10	1:3584

INTERPRETATION

With serum absorbed with guinea pig kidney, a positive test for infectious mononucleosis consists of a 3-tube or smaller decrease in titer from the presumptive value. In addition, serum absorbed with boiled-beef erythrocytes should show a 4-tube decrease in titer.

CRITERIA FOR POSITIVE DIFFERENTIAL TESTS

Tested with Washed Sheep Erythrocytes	Decrease of Titer after Absorption in Number of Tubes
Serum absorbed with guinea pig kidney	0 1 2 ③ maximum
Serum absorbed with beef erythrocytes	④ 5 6 . . . minimum

REFERENCE

Davidsohn, I., and Stern, K., and Kashiwagi, C., The Differential Test for Infectious Mononucleosis. Amer. J. Clin. Pathol., *21*, 1101, 1951.

Fluorescent Test for Antinuclear Factor

PRINCIPLE

An antibody against a nuclear constituent can be detected in a patient's serum by the indirect fluorescent-antibody technic; i.e., antigen-antibody complex plus fluorescein-labeled anti-human globulin yields antigen-antibody, anti-human globulin, fluorescent complex (visible under the fluorescent microscope).

SPECIMEN

Serum.

SPECIAL EQUIPMENT

1. Cryostat
2. Liquid-nitrogen flask
3. Freezer (−70°C)
4. Fluorescent microscope with high-pressure mercury-arc light source.

REAGENT

1. Phosphate-buffered saline (pH 7.3)

   Dissolve 9.23 g of FTA hemagglutination buffer (BBL) in 1 liter of distilled water.
2. Fluorescein-labeled anti-human globulin serum
3. Liquid nitrogen
4. Mounting medium

   Add 1 part phosphate-buffered saline to 9 parts glycerine.
5. Tissue

   Surgical material is preferred. The choice of tissue to be used is up to the individual laboratory. Spleen imprints and cryostat sections of normal thyroid, normal stomach and rat kidney have been used satisfactorily.

PROCEDURE

1. Obtain tissue and freeze it for 30 seconds in liquid nitrogen. Keep at −70°C until ready to use.
2. Cut tissue sections at 5 microns on a cryostat microtome.
3. Allow the tissue sections to dry at room temperature for at least 1 hour.
4. Overlay the tissue section with the patient's serum (not inactivated) and incubate in a closed moist chamber for 20 minutes at room temperature. A flat covered tray with wet paper towels on the bottom will serve as a moist chamber.
5. Rinse the slides in 3 changes of phosphate-buffered saline, then place in a 4th change for 15 minutes, with another change of buffer during this time.
6. After removing excess buffer from around the sections, overlay them with appropriate dilutions of fluorescent anti-human globulin (see Note 6). Incubate the slides in the moist chamber for 20 minutes at room temperature.
7. Rinse the slides as in step 5.

8. Remove excess buffer from around the sections, then mount them in buffered glycerine.
9. If the patient's serum contains antinuclear factor, the nuclei will give an apple-green fluorescence.

SIGNIFICANCE

1. 99% of patients with systemic lupus erythematosus will demonstrate a positive antinuclear factor.
2. A positive antinuclear factor can be regarded as a "marker" for possible auto-immune diseases.

NOTES

1. Slides should be read the day they are processed.
2. A positive and negative control should always be included in the test run.
3. Tissue obtained from surgery or from any other source should be frozen as soon as possible.
4. Always run a slide with just the fluorescein-labeled anti-human globulin as a guide line for the presence of nonspecific staining.
5. It must be remembered that different types of nuclear staining may be seen, such as homogeneous, speckled and nucleolar. All constitute a positive anti-nuclear-factor reaction.
6. The most appropriate dilution of fluorescein-labeled anti-human globulin is determined by making serial twofold dilutions and testing these dilutions against a known reactive serum. The greatest dilution giving a strong reaction is selected for future use. Each batch of fluorescein-labeled anti-human globulin must be evaluated in this manner.

REFERENCE

Mackay, I. R., and Burnet, F. M., Autoimmune Diseases: Pathogenesis, Chemistry, and Therapy. Charles C Thomas, Springfield, Illinois, 1963.

Colloidal-Gold Test

Method of Lange

PRINCIPLE

Cerebrospinal fluid is mixed with a colloidal suspension of gold. In normal cerebrospinal fluid no change occurs. In certain pathologic conditions of the nervous system, however, cerebrospinal fluid causes a color change that varies with the amount of dilution of the fluid. This is due to an abnormal albumin/globulin ration and has considerable diagnostic significance.

NORMAL VALUES

No color change in the tubes.

SPECIMEN

Cerebrospinal fluid.

REAGENTS

1. Saline solution (0.4%), sterile
2. Saline solution (1.0%), sterile
3. Colloidal-gold solution

   Add 1 ml of a 1% solution of gold chloride to 95 ml of distilled water. Heat to 90°C on an electric hot plate (no flame). Add 5 ml of 1% solution of sodium citrate. Boil the solution for 1 to 3 minutes. This reagent is stable for several months.

PROCEDURE

1. For each test fluid arrange twelve clean test tubes in a rack.
2. Place 1.8 ml of fresh sterile 0.5% sodium chloride in the first tube, and 1 ml in each of the others, except the twelfth.
3. In the twelfth tube place 1.7 ml of sterile 1% sodium chloride.
4. Add 0.2 ml of the cerebrospinal fluid to the first tube. Mix well by sucking the fluid up into the pipette and expelling it.
5. Transfer 1 ml of this mixture to the second tube and mix.
6. Transfer 1 ml to the next tube, and so on through the tenth tube, discarding the last 1-ml portion.
7. Use the eleventh and twelfth tubes as saline controls.
8. Add 5 ml of the colloidal-gold solution to all twelve tubes.
9. Let stand at room temperature for 1 hour or longer, then record the results.
10. Report the action of each tube in the series individually as follows:

complete decolorization	5
pale blue	4
blue	3
lilac or purple	2
red-blue	1
brilliant red-orange	0

INTERPRETATION

In a positive reaction, the solution in some of the tubes will have changed from red to purple, deep blue, or pale blue, or will have become colorless. If the fluid is normal, no color change will have occurred. The eleventh and twelfth control tubes should be red-orange or colorless respectively. Characteristic types of reactions would be:

normal	0	0	0	0	0	0	0	0	0	0
paretic	5	5	5	5	5	4	2	1	0	0
syphilitic or tabetic	0	1	2	3	3	2	0	0	0	0
meningitic	0	0	0	1	2	2	4	5	3	1

REFERENCE

Davidsohn, I., and Wells, B. B., Clinical Diagnosis by Laboratory Methods, 13th ed., p. 992. W. B. Saunders, Philadelphia, 1962.

MISCELLANEOUS

Sectional Directory

Gastric Acidity

PRINCIPLE

Gastric juice is an acid solution of electrolytes and digestive enzymes, with small amounts of protein and phosphates. Clinically the concentration of acid is of main interest, as this is a useful index of gastric function. The juice is first stimulated with a special feeding, then aspirated from the stomach. With the use of indicators of different pH ranges, the concentration of free and combined acid of the aspirate is measured titrimetrically. Recently interest has been raised in the pH value of the gastric juice, as this is felt to be a more useful measurement than titration values.

NORMAL VALUES

A. Free Hydrochloric Acid (After First Titration)

1. Fasting: 5—20 degrees.*
2. 1 hour after alcohol meal: 30—70 degrees.
3. 1 hour after histamine: 30—85 degrees.

B. Total Acid

1. Fasting: 15—45 degrees.
2. 50-minute histamine stimulation: 50—75 degrees.

PROCEDURE

1. Add 4 drops of Töpfer's reagent to 10 ml of centrifuged gastric contents in a beaker.
2. Add 0.1*N* sodium hydroxide from a burette until the initial red color has been replaced by a salmon-pink color (first titration).
3. Record the amount of sodium hydroxide used.
4. Add 4 drops of phenolphthalein.
5. Add 0.1*N* sodium hydroxide until the first permanent pink (not red) color appears (second titration).
6. Record the amount of sodium hydroxide used.

CALCULATION

1. After first titration:

$$\text{ml of } 0.1N \text{ NaOH used} \times 10 = \text{degrees or mEq of free HCl/liter contents}$$

2. After second titration:

$$\text{ml of } 0.1N \text{ NaOH used} \times 10 = \text{degrees or mEq of combined acid/liter contents}$$

3. For total acid:

$$\text{free HCl} + \text{combined acid} = \text{total acidity}$$

NOTES

1. A degree of acidity is defined as the amount of 0.1*N* sodium hydroxide that is

*See note

required to neutralize the acid content of 100 ml of gastric juice. This happens to be equal to milliequivalents per liter.

REAGENTS

1. Töpfer's reagent (alcoholic solution of *p*-dimethylaminiazobenzene, 0.5%)
2. Sodium hydroxide (0.1*N*)
3. Alcoholic solution of phenolphthalein (1%)

REFERENCE

Hepler, O. E., Manual of Clinical Laboratory Methods, 4th ed., p. 100. Charles C Thomas, Springfield, Illinois, 1965.

Gastric Analysis

Tubeless Method

PRINCIPLE

The use of a test for gastric acidity that does not require intubation has many advantages when dealing with nervous patients and in other special circumstances. A commercial test of this type is now available. Resin-dye (Diagnex Blue®*) reagent is administered orally to the patient. In the presence of gastric juice containing free hydrochloric acid, the dye in the resin-dye complex will dissociate and will be absorbed by the patient and excreted in the urine. Conversely, when free acid is not present in the gastric juice, the dye is not released until the complex enters the intestines, and urinary excretion of the dye is delayed. The amount of dye present in the specimen becomes a measure of the presence or absence of free hydrochloric acid in the stomach.

SPECIMEN

Urine collected over a 2-hour period immediately after administration of the reagent.

PROCEDURE

Preparation of Patient

The test should be done on the patient in the morning. He should not have had breakfast, but in order to be properly hydrated, he may be allowed water and black coffee or tea up until the time he is sent to the laboratory.

Test

1. The patient empties his bladder immediately before he is sent to the laboratory. This urine is discarded.
2. Give the patient 1 ml of Histalog®† subcutaneously and instruct him to wait for 50 minutes. He may smoke during this period, but not eat or drink.
3. At the end of this period, administer to the patient orally an entire packet of Diagnex Blue® accompanied by a glass (200 ml) of water.
4. Collect all urine over a 2-hour period, emptying the bladder at the end of this time and pooling all the urine as the test specimen. Dilute the entire urine collection to 300 ml.
5. Prepare three tubes of the test urine. Use two as controls, emptying a capsule of ascorbic acid (furnished with the kit) into each control urine and shaking the stoppered tubes. This removes any color present due to the dye, but does not interfere with the normal color of the urine. Thus the color background is the same for both the test urine and the controls.
6. Ascertain the pH of the urine, using paper to determine how much copper sulfate should be used (1 to 3 drops) to bring the pH to the acid side.
7. Place the test specimen in the central well of the comparator and the controls in each of the lateral wells. If the test urine contains more than 0.6 mg per 300 ml, the test is complete and is reported as positive for free hydrochloric acid.

*E. R. Squibb and Sons, Division of Olin Mathieson Chemical Corporation.

†Eli Lilly and Company, P.O. Box 618, Indianapolis, Indiana 46206. This preparation is available in a solution of 50 mg per ml. If desired, a dose of 0.5 mg per kilogram of bodyweight may be used.

8. If the test specimen contains less than 0.6 mg per 300 ml, develop the color further by acidifying 10-ml aliquots of the urine with 3 drops of the copper sulfate acid reagent supplied with the test material and boiling in a water bath for 10 minutes. If the pH is below 6, use only 2 drops of copper sulfate acid reagent.
9. Allow the boiled tubes to cool to room temperature, then read in the comparator as before. If the content of the urine is 0.6 mg above level, report as positive for free hydrochloric acid. If the content is more than 0.3 mg, but less than 0.6 mg, report as indicative of hypochlorhydria. If the content is below 0.3 mg, report as negative and as presumptive evidence of achlorhydria.

INTERPRETATION

1. 0.6 mg or more: positive.
2. 0.3 mg or less: negative or indicative of achlorhydria.

NOTES

1. The procedure given here differs from the original only in the use of Histalog® in place of the caffeine. In practice it has been found that the patients for whom the tests are ordered in place of conventional gastric analysis are usually nursing problems and that specimens can be more easily collected in the hospital than in the laboratory. The patients are returned to the ward immediately after receiving the resin, and the 2-hour collection is also made there.
2. The resin granules can best be administered by suspending them in a small amount of water and having the patient drink them as rapidly as possible. Granules remaining in the mouth may be washed down with the rest of the water prescribed.
3. The patient will continue to excrete dye in his urine for several days following the test. This is of no significance, but he should be told that this will happen, as some patients are distressed by this.
4. False negative tests may be found in patients who do not form sufficient urine to excrete the dye adequately. It is therefore necessary to give the patient enough fluid to permit this. This is the reason clear fluids are permitted prior to the test, as it is felt that adequate hydration is more important to the proper conduct of the test than keeping the stomach completely empty. The control specimen is no longer used in the test, but is collected to make sure that the patient can void and produce an adequate specimen.
5. Gastrectomized individuals and patients with vomiting, pyloric obstruction, severe kidney or liver damage, malabsorption syndromes (such as sprue), marked cardiac failure, or urinary retention are not good candidates for this test.

REAGENTS

1. Diagnex® Blue test unit

   Diagnex Blue® is supplied in single-dose packets accompanied by a caffeine capsule to use as a gastric stimulant. Our preference has been to discard the caffeine and to use 1 ml of Histalog® instead. The reagent is supplied with a comparator block that provides glass standards representing 0.3 and 0.6 mg of dye per 300 ml of urine.

REFERENCES

Anonymous, Diagnex Blue: A Tubeless Test for Gastric Acid. E. R. Squibb and Company, New York, 1958.

Galambos, J. T., and Kirsner, J. B., Tubeless Gastric Analysis. Arch. Internal Med., *96*, 752, 1955.

Measurement of Urine Specific Gravity

PRINCIPLE

The urinometer is a hydrometer adapted to the observation of specific gravity of urine at 20°C. Urinometers should be calibrated by floating in distilled water. They are usually accurate to within ±0.002.

NORMAL VALUES

1.015–1.025

PROCEDURE

1. Fill a cylinder three-fourths full of well-mixed urine.
2. Float the urinometer with a spinning motion to keep it from adhering to the side of the cylinder.
3. The specific gravity is read at the graduation on the stem of the urinometer at the lower level of the meniscus.
4. If the quantity of urine is small, the urine may be diluted with distilled water. To obtain the specific gravity, multiply the last figures of the reading by the amount of dilution.
5. Correct observed values as follows.
   (a) For temperature, add 0.001 for each 3°C that the urine temperature is above the calibration temperature, and subtract 0.001 for each 3°C that it is below the calibration temperature.
   (b) For glucose, subtract 0.001 for each 270 mg/100 ml.
   (c) For protein, subtract 0.001 for each 400 mg/100 ml.

Semen Examination

PRINCIPLE

Any study of a sterility problem must begin with an examination of the husband's semen. Not only is this test the easiest to do, but it is also one of the easiest to interpret. Absence of spermatozoa effectively precludes the possibility of a man becoming a father and thus eliminates the need for making extensive and often uncomfortable tests on the wife.

SPECIMEN

Semen may be collected by the patient at home following normal sexual relations or by masturbation. The specimen should be ejaculated directly into a clean, dry jar and transported at room temperature to the laboratory, arriving there not later than one hour after collection. The entire specimen should be submitted, since the determination of semen volume is an important part of the test. If split specimens are desired, the patient is given two containers and directed to collect part of the specimen into one container and the remainder into the other. The fractions should be labeled accurately.

Studies have shown that, in the normal male, maximum sperm activity is seen in specimens collected after three and not more than seven days of abstinence from sexual intercourse. However, the fact that this condition cannot always be met should not preclude doing the test. No lubricants or contraceptive preparations should be used, as these may adversely affect the test.

PROCEDURE

The examination should begin 1 hour after collection, if possible.

A. Volume

1. Pour the specimen into a centrifuge tube.
2. Add 0.6 ml to the total volume of semen to compensate for specimen retained on the sides of the bottle.

B. Color

The color of the specimen should be reported. Normal specimens are usually whitish-gray, but abnormal specimens may be yellow or vary in color.

C. Turbidity

Normal specimens are usually opaque. Large clumps that readily fall out of suspension are abnormal and should be noted.

D. Consistency

Consistency is homogeneous, without strands or stringy material. It is viscid, comparable to whole blood.

E. Chemical Examination

Normal semen is alkaline (pH 7.0—9.0). The pH of most semen is approximately

7.5. Alkalinity or acidity is of little value in determining the pathology, but it does serve as a check of contamination.

F. Microscopic Examination (Wet-Mount) for Motility and Viability

1. Place a drop of specimen on a clean slide, using a pipette with a rubber bulb, and cover with a cover slip.
2. Examine the slide under high dry magnification for the grade and percent of motility.

Grade of Motility

Although estimation of the rate of movement is difficult without experience, the following is an approximate description of motility:

no movement	0
sluggish	1+
medium	2+
active	3+
rapid	4+

Percent of Motility

With focus still on high dry magnification, use a limited-field ocular and determine the number of motile sperm per 100 sperm seen. Use two counters: one for a total of 100 sperm, the other for nonmotile sperm only. This count should be repeated. If the second count approximates the first, take the average of the two counts; if the second count is not similar to the first, a third count should be made. A fresh drop of semen should be taken for each count, since the motility of the sperm is quickly decreased when the sperm is allowed to remain on the slide for more than a few minutes.

G. White-Cell Count

Approximate the number of white cells present, counting them on the basis of their number per high-power field. Count several fields, then average the number of pus cells in all fields counted.

H. Sperm Count

Counting Technic

1. Mix the specimen thoroughly.
2. Draw seminal fluid to the 0.5 mark in a white-cell counting pipette, then draw in diluting fluid to the 11 mark. This makes a dilution of 1:20.
3. Shake the pipette for 2 minutes, then fill both sides of a counting chamber. Focus until the spermatozoa are sharply defined and the ruling appears as black lines. If the specimen is very viscid, a more accurate dilution can be made by using 1 ml of semen and 19 ml of diluting fluid in a test tube.
4. Count the sperm in the four corner squares and in one of the middle squares of the central (erythrocyte) ruled area, then count the other half of the chamber. Take the average of the two counts.

Calculation of Totals

Since the central ruled area has a surface of 1 mm^2 and one fifth of this area is counted, and since the depth of the chamber is 0.1 mm and the dilution is 1 : 20, the number of sperm per mm^3 would be as follows: sperm counted $\times 5 \times 10 \times 20$ would equal the number per mm^3; since there are 1000 mm^3 in 1 cm^3, multiply by 1000 to determine the sperm in 1 ml.

Example

Volume is 3.5 ml; average of the two sides of the counting chamber is 82.

$$82 \times 5 = 410 \text{ (number of sperm in 1 mm}^2\text{);}$$
$$410 \times 10 = 4{,}100 \text{ sperm in 1 mm}^3 \text{ (diluted);}$$
$$4{,}100 \times 20 = 82{,}000 \text{ sperm in 1 mm}^3 \text{ (undiluted);}$$
$$82{,}000 \times 1000 = 82{,}000{,}000 \text{ sperm in 1 ml;}$$
$$82{,}000{,}000 \times 3.5 = 287{,}000{,}000 \text{ sperm in specimen.}$$

If the sperm are few in number, count the large corner squares, 1 mm^2, as for counting white blood cells. The count in this case would be the total in 4 mm^2 divided by 4 and multiplied first by 10, then by 20.

Interpretation

The number of sperm in a normal specimen varies greatly. Total count in 1 ml is 100 million or more, and the total number in the specimen should be approximately 500 million. Counts below 60 million suggest abnormality, but must be interpreted along with other information in judging sterility.

I. Differential Count

A modified Papanicolaou technic may be used to stain the semen specimen. Smears are made and dropped wet into the alcohol-acetic acid fixation solution (see p. 234). Differentiate 100 stained sperm, using the oil-immersion objective. Normal, immature, and teratoid forms are counted.

Normal Forms. These have oval heads, somewhat pear-shaped, 4 to 6 micra in length, with a clear or weakly staining anterior and darkly staining chromatin mass (posterior); the tails are 10 times the length of the heads. Between head and tail is a middle piece, sometimes called the body or neck. This is slightly wider than the tail piece proper. Normal sperm shed cytoplasm, which may remain attached to the cell; this is no indication of immaturity.

Immature Forms. These are any form approaching a spermatoid, having large cells with a dark, round nucleus, diffuse staining, and an excess of attached cytoplasm around the head. A high immature count should correspond to a high spermatoid count in the fields observed. Few or no immature forms are found in normal semen specimens.

Teratoid Forms. These have abnormal shapes, abnormal chromatin, deformed heads, deformed centers, short or absent tails, and abnormal distribution of chromatin. Also characteristic are chromatin anterior, no center piece, more than one tail, multiple heads, pinheads, and megalosperm. The number of teratoid forms in normal semen will usually exceed the number of immature forms. Many abnormal-appearing sperm may be regarded as normal, since they are due to artifacts and the refractive index of the nucleus.

J. Bacteria Count

Bacteria should be reported on the basis of an estimation of the number present. If the patient has an infection, the number of white cells should correspond to the number of bacteria present. Otherwise, the bacteria in the specimen may be the result of contamination from the specimen jar or other external sources.

REFERENCES

Hotchkiss, R. S., Fertility in Men. J. B. Lippincott, Philadelphia, 1944.

Hotchkiss, R. S., Etiology and Diagnosis in the Treatment of Infertility in Men. Charles C. Thomas, Springfield, Illinois, 1952.

Sperm Agglutination Test

PRINCIPLE

Some infertility problems can be explained by the demonstration of antibodies against spermatozoa in the serum of the woman. These antibodies are not specific against the husband's spermatozoa, but appear to react with any sperm specimen. The test involves the observation of mixtures of normal spermatozoa and serum dilutions to observe the possible development of aggregates that are indicative of the antibody reaction.

SPECIMEN

Blood is obtained from the patient and the patient's husband, who serves as a control. As the test is done on serum, clotted blood is required.

PROCEDURE

1. Dilute a normal semen specimen with Baker's buffered-glucose saline solution to give a final concentration of 40,000,000 cells per ml.
2. Mix an aliquot of the standardized semen dilution with an equal part of 10% gelatin in Baker's solution.
3. Set up dilutions of patient's and control sera to give dilutions of 1 : 2, 1 : 4, 1 : 8, 1 : 16, 1 : 32, and 1 : 64. Use physiological saline as the serum diluent.
4. Dispense 0.2 ml of each serum dilution into 10 × 75 mm tubes and add an equal volume of semen reagent from step 2. Also set up the undiluted serum against the antigen.
5. Incubate the serum-semen mixture at 37°C for 2 hours.
6. Read after the first and second hour without centrifugation.

REAGENTS

1. Semen specimen, antigen

   The semen specimen used as the antigen must be normal by the parameters of routine sperm count. Unfortunately, such specimens are not always available, as most specimens are sent to the laboratory because of infertility problems and thus may not be normal.

2. Semen specimen, sperm source

   A complete semen analysis is done on the specimen to be used as the sperm source, and a portion of the specimen is diluted to give a final concentration of 40,000,000 spermatozoa per ml.

3. Baker's buffered-glucose saline solution

glucose	3.00 g
sodium phosphate, dibasic, dodecahydrate	0.60 g
sodium chloride	0.20 g
potassium hydrogen phosphate	0.01 g

   Dissolve and add enough distilled water to make 100 ml. The 10% gelatin solution is made by adding 10 g of gelatin to 100 ml of this mixture.

REFERENCE

Franklin, R. R., and Dukes, C. D., Antispermatozoal Antibody and Unexplained Infertility. Am. J. Obstet. Gynecol., *89*, 6, 1964.